Pathology of Infertility

Pathology of Infertility

Ivan Damjanov, M.D., Ph.D.
Professor of Pathology
Department of Pathology and Cell Biology
Jefferson Medical College
Thomas Jefferson University
Philadelphia, Pennsylvania

with illustrations by Ira Grunther

with 231 illustrations

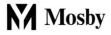 Mosby

St. Louis Baltimore Boston Chicago London Philadelphia Sydney Toronto

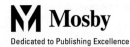

Mosby

Dedicated to Publishing Excellence

Publisher: George Stamathis
Editorial Assistant: Lauranne Billus
Project Manager: Arofan Gregory

Printed in the United States of America

Mosby–Year Book, Inc.
11830 Westline Industrial Drive
St. Louis, Missouri 63146

Library of Congress Cataloging in Publication Data

Damjanov, Ivan.
    Pathology of infertility / Ivan Damjanov ; with illustrations by
Ira Grunther. — 1st ed.
        p.   cm.
    Includes bibliographical references and index.
    ISBN 0-8016-0219-X
    1. Infertility—Pathophysiology.   I. Title.
    [DNLM: 1. Infertility—etiology.   WP 570 D161p]
RC889.D27   1993
618.1′78071—dc20
DNLM/DLC   92-49257
for Library of Congress   CIP

92 93 94 95 96 CL/MY 9 8 7 6 5 4 3 2 1

Dedicated to the memory of Petar Drobnjak (1924–1984), Professor of Obstetrics and Gynecology, University of Zagreb School of Medicine, Zagreb, Yugoslavia; and to those wonderful days of my youth we spent together in a godforsaken country; which, like my professor, has turned since then into dust bestrewn among the asphodels.

PREFACE

A few years ago an erudite friend of mine taught me that the adjective, *complete,* was in old times spelled *compleat* as in *The Compleat Angler.* Subsequently I found this book by Izaak Walton, published in 1653, and an advertisement for it that read: "An interesting discourse on fish and fishing, not unworthy of the perusal of most anglers." I began thinking about the meaning of *complete* (Can anything be complete? Can one provide complete coverage of a subject? What are the criteria for calling anything complete?, etc.). Thus I became sensitized to the concept of that elusive word which again came to my mind while writing this book. I tried to make it compleat, but I leave it to the reader to make his or her own conclusions about the final outcome of my endeavor.

In contrast to Izaak Walton's opus, this book is not on fish or fishing, although I hope that anglers of another kind will find it not unworthy of their perusal. It deals with material that a pathologist acting as a consultant for the infertility team might see in his or her practice.

Primarily I have addressed pathologic lesions that cause infertility. In addition, I have attempted to touch upon the common and not-so-common lesions of human male and female genital organs that may not be related to infertility but could be important in the differential diagnosis.

I have written primarily for the pathologist, and the book's primary emphasis is on morphology, that is, anatomic pathology. However, since pathologists do not work in a vacuum, and since they converse with clinicians of different profiles, I think that it is important for my colleagues to learn the clinical glossary and understand the basic clinical features of various diseases causing infertility. I have thus devoted some space in my book to basic definitions, concepts, and terms used in infertility, gynecology, and urology clinics and wards. I have tried to explain the significance of the clinical work-up of the infertile couple, and I have therefore outlined the principal approaches to evaluating the reproductive potential of men and women.

The recent contributors of developmental biology, genetics, and endocrinology relevant for the understanding of infertility have also been reviewed.

The diseases and processes included in this book have been grouped under conventional headings such as genetic, endocrine, and infectious disorders. I tried to be systematic in my approach and thus fulfill my didactic function. For each of the more important diseases I have reviewed the etiology and pathogenesis and, if known, the pathophysiology of the process. The pathology and clinical presentations are then correlated.

In most instances the pathologist will examine tissues removed from the genital tract; therefore, this book deals mostly with lesions involving the internal and external male and female genital organs. Occasionally the pathologist will see extragenital lesions of the hypothalamic-pituitary-adrenal-gonadal axis and the conceptus itself. These lesions are reviewed "for the sake of completeness" but have received less attention and space within the text. Obviously this approach reflects more my own perception of what is important for the pathologist than the actual prevalence of various diseases. The "bread and butter" lesions, such as pelvic inflammatory disease (a major cause of infertility in women) or gonadal tumors, are described in a sketchy form— not because these lesions are unimportant, but because they are covered in greater detail in standard textbooks of pathology. Likewise, very little space was devoted to abortions or placental diseases in the early embryos since these topics have been extensively discussed in several recent books and monographs.

The reader interested in pathology of infertility may find it prudent to consult the clinical textbooks devoted to infertility, endocrinology, gynecology, or urology, which are all referenced in the present book.

As a single-authored book, *Pathology of Infertility* is by necessity more subjective than the multi-authored texts, and reflects my own views, prejudices, preferences, and biases. However I hope that the readers will find it more readable and manageable than large multi-authored, encyclopedic texts. I believe that it could be used as a source book and a compendium for diagnosis, but also as a primer and a basic introductory text depending on the needs and background of the reader. I have garnished my writing with up-to-date references, which should serve as a guide for additional reading.

As the sole author of this book I take full blame for all the unintentional—albeit unavoidable—omissions, deficiencies, occasional overinterpretations, or inaccuracies that might have crept into my writing. Having read recently the memoirs of the Nobel Prize laureate Rita Levi-Montalcini, aptly titled *In Praise of Imperfection,* I readily accept my own; I hope that it is not criticized too harshly.

Finally, I would like to acknowledge the tangible as well as the intangible contributions of my support team, which include several of my friends and colleagues, my secretaries, the staff of Mosby–Year Book, and members of my unconventional extended family who were always available when I needed them. Regrettably, one person whom I would have needed the most was not here: Professor Petar Drobnjak, my teacher, friend, and inspiration who died a few years ago. My book contains several photographs that I received posthumously from Professor Drobnjak's family. My dedication is a small token of gratitude to a man who profoundly influenced my professional life and whose memory I still cherish.

Ivan Damjanov

vii

CONTENTS

Pathology of Infertility

Chapter 1

BASIC CONCEPTS
OF INFERTILITY

Definition of infertility
Prevalence and incidence of infertility
Causes of infertility
Treatment of infertility

DEFINITION OF INFERTILITY

Infertility is empirically defined as the inability of a couple to conceive after 1 year of coital activity without contraception (Mosher and Pratt, 1991). Historically, the concepts of infertility have changed over time, and although the problems pertaining to procreation have been mentioned even in the Bible (Ober, 1984), it is only with the advent of modern biomedical research techniques that a fuller insight into various causes of infertility has been obtained. Significant progress in the treatment of infertility, primarily in women, has been made only during the last decade when various modalities of extracorporeal fertilization were introduced into clinical practice.

Approximately 15% of all marriages are childless in the United States and Western world (Mosher, 1985). However, the prevalence of infertility in the population is notoriously difficult to assess because it is confounded by various social, cultural, and political determinants of family planning, sexual mores, and conventions. Reports from different countries indicate that infertility is widespread and may be as high as 30% in sub-Saharan Africa (quoted by Rantala and Koskimies, 1986) or as low as 5% in China (Li et al., 1990). Nevertheless, one cannot conclude unequivocally that there are more infertile couples in highly developed, industrialized countries than in the Third World or that the amenities of modern civilization have reduced or increased infertility. Recent increasing concern with fertility (Aral and Cates, 1983) is probably related, at least in part, to the fact that many previously incurable conditions have become correctable.

The statisticians distinguish *infertility*, an objectively defined condition, from impaired *fecundity*, defined as a subjectively reported inability to conceive a baby or bring it to term (Mosher and Pratt, 1991). Fertility in populations is expressed as *fecundability*, a term denoting the probability of pregnancy in each menstrual cycle (Joffe, 1989), i.e., the monthly rate of conceptions in a defined population. Overall, the rate of fecundability is 0.2, indicating that every month 20 of 100 couples engaged in unprotected sexual intercourse conceive (Cramer et al., 1979). Longitudinal studies (e.g., Joffe, 1989) show that at least 60% of couples conceive during the first 6 months of unprotected intercourse and the vast majority during the first year (Fig. 1-1).

Couples with low fecundability due to unknown causes, "bad luck," or a treatable condition are called *subfertile*.

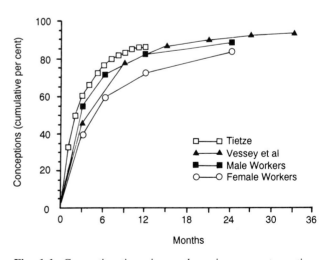

Fig. 1-1. Conception times in couples using no contraception. At least 60% of all women have become pregnant during the first 6 months, and most couples have recorded pregnancy during the first year. (Modified with permission from Joffe M. Feasibility of studying subfertility using retrospective self reports. J Epidemiol Community Health 1989; 43:268.)

Subfertile couples may conceive spontaneously over the years or with medical assistance. If one or both partners suffer from an irreversible, untreatable cause of infertility, the couple is labeled *sterile*. Obviously, such operational subdivisions are arbitrary and the progress of medical sciences may call for reassessment of various forms of infertility, e.g., some conditions classified as representing sterility today may become treatable in the near future.

PREVALENCE AND INCIDENCE OF INFERTILITY

The prevalence and incidence of infertility or subfertility are often considered together, although from the point of epidemiology these two indexes measure different parameters. The issue is confused even more by the multitude of approaches to assessing or estimating infertility, to defining infertility, and to collecting data (Marchbanks et al., 1989).

The rate of infertility in the same population may be as low as 6.1% if the study is based on doctors' reports, or as high as 32.6% if the data are derived from patient-oriented questionnaires. The results may differ depending on whether the period of infertility is defined in terms of 12 or 24 months of unprotected intercourse (Marchbanks et al., 1989).

The incidence and prevalence of *primary* versus *secondary* infertility are treated separately in some studies and as a single entity in others. Because most infertile couples ultimately solve their problem spontaneously, with or without medical assistance, some reports distinguish terminal *(unresolved)* from temporary *(resolved)* infertility (Greenhall and Vessey, 1990). Political, religious, social, and psychological aspects of human reproductive biology confound the issues even more, making a realistic assessment of infertility almost impossible.

The *prevalence* of infertility is the number of women of reproductive age, usually 15 to 45 years old, who have been engaged in unprotected sexual intercourse without conception for more than 1 year, divided by the number of married or heterosexual cohabitants of the same age in the population studied (Page, 1989). The *incidence* of infertility is the number of registered women of reproductive age who reach the point at which they have been trying unsuccessfully for 12 months to conceive, divided by the num-

ber of married or heterosexual cohabitants of the same age. Incidence is a measure of new cases of infertility reported in a population every year. Using these definitions and surveying the population of women between 20 and 44 years of age, Page (1989) reported the prevalence of primary infertility in Sheffield, United Kingdom, at 5.9%, noting that 28% of all couples experienced infertility at some time. The vast majority of couples (78%) conceived during the first year of unprotected intercourse; 88.8% conceived in 2 years and 94.6% within 3 years; and 5.3% remained childless for more than 3 years. Mosher (1985) recorded that in the United States 8.4% of couples, in which the woman was 15 to 44 years old, did not conceive during the year in which they used no contraception. These reports compare favorably with the data from similar studies listed in Table 1-1.

Greenhall and Vessey (1990) estimate that 24% of all women attempting to conceive will have an episode of infertility (subfertility) in their life. In their Oxford general practice and hospital data–based study, they found that 13% of women will have problems conceiving the first child and 17% the subsequent children. If the same results are analyzed in terms of how many cases of subfertility were "resolved" and how many remained "unresolved," the prevalence rates for unresolved primary and secondary subfertility are 3.3% and 5.9%, respectively, and for resolved primary and secondary subfertility 10% and 12.4%, respectively. These data are consistent with the ranges reported from several countries, as reviewed in the paper of Greenhall and Vessey (1990).

The claims that infertility has become more prevalent in recent years (Aral and Cates, 1983) have been difficult to confirm, although it appears that the number of women who remain childless has increased during the last decades (Johnson et al., 1987). Johnson et al. (1987) found in England that 7.7% of women born in 1935 and 14.3% of women born in 1950 were childless by the time they had reached 35 and 50 years of age, respectively. Of these women, 3.2% born in 1935 and 11% of those born in 1950 were considered childless by choice. Although this in part may reflect changing attitudes and less stigma attached to childlessness, and although the various reasons for remaining childless are difficult to assess objectively, the trend in Western countries seems to be toward smaller families; the

Table 1-1. Prevalence rates of unresolved infertility in women

Author	Country	Age	Total (%)	Primary infertility (%)	Secondary infertility (%)
Mosher (1985)	United States	15–44	8.4	3.8	4.6
Mosher and Pratt (1991)	United States	25–44	10.1	4.0	6.1
Greenhall and Vessey (1990)	England	25–44	9.2	3.3	5.9
Templeton et al. (1990)	Scotland	<50	6.0	4.0	2.0
Page (1989)	England	20–40	13.1	5.9	7.2
Rantala and Koskimies (1986)	Finland	30–50	11.5	4.8	6.7

number of voluntarily childless women is increasing and parallels the trend toward smaller families.

Any discussion about infertility as a social or medical problem would benefit from some historical and transcultural data that could provide a broader perspective and shed light on the issue from a different angle. In this context, it should be kept in mind that for many health authorities it is a more daunting task to reduce population growth and reduce fertility in population than to resolve the problems of infertile couples, who constitute only one sixth of the populace. Further, the modern concept of "ideal family" with two or three children has evolved in the Western world only recently, and although it may be related to social factors, it may also be due to some other poorly understood environmental influences that have reduced the birth rate in Europe in the nineteenth century (Fig. 1-2) (Matossian, 1991). Finally, the Western concept of reproduction and marital life, which we accept as the optimal model for maintaining the stability and growth of society, is not shared in other cultures, which, however, form the majority of humankind (Bittles et al., 1991). Hence it is best to refrain from all-encompassing statements and generalizations and keep an open mind while observing the ever-changing aspects of human reproduction.

Infertility is treated medically as a problem affecting heterosexual couples. However, unmarried women and men may also request infertility evaluation and/or treatment. For simplicity, the term *infertile couple* is used in this book for heterosexual pairs engaged in procreational sexual intercourse irrespective of their legal status. It is understood that most of these couples will not be registered for statistical purposes unless they live in family units equivalent to marriage. No attempt is made to analyze infertility in various settings, especially because most of the published data refer to the standard family of the Western world.

CAUSES OF INFERTILITY

According to most estimates, infertility is caused by a male factor in one third of all couples. In another 20% of couples both partners have medical problems, whereas in the remaining 50% of cases the cause of infertility resides in the woman (Lipshultz and Howards, 1984; Swerdloff et al., 1988). However, the views of various authors vary considerably, reflecting both objective differences in samples studied as well as the observer's biases (Table 1-2).

Table 1-2. Causes of infertility*

Cause	Rowland (1980)	Katayama et al. (1979)	Hull (1990)
Male	13	18	26
Female			
Ovulation	18	16	21
Tubal disease	33	12	14
Endometriosis	—	25	6
Uterine factor	3	2	—
Cervical factor	25	5	3
Coital failure	—	—	6
Luteal phase defect	5	7	—
Others	—	15	11
Unexplained	3	—	28

*The data are expressed as approximate percentage of the total number of cases.

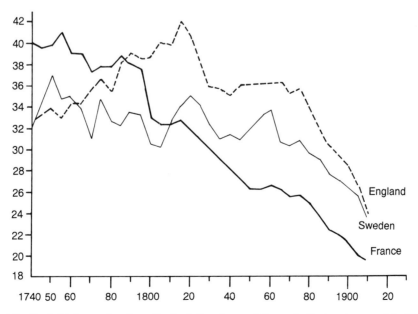

Fig. 1-2. Crude birth rate data from England, Sweden, and France indicate a decreased fertility in the nineteenth century. The reasons for this event are not fully understood. (Used with permission from Matossian MK. Perspect Biol Med 1991; 134:604, and the University of Chicago Press.)

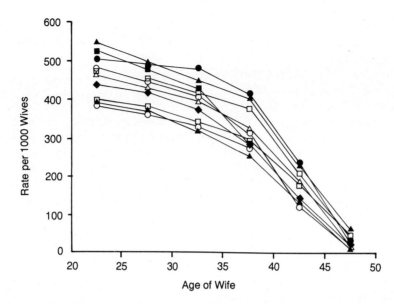

Fig. 1-3. Age-related decrease in fertility of women. The different populations were analyzed by 5-year age groups, and a decreased fertility was noted in all groups even though the data stem from records compiled as early as 1600 or as recently as 1950. (From Mencken J, Trussell J, Larsen U. Science 1986; 233:1389 with permission.)

Age affects the fertility of women. The survey of Menken et al. (1986) shows that marital fertility rates decrease gradually with aging of the female consort (Fig. 1-3). In the age group 20 to 24 years, 6% of women are infertile. The rate of infertility increases to 9% in women who married between the ages 25 to 29, to 15% in those married between ages 30 and 35, and to more than 60% in those married between 40 and 44 years of age. Navot et al. (1991) have shown that the age-related decline in female fertility is a consequence of diminished quality of oocytes in older women. Fertility of men is not affected by age.

Male infertility of old age is related to the overall decline in spermatogeneic, metabolic, vascular, and endocrine functions; these changes have been poorly documented because they are rarely brought to medical attention with respect to fertility. Testes involute with age (Paniagua et al., 1987), but the consequences of this are difficult to assess. The effect of age on testes may be confounded by nutritional factors and disease (Handelsman and Staraj, 1985). An age-related attrition of Leydig's cells has been recorded (Kaler and Neaves, 1978). Reduced levels of serum testosterone and inhibin in older men are associated with altered neuroendocrine regulation of pulsatile luteinizing hormone release and decreased gonadotropic and Leydig cell secretory reserve (Urban and Veldhuis, 1988), but the reproductive consequences of these age-related changes have not been established. Semen quality may deteriorate with age (Schwartz et al., 1983); fertility in men over 90 has been documented, although it is not known how many men remain fertile into old age.

Nutrition may affect sexual functions and reproduction in several ways. Sexual maturation may be delayed because of malnutrition by delaying overall growth and by inhibiting gonadotropin secretion at the level of gonadotropin-releasing hormone in the hypothalamus as seen in anorexia nervosa (Yen, 1991). To a greater extent, nutritional factors affect women more than men, but the effect of starvation on male sexual functions, including spermatogenesis, has been documented. Strenuous exercise combined with nutritional factors largely accounts for amenorrhea in female athletes (Henley and Vaitukaitis, 1988).

Obesity may cause hormonal disturbances in men and women. In men, obesity has been associated with reduced serum testosterone levels and elevated estrogen (E_2), probably because of increased conversion of testosterone to E_2 in adipose tissue (Glass et al., 1977). The effects of obesity on women may be less evident, although it is known that obese women, like obese men, show peripheral aromatization of androgens to estrogens, decreased levels of sex hormone binding–globulin and concomitantly increased levels of free estradiol and testosterone, and increased levels of insulin, which may stimulate ovarian production of androgens (Speroff et al., 1989). These hormonal changes could but often do not interfere with ovulation.

Alcohol induces testicular atrophy in animals and may be associated with temporary subfertility in men owing to a reversible depression of the hypothalamic-pituitary function (Van Thiel et al., 1982). Experimentally induced zinc deficiency may alter testicular function (Abbasi et al., 1980), but the clinical relevance of these data has not been

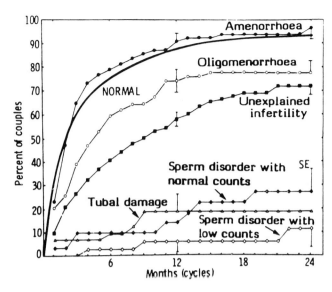

Fig. 1-4. Cumulative conception rates resulting from conventional management in couples with a single cause of infertility as compared with normal. (From Hull MGR. Br Med Bull 1990; 46(3):580 with permission.)

proved. Hypothetical deficiency of zinc has been proposed as one of the possible causes for the decline of birth rates that occurred in the nineteenth century in Europe (Matossian, 1991).

Environmental factors affect fertility, although it is not known precisely to what extent. Sexually transmitted infections are the most important exogenous factor and account for a significant number of infertility problems in women (Cates et al., 1990) and to a lesser extent in men (Berger et al., 1982). Occupational reproductive risks are more difficult to assess (Thomas and Ballantyne, 1990). Chemicals in the environment may affect reproductive organs directly or indirectly through their action on the hypothalamo-hypophysial-gonadal axis (Steeno and Pangkahila, 1984). Pesticides, such as 1,2-dibromo 3-chloropropane, affect testicular function (Levine et al., 1983). Radiation may cause dose-related gonadal changes that appear to be irreversible in women and are either reversible or irreversible in men (MacLeod et al., 1964). Subfertility was reported in male welders (Bonde, 1990). Other occupational epidemiologic reports indicate that adverse conditions in the workplace could influence fertility but these sporadic publications are far from conclusive.

Drugs are well-known causes of iatrogenic fertility (Driffe, 1982). Cytotoxic drugs used in the treatment of malignant tumors such as those included in the cyclophosphamide, vincristine, procarbazine, and prednisolone (COOP) treatment regimen for Hodgkin's disease lead to destruction of germinal epithelium of the testis (Charak et al., 1990). The female gonads are affected to a lesser extent (Mattison et al., 1990).

Systemic diseases are important causes of infertility. These include metabolic disorders such as diabetes, renal disease (Holdsworth et al., 1977; Chopp and Mendez, 1978), liver failure (Gluud et al., 1988), and sickle cell anemia (Abbasi et al., 1976); Endocrine and endocrine disturbances involving the hypophysial-gonadal axis are well-defined but rare causes of infertility. Immune mechanisms possibly play an important role in infertility (Haas and Beer, 1986; Tung, 1987).

Developmental, chromosomal, and *genetic* disorders, especially those involving sex chromosomes, affect the reproductive functions of men and women. These disorders are often associated with abnormalities of the gonads and/or primary and secondary sex organs (Ferguson-Smith, 1991).

Primary diseases of the male and female reproductive organs are the immediate cause of infertility in most patients seeking medical treatment. This book deals predominantly with these disorders and illustrates various pathologic conditions of the male and female reproductive systems as seen by the pathologist.

TREATMENT OF INFERTILITY

Various modalities of treatment of infertile couples have been extensively reviewed (Seibel, 1990; Mishell et al., 1991) and are beyond the limits of this text. Major advances have been made in treating infertile women, and the introduction of extracorporeal fertilization and assisted conception has revolutionized the entire reproductive medicine. In this context, suffice it to say that the results of classic medical or surgical treatment of infertility are less spectacular, although some causes of infertility seem to be more amenable to therapy than others (Fig. 1-4). As stated by Hull (1990), even with conventional treatment, female infertility has been more curable than male infertility.

Medical and surgical treatment and assisted conception are not without potential mishaps and complications. Ovarian hyperstimulation syndrome secondary to hormonal induction of ovulation is the most salient example of such iatrogenic abnormality (Buttendorf and Lindner, 1987). Treatment-related pathologic changes induced in men and women treated for infertility, as well as those induced by various contraceptive methods that could cause secondary infertility, and systemic or local therapeutic interventions that may affect fertility are discussed fully.

REFERENCES

Abbasi AA, Prasad AS, Ortega J, Congco E, Oberleas D: Gonadal function abnormalities in sickle cell anemia: Studies in adult male patients. Ann Intern Med 1976; 85:601.

Abbasi AA, Prasad AS, Rabbani P, DuMouchelle E: Experimental zinc deficiency in man: Effect on testicular function. J Lab Clin Med 1980; 96:544.

Aral SO, Cates W: The increasing concern with infertility—why now? JAMA 1983; 250:2327.

Berger RE, Karp LE, Williamson RA, Loenler J, Moore DE, Holmes KK: The relationship of pyospermia and seminal fluid bacteriology to sperm function as reflected in the sperm penetration assay. Fertil Steril 1982; 37:557.

Bittles AH, Mason WM, Greene J, Rao NA: Reproductive behavior and health in consanguineous marriages. Science 1991; 252:789.

Bonde JPE: Subfertility in relation to welding. A case reference study among male welders. Dan Med Bull 1990; 37:105.

Buttendorf G, Lindner C: The ovarian hyperstimulation syndrome. Horm Metab Res 1987; 19:519

Cates W Jr, Rolfs RT Jr, Aral SO: Sexually transmitted diseases, pelvic inflammatory disease, and infertility: An epidemiologic update. Epidemiol Rev 1990; 12:199.

Charak BS, Gupta R, Mandrekar P, Sheth NA, Banavali SD, Salkia TK, Gopal R, Dinshaw KA, Advani SH: Testicular dysfunction after cyclophosphamide-vincristine-procarbazine-prednisolone chemotherapy for advanced Hodgkin's disease. Cancer 1990; 65:1903.

Chopp TR, Mendez R: Sexual function and hormonal abnormalities in uremic men on chronic dialysis and after renal transplantation. Fertil Steril 1978; 29:661.

Cramer DW, Walker AM, Schiff I: Statistical methods in evaluating the outcome of infertility therapy. Fertil Steril 1979; 32:80.

Driffe JO: Drugs and sperm. BMJ 1982; 284:844.

Ferguson-Smith MA: Genotype phenotype correlations in individuals with disorders of sex determination and development including Turner's syndrome. Semin Dev Biol 1991; 2:265.

Glass AR, Swerdloff RS, Bray GA, Dahms WT, Atkinson RL: Low serum testosterone and sex-hormone-binding-globulin in massively obese men. J Clin Endocrinol Metab 1977; 45:1211.

Gluud C, Wantzin P, Ericksen J, and the Copenhagen Study Group for Liver Diseases: No effect of oral testosterone treatment on sexual dysfunction in alcoholic cirrhotic men. Gastroenterology 1988; 95:1582.

Greenhall E, Vessey M: The prevalence of subfertility: A review of the current confusion and a report of two new studies. Fertil Steril 1990; 54:978.

Haas GG, Beer AE: Immunologic influences on reproductive biology: Sperm gametogenesis and maturation in the male and female genital tracts. Fertil Steril 1986; 46:753.

Handelsman DJ, Staraj S. Testicular size. The effect of aging, malnutrition and illness. J Androl 1985; 6:144.

Henley K, Vaitukaitis JL: Exercise-induced menstrual dysfunction. Annu Rev Med 1988; 39:443.

Holdworth S, Atkins RC, deKretser DM: The pituitary-testicular axis in men with chronic renal failure. N Engl J Med 1977; 296:1245.

Hull MGR: Indications for assisted conception. Br Med Bull 1990; 46:580.

Joffe M: Feasibility of studying subfertility using retrospective self reports. J Epidemiol Community Health 1989; 43:268.

Johnson G, Roberts D, Brown R, Cox E, Evershed Z, Goutam P, Hassan P, Robinson R, Sahdev A, Swan K, Sykes C: Infertile or childless by chance? A multipractice survey of women aged 35 and 50. BMJ 1987; 294:804.

Kaler LW, Neaves WB: Attrition of the human Leydig cell population with advancing age. Anat Rec 1978; 192:513.

Katayama KP, Ju K-S, Manuel M, Jones GS, Jones HW Jr: Computer analysis of etiology and pregnancy rate in 636 cases of primary infertility. Am J Obstet Gynecol 1979; 135:207.

Levine RJ, Blunden PB, Dalcorso RD, Starr TB, Ross CE: Superiority of reproductive histories to sperm counts in detecting infertility at a dibromiochloropropane manufacturing plant. J Occup Med 1983; 25:591.

Li Y, Wang JL, Quian SZ, Gao ES, Tao JG: Infertility in a rural area of Jiangsu province: An epidemiologic survey. Int J Fertil 1990; 35:34.

Lipshultz LI, Howards SS: Evaluation of the subfertile man. Semin Urol 1984; 2:73.

MacLeod J, Hotchkiss RS, Sitterson BW: Recovery of male fertility after sterilization by nuclear radiation. JAMA 1964; 187:637.

Marchbanks PA, Peterson HB, Rubin GL, Wingo PA, and the Cancer and Steroid Hormone Study Group: Research on infertility: Definition makes a difference. Am J Epidemiol 1989; 130:259.

Matossian MK: Fertility decline in Europe, 1875–1913. Was zinc deficiency the cause? Perspect Biol Med 1991; 34:604.

Mattison DR, Plowchalk DR, Meadows MJ, Al-Juburi AZ, Gandy J, Malek A: Reproductive toxicity. Male and female reproductive systems as targets for chemical injury. Med Clin North Am 1990; 74:391.

Menken J, Trussell J, Larsen U: Age and infertility. Science 1986; 233:1389.

Mishell DR Jr, Davajan V, Lobo RA (Eds): Infertility, Contraception and Reproductive Endocrinology. 3rd ed. Boston, Blackwell Scientific, 1991.

Mosher WD: Reproductive impairments in the United States, 1965–1982. Demography 1985; 22:415.

Mosher WD, Pratt WF: Fecundity and infertility in the United States: Incidence and trends. Fertil Steril 1991; 56:192.

Navot D, Bergh PA, Williams MA, Garrisi GJ, Guzman I, Sandler B, Grunfield L: Poor oocyte quality rather than implantation failure as a cause of age-related decline in female fertility. Lancet 1991; 337:1375.

Ober WB: Reuben's mandrakes: Infertility in the Bible. Int J Gynecol Pathol 1984; 3:299.

Page H: Estimation of the prevalence and incidence of infertility in a population: A pilot study. Fertil Steril 1989; 51:571.

Paniagua R, Martin A, Nistal M, Amat P: Testicular involution in elderly men: Comparison of histologic quantitative studies with hormone patterns. Fertil Steril 1987; 47:671.

Rantala M-L, Koskimies AL: Infertility in women participating in a screening program for cervical cancer in Helsinki. Acta Obstet Gynecol Scand 1986; 65:823.

Rowland A: Infertility therapy: Effect of innovations and increasing experience. J Reprod Med 1980; 25:42.

Schwartz D, Mayaux MJ, Spira A: Semen characteristics as a function of age in 833 fertile men. Fertil Steril 1983; 39:530.

Seibel MM: Infertility: A Comprehensive Text. Norwalk, Conn, Appleton & Lange, 1990.

Speroff L, Glass RH, Kase NG: Clinical Gynecologic Endocrinology and Infertility. Baltimore, Williams & Wilkins 1989.

Steeno OP, Pangkahila A: Occupational influences on male fertility and sexuality. Andrologia 1984; 16:5.

Swerdloff RS, Wang C, Kandeel FR: Evaluation of the infertile couple. Endocrinol Metab Clin North Am 1988; 17:301.

Templeton A, Fraser C, Thompson B: The epidemiology of infertility in Aberdeen. BMJ 1990; 301:148.

Thomas JA, Ballantyne BL: Occupational reproductive risks: Sources, surveillances, and testing. J Occup Med 1990; 32:547.

Tung K: Immunologic basis of male infertility. Lab Invest 1987; 57:1.

Urban RY, Veldhuis JD: Hypothalamo-pituitary concomitants of aging. In Endocrinology of Aging, edited by Sowers JR, Felicetta JV. New York, Raven Press, 1988, p 41.

Van Thiel DH, Gaveler JS, Sanghvi A: Recovery of sexual function in abstinent alcoholic men. Gastroenterology 1982; 85:677.

Van Thiel DH, Gaveler JS, Lester R, Goodman MD: Alcohol-induced testicular atrophy. Gastroenterology 1975; 69:326.

Yenn SSC: Chronic anovulation due to CNS-hypothalamic-pituitary dysfunction. In Reproductive Endocrinology, edited by Yen SSC, Jaffe RB. Philadelphia, WB Saunders, 1991, p 631.

Chapter 2

CLINICAL EVALUATION OF
THE INFERTILE COUPLE

Clinical evaluation of infertility is based on the assumption that reproductive problems affect *couples* and that the cause of reproductive failure may lie with the man, woman, or both. Hence the infertile couple has to be examined as a single unit. An algorithm for the evaluation of infertile couples is given in Algorithm 2-1. A more detailed discussion of the clinical work-up of infertile patients may be found in recent clinical monographs (Spark, 1988; Lipshultz and Howards, 1990; Seibel, 1990; Mishell et al., 1991), which also deal with hormonal and therapeutic aspects of infertility.

CLINICAL EVALUATION OF THE MALE PATIENT

Clinical evaluation of infertile men includes:

1. History
2. General physical examination and routine laboratory tests
3. Semen analysis
4. Hormonal studies

On the basis of these findings, assuming that the female partner is fertile, it is customary to classify the causes of male infertility as *pretesticular* (hormonal, metabolic, pharmacologic), *testicular,* and *posttesticular* (box on p. 9).

Swerdloff et al. (1985) consider 70% to 75% of all male infertility problems as idiopathic since they cannot be adequately explained on the basis of current medical knowledge. All forms of isolated oligospermia, asthenospermia, and teratospermia belong to this category. Infertility associated with varicocele is also included in his group since there is an ongoing debate as to whether surgery on the internal spermatic vein will correct the abnormalities in sperm morphology (Ayodeji and Baker, 1986) and increase male fertility (Nilsson et al., 1979; Cockett et al., 1984; Acosta et al., 1990). Of the remaining 25% to 30% of cases with an identifiable cause, 1% are related to hypothalamic-pituitary disorders, 10% to 15% to testicular disease, 4% to 6% to sperm autoimmunity, 8% to 10% to posttesticular genital diseases, and 1% to copulatory and ejaculatory dysfunctions.

History

A complete past and present history should be taken; past history should include questions about childhood, with special emphasis on timing of development of genital organs and virilization. The patient should be asked about previous surgeries in the genital area, including hernia repair and cryptorchidism or evidence of late or incomplete testicular descent into the scrotum. A history of childhood diseases with special emphasis on mumps should be elicited. Mumps is a relatively innocuous disease of early childhood; however, in postpubertal males, mumps may cause orchitis with significant tissue destruction and subsequent oligospermia, especially in patients in whom both testes were affected (Werner, 1950; Scott, 1960).

Inquiries about sexually transmitted disease should be made, including the mode of infection, symptomatology, complications, treatment, and duration of disease (Fowler

7

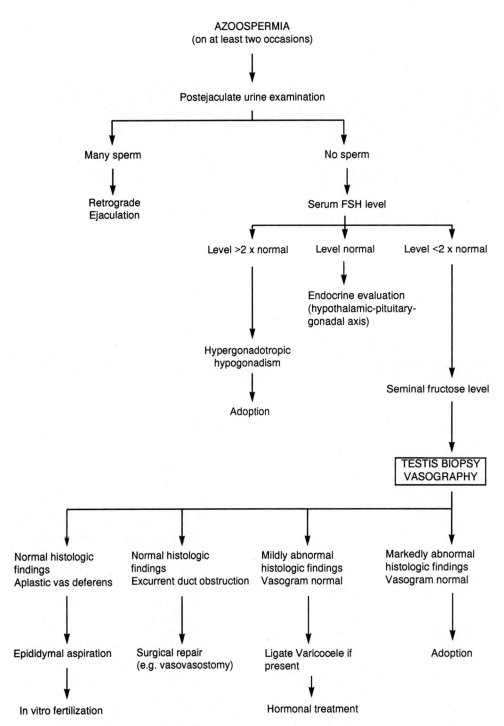

Algorithm 2-1. Evaluation of azoospermia. (From DeCherney et al., 1988.)

and Kessler, 1990). Residual complications pertaining to sexually acquired diseases should be recorded. Urinary tract infections, especially if recurrent and associated with extension into the epididymis, should be noted.

Acute viremia of recent origin may depress spermatogenesis (MacLeod, 1951) and should not be overlooked. A full recovery may take a few months because the spermatogenic cycle in man lasts approximately 75 days from

its initiation to the appearance of mature spermatogonia in the ejaculate (Heller and Clermont, 1964). Metabolic disorders such as diabetes, renal disease, and liver disease may contribute to infertility. Diabetes is associated with disturbances of erection and ejaculation; it may also affect spermatogenesis (Lipson, 1984). Cirrhosis causes profound endocrine changes (Baker et al., 1976) especially if related to alcoholism (Gavaler and Van Thiel, 1988). Ure-

---

Etiologic classification of male infertility

A. Systemic pretesticular causes

1. Disorders of the hypothalamo-pituitary-gonadal or adrenal axis
2. Endocrine diseases of the thyroid, adrenal, diabetes
3. Metabolic disorders due to renal, liver, or lung diseases
4. Chronic infectious and debilitating diseases
5. Pharmacologic
6. Substance abuse

B. Testicular causes

1. Idiopathic hypospermatogenesis
2. Developmental and genetic disorders affecting testes
3. Inflammatory lesions—infectious and immune
4. Iatrogenic—chemical, radiation, surgical
5. Environmental

C. Genital, posttesticular causes

1. Congenital anomalies of excretory ducts, accessory glands, and external genitalia
2. Inflammatory lesions of the excretory ducts and accessory glands
3. Iatrogenic or posttraumatic lesions of the excretory ducts, accessory glands, and ejaculatory nerve plexus

---

mia is known to reduce fertility, but even long-term hemodialysis may be associated with endocrine disturbances (Gomez et al., 1980). Uncontrollable obesity may be a sign of a pituitary disorder, although it has been reported that obesity in itself may be associated with relative hyperestrinism and subfertility in males (Glass et al., 1977).

The patient should be questioned about gonadal as well as extragonadal neoplasia and whether he ever received chemotherapy or was exposed to radiation. Radiotherapy and chemotherapy may adversely affect spermatogenesis (Schilsky et al., 1980; Rivkees and Crawford, 1988). Treatment of childhood malignancy may cause azoospermia or oligospermia, especially if the therapy involved cranial and testicular irradiation and cyclophosphamide (Siimes and Routonen, 1990). Radical surgery in the urogenital area and lymph node dissection may affect the excretory ducts or cause neurogenic and vascular disturbances of erection and ejaculation. Treatment of testicular cancer is often associated with temporary infertility and azoospermia, which persist in 20% of patients 2 to 5 years after treatment (Hansen et al., 1989).

Social habits of the patient should be discussed to determine whether he is abusing alcohol, recreational drugs, or hormones. Adverse effects of alcohol on spermatogenesis are well known (Gavaler and Van Thiel, 1988). The potentially harmful influences of recreational drugs such as

marijuana have not been unequivocally established, although reports suggest that these substances affect spermatogenesis (Smith and Asch, 1987). Cigarette smoking has been implicated as a cause of low sperm count and sperm abnormalities (Evans et al., 1981), although such data are not unequivocally accepted as important (Howe et al., 1985; Stillman et al., 1986; Vogt et al., 1986; Klaiber et al., 1987). The history of smoking should be recorded. Hormones, such as steroids used by athletes, may suppress spermatogenesis by suppressing gonadotropin release (Wong et al., 1978). Other drugs used for treatment of conditions not necessarily related to infertility, such as cimetidine (Van Thiel et al., 1979), nitrofurantoin and sulphasalazine (Toovey et al., 1981) should also be noted as they may have effects on the hormonal status of the patient and thus affect male reproductive function as well (Jenson et al., 1983; Schlegel et al., 1991).

Occupational exposure to radiation, extraneous heat, and potentially toxic chemicals should be taken into account. Adverse effects of iatrogenic radiation are fully documented (Clifton and Bremmer, 1983; Fossa et al., 1989), and it is quite possible that radiation in the workplace could have the same outcome. Heat may affect spermatogenesis (Kandeel and Swerdloff, 1988), but claims that heat in the workplace reduces fertility, as reported in steelworkers and welders (Mortensen, 1988; Bonde, 1990), remain to be proved. Herbicides and pesticides have been shown to reduce the sperm counts in agricultural workers (Whorton et al., 1977).

A history of scrotal trauma may be important and should include, if available, the surgical report detailing the extent of injury, the approach to repair, and the consequences, perceived or actual. Torsion of one testis may affect the contralateral testis (Nagler and White, 1982) and may even have systemic consequences that affect fertility (Bartsch et al., 1980). A patient's sexual history should include specific questions about the onset of puberty, libido, frequency of intercourse, and general questions to test his understanding of and attitude toward sexuality and the desire to have children.

Salient features of a history taken for evaluation of an infertile man are listed in the box on p. 10.

Physical examination

A complete physical examination should be performed to determine general health, the presence of specific single-organ or multiorgan diseases, and endocrine disturbances. The extent of masculinization, general body habitus, length of extremities, and any grossly visible anomalies should be noted.

Typical eunuchoid features of Klinefelter's syndrome are readily recognizable. Any debilitating chronic disease may temporarily impair the quality of semen. Autoimmune diseases, especially those affecting endocrine organs, such as the pluriglandular autoimmune diseases, deserve scru-

---

Important points to be covered in the medical history of the male partner of an infertile couple

Childhood events

Development
Diseases (mumps)
Surgery (hernia, cryptorchidism)
Malignancy (chemotherapy or radiation therapy)

Infectious diseases

Sexually transmitted
Recent systemic infections

Metabolic disorders

Diabetes mellitus
Obesity

Other diseases

Ulcer; liver, kidney, lung disease

Malignancy

Extragonadal
Gonadal

Drugs

Psychotropic drugs
Cimetidine
Antibiotics
Hormones

Social habits

Tobacco
Alcohol
Substance abuse (marijuana, cocaine)

Occupational exposure

Radiation
Heat
Pesticides

Trauma

Testicular torsion
Spinal cord injury

Sexual history

Puberty
Libido
Pattern of sexual activity
Sexual habits and preferences

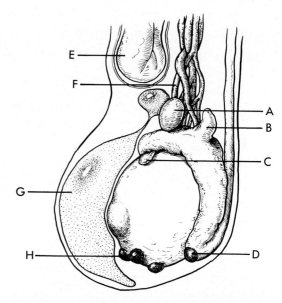

Fig. 2-1. Intrascrotal structures. *A*, Appendix testis. *B*, Appendix epididymis. *C*, Abberaut ducts. *D*, Paradidymis. *E*, Hernia. *F*, Varicocele. *G*, Hydrocele. *H*, Testicular tumor. (Redrawn from Baker HWG. Clinical evaluation and management of testicular disorders in the adult. New York, Raven Press; 1981, p. 360 with permission.)

linization combined with obesity may be a sign of pituitary disease. Anosmia occurs in Kallmann's syndrome (Males et al., 1973). Gynecomastia may be a sign of estrogen-producing tumors or relative hyperestrinism (Elias et al., 1990).

A genital examination should assess the development of the penis and the presence of epispadias or hypospadias, penile curvatures, or Peyronie's disease (Spark, 1988). These abnormalities may hinder normal intercourse or prevent proper ejaculation. Scrotal contents should be palpated to determine the size of the testis. The normal testis measures approximately 4 to 5 cm in length; any reduction in size may indicate a problem that needs further evaluation and even a biopsy. It should be noted that Orientals have smaller testes than whites and blacks.

Anorchia, polyorchia (Leung, 1988), inguinal ectopia, or retractile testes (Nistal and Paniagua, 1984) can be readily diagnosed on physical examination. Cryptorchidism should be noted and if present should be classified according to current medical views (Hadziselimovic, 1983).

Paratesticular structures should also be palpated and identified (Fig. 2-1). The consistency, shape, and sensitivity to palpation of the epididymis and vas deferens should be noted. Any nodularity, cysts, or indurations should be recorded. Palpation of the vas deferens could identify developmental anomalies such as discontinuity or absence of the vas (Dubin and Amelar, 1971). The pampiniform plexus should be palpated and any signs of venous congestion or overt varicocele noted. Hydrocele and paratesticular cysts should be recorded.

Scrotal or inguinal hernia can be diagnosed readily by

tiny (Weinberg et al., 1976). The presence of chronic respiratory infections or bronchiectasis may be a sign of Kartagener's syndrome, characterized by immobility of spermatozoa, or Young's syndrome and ejaculatory duct obstruction (Handelsman et al., 1984). The extent and pattern of distribution of body hair are indicators of masculinization and should be carefully assessed. A lack of mascu-

palpation of the scrotum and insertion of the finger into the external orifice of the inguinal canal. During this examination the patient should strain and perform the Valsalva maneuver, which may expulse the hernia sac content. The Vasalva maneuver also increases the engorgement of the scrotal venous system and may facilitate the demonstration of varicocele.

No physical examination of a male patient is complete without rectal palpation of the prostate and seminal vesicles, which should be included also in the evaluation of infertility. Painful, swollen prostate may indicate infection. Overt pyospermia, the presence of bacteria, and an increased number of leukocytes are typical findings in sperm that correlate with prostatitis (Pryor, 1982).

Sperm analysis

The details of sperm analysis have been outlined in several manuals, including the widely used one prepared by the World Health Organization (1987).

Routine analysis of the ejaculate includes determination of:

1. Volume
2. Sperm count
3. Sperm motility
4. Sperm viability
5. Sperm morphology

None of these parameters has a strong predictive value individually, and in most instances even the most sophisticated analysis of the semen can give only a rough indication of the patient's status (Bostofte et al., 1984; Zaneveld and Jeyendran, 1988).

Sperm analysis rarely provides definitive proof of infertility, primarily because sperm parameters vary considerably from one individual to another (Osser et al., 1983; Krause, 1984). Sperm counts vary in the same individual from day to day, depending on the number and frequency of ejaculations or abstinence (Schwartz et al., 1979). The seasonal nature of spermatogenesis is another cause of variations (Lincoln, 1981; Tjoa et al., 1982). Levine et al. (1990) documented that during summer most men show a reduction in sperm concentration, total sperm count, and concentration of motile sperm. To prevent subjectivity and eliminate the effect of potentially confounding influences, it is therefore recommended to perform at least two examinations of the sperm and to standardize the collection of sperm as much as possible. The patient should be instructed to abstain from sex for 2-3 days before collection, to derive the specimen by masturbation and to bring it within 2 hours to the laboratory for examination in a clean wide-mouthed glass container (Lipshultz and Howards, 1990).

Mankveld and Kruger (1990) have studied close to 2,000 men and concluded that optimal semen quality is obtained after 3-5 days of abstinence. Abstinence for more than 10 days adversely influenced the morphology and mo-

---

Glossary of common semen abnormalities

Aspermia—Inability to produce semen
Hematospermia—Semen containing blood
Hyperspermia—Volume of ejaculate in excess of 6 ml
Hypospermia—Volume of ejaculate less than 1 ml
Pyospermia—Semen containing pus

---

tility of sperm. Thus the recommended period of abstinence varies, but should be in the range of 2-7 days. However, if this schedule is impractical, acceptable and interpretable results may still be obtained if sperm is collected systematically and in a consistent manner.

In most instances there is less than 20% variation between two samples of sperm from the same donor. However, if the variation is greater than 20% more than two ejaculates should be examined. In the vast majority of cases 3 ejaculates will usually suffice for an objective assessment (Poland et al., 1985). The volume of the ejaculate varies from one individual to another. If the volume is less than 1 ml or greater than 6 ml the patient is considered to be hypospermic or hyperspermic, respectively (Zaneveld and Polakoski, 1977). A small volume usually correlates with low sperm count and may be an indication of obstruction of the ejaculatory ducts. Inflammation of accessory glands or retrograde ejaculation (Pryor, 1981) may cause hypospermia and be associated with pyospermia.

Hyperspermic ejaculates reflect either long abstinence or overproduction of seminal fluid, which may be associated with subfertility (Dubin and Amelar, 1971). Close to two thirds of ejaculate fluid stems from seminal vesicles, one third is from the prostate, and less than 5% is the sperm-containing epididymal fluid. An excess of seminal vesicular secretion could presumably dilute the sperm too much and affect its fecundity.

Common terms pertaining to semen are listed in the box above.

Physical properties of sperm are routinely recorded, although these parameters have little diagnostic significance. After ejaculation the sperm coagulates, but the coagulum liquefies within the first 5 to 30 minutes. Coagulum does not form if the vas deferens and/or the seminal vesicles are absent (Menkveld and Kruger, 1990). Impaired liquefaction and increased viscosity occur occasionally with prostatitis, but in the absence of prostatic inflammation the significance of this phenomenon is not known. Increased viscosity may interfere with counting of sperm.

The pH of seminal fluid is usually 7.2 to 7.6. In acute prostatitis the sperm may become more alkaline (Blacklock and Beavis, 1974), whereas chronic infections contribute to an acidification of seminal fluid to a pH below 7.0. The obstruction of ducts also increases the acidity of sperm (Ludwig and Frick, 1990).

Sperm count is important for the assessment of the

quality of sperm, even though this test has a 20% margin of error. The mean sperm count for normal males is 60 to 80 million per milliliter, but the variation is extremely high and the lower limits of normality are difficult to determine unequivocally (MacLeod and Gold, 1953; Poland et al., 1985; Menkveld and Kruger, 1990). Sperm counts over 40 million per milliliter are generally considered normal, and those below 20 million per milliliter are classified as oligozoospermia (Pryor, 1982). Polyzoospermia denotes sperm counts over 250 million per milliliter (Glezerman et al., 1982).

Low sperm count should be interpreted together with data on sperm viability, motility, and morphology, as it was repeatedly shown that low count does not by itself preclude fertilization. Oligoasthenozoospermic semen is, however, definitely associated with decreased male fertility even if one were to use such sperm for intrauterine insemination (Ito et al., 1989). For fertilization *in vitro* less than 1 million sperm are considered adequate (Acosta et al., 1990). Successful *in vitro* fertilization has been reported using spermatozoa from donors with low-density sperm counts but the results may be considerably improved with techniques that facilitate the penetration of spermatozoa into the oocyte (Cohen et al., 1989).

Sperm motility and viability are determined by estimating the number of motile spermatozoa and the direction of their movement or by supravital staining. In the normal specimen examined 1 to 2 hours after ejaculation, 50% to 70% of the spermatozoa are motile, and the specimens showing less than 50% motile spermatozoa are considered abnormal. Most spermatozoa show vigorous forward movement.

On the basis of subjective assessment, spermatozoal motility can be graded on a scale of 0 to 4 (Spark, 1988) or 0 to 10 (Freund, 1966). Alternatively, the motility of sperm may be expressed as a percentage of motile spermatozoa per milliliter of ejaculate (Acosta et al., 1990).

Sperm motility also can be estimated objectively or by multiple-exposure photography and computer-based videomicrography (Makler et al., 1980; Mortimer and Mortimer, 1990). The clinical value of these tests remains controversial, and it is not clear whether the sophisticated technology makes the assessment more objective (Knuth et al., 1987) and whether it contributes to predicting the fertility of the semen more accurately than subjective appraisal.

The term *asthenozoospermia* is used for hypomotile sperm and *necrozoospermia* for nonviable spermatozoa. The diagnosis of necrozoospermia should always be confirmed by supravital staining with eosin, which allows the distinction between immotile and dead spermatozoa (Eliasson, 1977). These and other terms frequently used in andrologic practice are listed in the box above right.

In practical terms, there are three causes of azoospermia or severe oligospermia:

Glossary of common abnormalities of spermatozoa*

Azoospermia—Absence of spermatozoa in the ejaculate
Asthenozoospermia—Reduced motility of spermatozoa
Necrozoospermia—Dead spermatozoa. The term should be used only for nonviable spermatozoa proven to be so by supravital staining. In practice, the term is often used erroneously to denote immotile spermatozoa.
Oligozoospermia—Less than 20 million spermatozoa per milliliter of ejaculate
Polyzoospermia—More than 250 million spermatozoa per milliliter of ejaculate
Teratozoospermia—More than 60% abnormal spermatozoa without a reduction of sperm count

*Abnormal ejaculates often show more than one abnormality (e.g., oligo-asthenozoospermia).

Etiology of oligospermia and azoospermia

1. Genetic and chromosomal disorders (e.g., Klinefelter's syndrome, Noonan's syndrome)
2. Hypothalamic and pituitary disorders (e.g., hypogonadotropic hypogonadism)
3. Testicular disease
   Developmental (e.g., cryptorchidism)
   Infectious (e.g., mumps)
   Iatrogenic (e.g., cancer chemotherapy)
   Idiopathic (e.g., germinal cell aplasia)
4. Obstruction or aplasia of the ductal system
   Congenital (e.g., aplasia of vas deferens)
   Inflammatory (e.g., sexually transmitted diseases)
   Traumatic/iatrogenic (e.g., vasectomy, torsion)
5. Retrograde ejaculation (e.g., autonomic disturbances, ganglionic blockers)

---

1. Disturbance of spermatogenesis
2. Ejaculatory duct obstruction
3. Retrograde ejaculation

Etiologically, various diseases causing sperm abnormalities may be further subclassified, as shown in the box directly above.

The morphology of sperm in air-dried, routinely stained cytology slides may be scrutinized readily. The early reports of MacLeod and Gold (1953) found good correlations between abnormal sperm morphology and infertility. Others, such as Pryor (1981), dispute the value of morphologic evaluation of sperm, because of considerable variation in the morphology of normal human sperm. Several attempts were made to introduce strict criteria (Freund, 1966; Eliasson, 1971) but without general consensus. Nevertheless, careful evaluation of well-prepared specimens using criteria seems to yield reproducible data with a good predictive value for in vivo or in vitro fertilization (Kruger et al., 1986 and 1988). There is a correlation between abnormal sperm morphology and oligozoospermia (Singer et al., 1980) and abnormal spermatozoal motility (Katz et al., 1982). Hence, morphologic examination of the semen remains an important aspect of evaluation of infertility.

Normal spermatozoa have an oval head. Other forms include amorphous small and large spermatozoa and tapered, duplicated forms (Ludwig and Frick, 1990). Immature forms account for less than 3% of all live spermatozoa. Other spermatogenic cells may be found in the ejaculate but should be distinguished from lymphocytes and clumped leukocytes.

A more detailed analysis and more elaborated classification of abnormal spermatozoa may be used, although there is no agreement whether this investment of time and effort is always justified.

The ten most common sperm abnormalities, according to Ali and Grimes (1989), include:

1. Acrosomal cap defects
2. Vacuolated head
3. Tapered head
4. Elongated head
5. Bent head
6. Coiled tail piece
7. Absence of tail
8. Macrocephaly
9. Microcephaly
10. Presence of spermatocytes

Duplicate heads, acephaly, duplicate tail, cytoplasmic extrusions, cytoplasmic droplets, round head, and short tail are found in less than 5% of both fertile and infertile men. A similar detailed classification of abnormal spermatozoa, introduced by Hammen (1944) and used in the laboratory of Bostofte et al. (1985) lists the following (Fig. 2-2):

1. Piriform heads
2. Narrow heads
3. Round heads
4. Pinheads
5. Small heads
6. Giant heads
7. Amorphous heads
8. Staining abnormalities
9. Vacuoles
10. Belted heads
11. Irregular heads
12. Various rare head forms
13. Double forms
14. Abortive forms

Bostofte et al. (1984 and 1985) admit that such a detailed analysis does not provide useful predictors of fertility. Hence these authors restrict their assessment to a ratio of normal to abnormal spermatozoa, noting that the percentage of normal spermatozoa provides the best index of fertility.

The morphology of spermatozoa should be examined also in the cervical mucus obtained for the postcoital test. The approach advocated by Menkveld and Kruger (1990) has the advantage over other methods in that it is relatively simple, has been proved to be reproducible (Ayodeji and Baker, 1986), and has a good correlation with successful in vitro fertilization (Kruger et al., 1986 and 1988). These authors emphasize that the morphology of spermatozoa can be examined only in technically good smears and that a good reference point, derived from normal sperm, always should be available for comparison.

According to the criteria of Menkveld et al. (1990), a normal spermatozoon has an oval head of smooth contour and an acrosome that composes 40% to 70% of the total surface (Fig. 2-3). No abnormalities of the neck, midpiece, or tail should be evident, and the cytoplasmic droplets should not occupy more than half of the head. Acrosomal abnormalities and amorphousness or elongation of the head should be noted, and all borderline normal spermatozoa should be considered abnormal. The dimensions of the head vary from 3 to 5 by 2 to 3 μm to 5 to 6 by 2.5 to 3.5 μm, depending on the staining technique used. The method for sperm evaluation should be standardized for each laboratory, although variation in the size and shape of spermatozoal heads does not seem to be critical in most cases.

Using strict morphologic criteria, Kruger et al. (1986) reported that semen with more than 15% normal spermatozoa has essentially the same capacity for in vitro fertilization as normal semen. No pregnancy occurred with ova exposed to semen with less than 15% normal spermatozoa. New techniques of in vitro fertilization, such as zone splitting, may enhance the fertilization by spermatozoa that are inadequate for reproduction in vivo (Simon et al., 1991).

Electron microscopy has been used extensively for detailed analysis of human spermatozoa (Zamboni, 1987 and 1991). Typical abnormalities recognized by electron microscopy can be classified as those involving either the head, connecting piece, or tail of spermatozoa (Fig. 2-4). Among the head defects, the most important and most common are various structural abnormalities that frequently occur conjointly. Abnormalities of the connecting piece result in the so-called bent head defect or decapitation, i.e., separation of the head from the tail (Baccetti et al., 1989). Tail abnormalities, such as fibrous sheath defects and microtubular derangements, may affect sperm motility (Afzelius, 1981; Williamson et al., 1984). Scanning electron microscopy has been used less frequently, although it seems to provide more reliable data (Badenoch et al., 1990).

Chemical analysis of ejaculates is of relatively limited value in the evaluation of infertility. The measurement of seminal fluid fructose as a test for evaluation of seminal

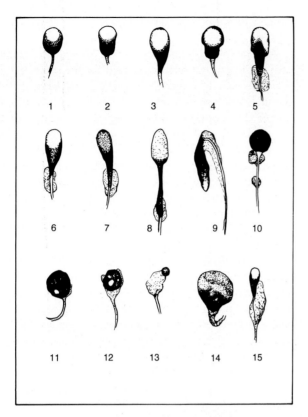
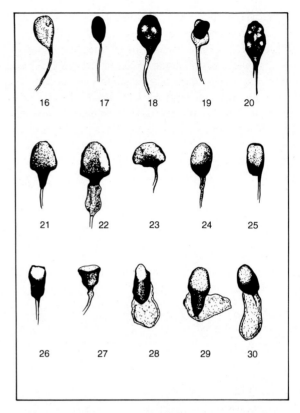
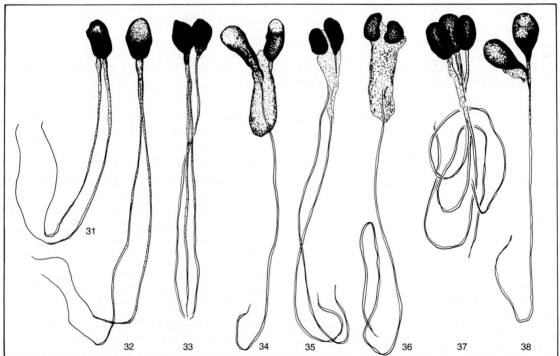

Fig. 2-2. Morphology of normal and abnormal human spermatozoa. *1*. Normal spermatozoa; *2*. normal piriform head; *3–8*. various forms of piriform heads; *9*. narrow head; *10–12*. round head; *13*. pin head, giant head; *14*. giant head; *15*. small head; *16–18*. staining abnormalities; *19*. amorphous head; *20*. vacuolated head; *21–23*. belted heads; *24*. stalked head; *25*. head with abaxial implantation of the middle piece; *26*. acrosomal defect; *27*. bell-shaped head; *28–30*. abortive forms with abnormal and normal heads; *31–38*. various double forms. (Redrawn from Hammen R. Studies on Impaired Fertility in Man with Special Reference to the Male. Copenhagen-London, Munksgaard & Milford; 1944.)

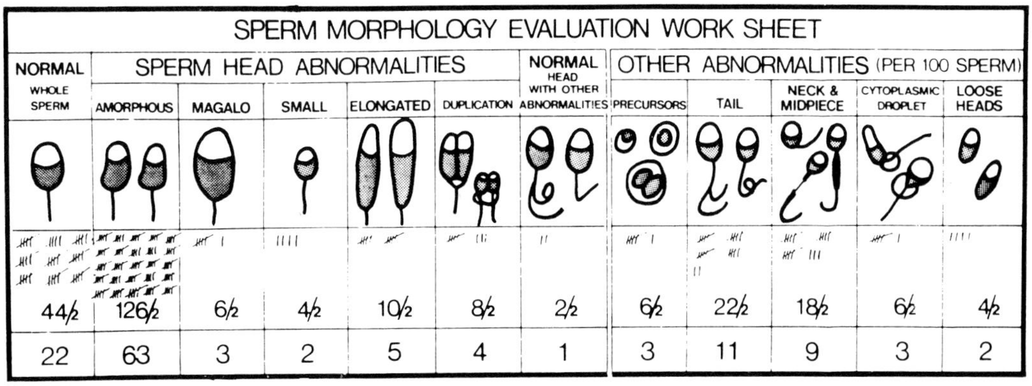

SPERM MORPHOLOGY EVALUATION WORK SHEET

NORMAL WHOLE SPERM	AMORPHOUS	MAGALO	SMALL	ELONGATED	DUPLICATION	NORMAL HEAD WITH OTHER ABNORMALITIES	PRECURSORS	TAIL	NECK & MIDPIECE	CYTOPLASMIC DROPLET	LOOSE HEADS
	SPERM HEAD ABNORMALITIES						OTHER ABNORMALITIES (PER 100 SPERM)				
44½	126½	6½	4½	10½	8½	2½	6½	22½	18½	6½	4½
22	63	3	2	5	4	1	3	11	9	3	2

Fig. 2-3. Schematic illustrations of seven main classes of spermatozoa. (From Menkveld et al., Hum Reprod, 1990; 5:586, by permission of Oxford University Press.)

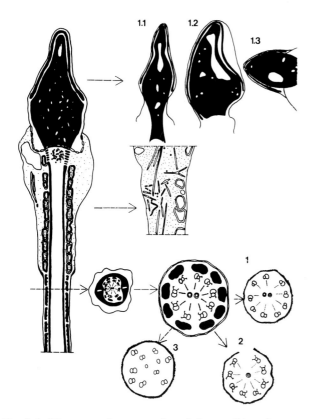

Fig. 2-4. Diagrammatic presentation of abnormalities of spermatozoa detected by electron microscopy. The abnormalities of the head include elongation, structural abnormalities, and angulation. The neck area abnormalities include rupture ("decapitation") and internal disorganization. The tail abnormalities include loss of the dynein arm (as in Kartagener's syndrome), loss of the normal 9+2 pattern of microtubular doublets, and complete disorganization of microtubules. (Drawn from data of Zamboni, 1991.)

vesicles and spermatic duct patency has achieved the greatest popularity (Ludwig and Frick, 1990). Fructose is secreted by seminal vesicles, and the lack of fructose in the ejaculate suggests either seminal vesicle disease or an obstruction. Transrectal ultrasonography may be per-

Table 2-1. Principal parameters of semen analysis

Parameter	Normal values
Volume of ejaculate	1–6 ml
Sperm count	20–100 million/ml
Sperm motility	50–70%
Forward progression	Most sperm move forward in a straight line.
Sperm morphology	> 60% normal
Other cells	< 3% immature spermatogenic cells or lymphocytes
	Occasional segmented leukocytes
Fructose	Present

formed for the same purpose and has proved to be a more reliable technique for detecting unilateral seminal vesicle disturbances and the sites of obstruction.

Seminal fluid alpha-glucosidase, an enzyme that originates primarily from the epididymis, may hold some promise for evaluating obstructive azoospermia (Casano et al., 1987; Guerin et al., 1990). Creatinine kinase activity of sperm may predict fertilizing potential as suggested by Huszar et al. (1990). The clinical value of these newer tests needs to be independently confirmed and correlated with other sperm parameters. The principal parameters of semen analysis are summarized in Table 2-1.

Hormonal studies

Hormonal studies are indicated to further evaluate azoospermia and to determine whether azoospermia is a symptom of primary or secondary hypogonadism. In most instances the first step in this evaluation is the measurement of serum follicle-stimulating hormone (FSH) followed by measurement of luteinizing hormone (LH) and prolactin (PRL) (Lipshultz and Howards, 1990). Some authorities advocate immediate measurement of LH, FSH, and testosterone initially in evaluating all azoospermic patients (Swerdloff et al., 1985).

Table 2-2. Hormonal profiles of infertile men with azoospermia or oligozoospermia

Testosterone	LH	FSH	PRL	Possible diagnosis
Low	Low	Low	Low	Hypothalamic or pituitary hypogonadism; pituitary tumor
Low	Low	Low	High	Prolactinoma
Low	High	High	Normal	Testicular failure (primary or secondary)
Normal	Normal	High	Normal	Germ cell aplasia
Normal	Normal	Normal	Normal	Idiopathic infertility

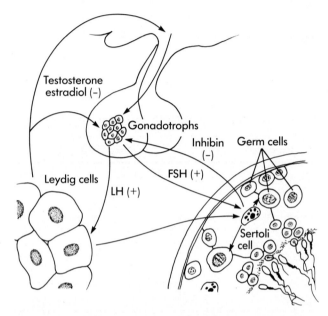

Fig. 2-5. Schematic drawing of the hormonal control of testicular function, illustrating the negative feedback of inhibin and testosterone on gonadotropin secretion. FSH acts on Sertoli cells and LH acts on Leydig cells. (Modified from Ying S-Y. Endocrine Reviews 1988; 9:267, © The Endocrine Society, and from Bardin CW. Hosp Pract 1988; Apr 15:89, with permission.)

LH secreted from the pituitary under the control of hypothalamic-releasing factor acts on Leydig cells and is the primary regulator of androgen synthesis in the testis (Ying, 1988). Lack of LH in serum suggests a primary pituitary problem. FSH stimulates Sertoli cells to release locally the androgen-binding protein (ABP), thus ensuring high concentration of androgens in seminiferous tubules essential for normal spermatogenesis. Inhibin, which is produced by Sertoli cells, inhibits the secretion of FSH, whereas activin has a stimulatory effect (Fig. 2-5).

The lack of negative feedback on pituitary gonadotrophs is typical of primary testicular disturbances and abnormal spermatogenesis. Low serum levels of FSH and LH associated with the low serum levels of other pituitary hormones, such as PRL, are indicative of a primary pituitary defect, such as panhypopituitarism (Table 2-2). Pituitary tumors, including prolactinomas and corticotropin- or somatotropin-secreting adenomas, may compress the gonadotrophs or the hypothalamic nuclei and thus suppress FSH and LH secretion. The most common pituitary tumors

are microscopic or macroscopic prolactinomas; these are typically associated with hyperprolactinemia. Other pituitary tumors such as those secreting adrenocorticotropic hormone (ACTH), thyroid-stimulating hormone (TSH), or growth hormone should be excluded if serum LH and FSH are low and there is no evidence of hyperprolactinemia.

Specialized and investigative studies

Immunologic studies are indicated if the sperm analysis reveals selective sperm motility problems or increased agglutinability (Bronson et al., 1984). The preferred test is based on detection of antisperm antibodies in the patient's serum or in the seminal fluid (Clarke, 1987). Immunobead test (IBT) has gained popularity because it shows the binding of antibodies to various parts of the sperm (Adeghe et al., 1986). With this test one can distinguish the motile from immotile spermatozoa and the effect of the bound antibody on sperm motility. The significance of a positive IBT, which usually means at least 20% spermatozoa are positively labeled with the beads, has not yet been fully evaluated and/or correlated with various treatment modalities. The usefulness of this test remains controversial, and additional immunologic tests are being introduced (Smithwick and Young, 1990).

Other special studies such as zona-free hamster oocyte sperm penetration assay, mucus migration tests, acrosome test (Kennedy et al., 1989), and hypoosmotic swelling test have been reviewed in Acosta et al. (1990). These tests are used with equivocal results and varying degrees of enthusiasm and are best relegated to highly specialized laboratories.

The standard work-up of infertile men may follow one of several typical algorithms outlined in clinical textbooks dealing with infertility (Lipshultz and Howards, 1990; Mishell et al., 1991). An algorithm for evaluation of infertility in men is shown in Algorithm 2-1.

Testicular biopsy

Testicular biopsy, introduced into clinical practice by Charny (1960), is performed as part of the surgical exploration of the scrotum and the evaluation of azoospermia or oligospermia (Pesce, 1987; Magid et al., 1990; Wheeler, 1991). Typically, the biopsy is indicated if the sperm findings cannot be explained in terms of endocrine abnormalities or clinical features indicative of a well-characterized syndrome (box on p. 17).

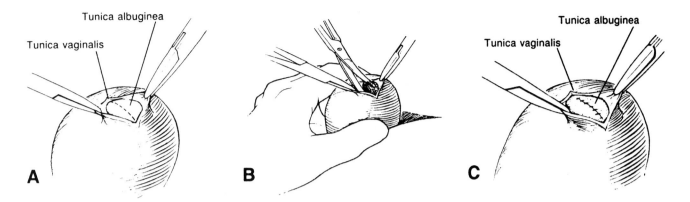

Fig. 2-6. "No-touch" testicular biopsy technique using the window approach. Method of testicular biopsy. **A,** The tunica vaginalis is incised, exposing the tunica albuginea. The edges of the tunica vaginalis are grasped with hemostats. **B,** A small bit of testicular stroma will extrude, and a 2-mm square portion is cut off with a small pair of scissors. **C,** The tunica albuginea is closed with 4-0 chromic atraumatic sutures. (Reproduced from deCherney et al., 1988.)

Indications for testicular biopsy*
Absolute
Azoospermia
Oligozoospermia
Teratozoospermia
Atypical cells in ejaculate
Relative
Varicocele
Cryptorchidism
Chronic infection

*Elevation of FSH three times over normal is considered sufficient evidence of primary hypogonadism to obviate a biopsy.

Table 2-3. Fixatives for testicular biopsy

Stieve's fixative		
Solution A:	Mercury chloride	90 g
	Distilled water	1430 ml
Solution B:	Formaldehyde (38%)	400 ml
	Acetic acid, glacial	80 ml
	Mix 38 ml of solution A and 12 ml of solution B. Mercury is corrosive, so gloves should be worn.	
	Fix for 24 to 36 hours.	
Bouin's solution		
	Picric acid, saturated	15 ml
	Formaldehyde (38%)	5 ml
	Acetic acid, glacial	1 ml
	Fix for 24 hours.	

Optimal results are obtained by open surgical incisional biopsy (Fig. 2-6). Transcutaneous biopsy and fine-needle aspiration biopsy provide reasonable alternatives (Papic et al., 1988) but are not widely used, mostly because the random sampling may result in undue damage and hematomas. Because there is significant variation of testicular morphology and uneven distribution of lesions (Posinovec, 1976), ideally both testes should sampled, although this may be impractical.

A specimen measuring 2 to 3 mm in largest diameter should be removed without much compression and immediately placed into Bouin's or Stieve's fixative (Table 2-3). Formalin is unsuitable because it causes excessive shrinkage of the tubules and poor preservation of nuclear details. The tissue may be processed routinely and embedded in paraffin or Paraplast. In specialized laboratories, biopsy samples may be processed for methacrylate or other hard plastic embedding. Routine hematoxylin and eosin staining suffices in most instances, but it may be supplemented with special stains such as periodic acid–Schiff (PAS) staining to demonstrate glycogen and the outlines of basement membranes, or one of the trichrome stains for evaluation of interstitial fibrosis.

The testicular biopsy specimen should be large enough to allow evaluation of at least 100 profiles of sectioned seminiferous tubules. The evaluation should take into account the following.

The overall morphology of the testicular tissue. The examiner should determine whether the normal architecture of the testis is preserved. If there are lesions, it should be established whether they are segmental, limited to a part of biopsy; multifocal or diffuse; unilateral or bilateral.

The size and structure of the seminiferous tubules. The contours of tubules and their size and distribution should be evaluated to determine the extent of atrophy, tubular loss, and basement membrane thickening.

Interstitial tissue. Connective tissue stroma should be examined and its texture and cellularity described. The ra-

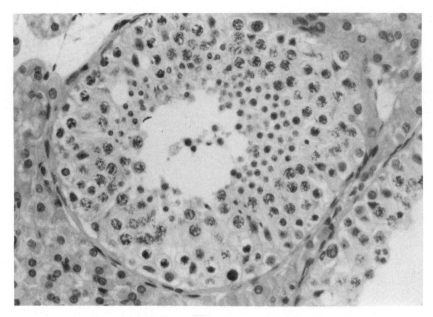

Fig. 2-7. Maturation arrest at the stage of round spermatids.

tio of tubules to interstitial tissue should be determined. Vascular changes should be noted. Leydig cells should be identified, and it should be noted whether they are aggregated in groups or scattered at random. The number and type of inflammatory cells should be recorded.

Spermatogenesis. Cell types lining the seminiferous tubules should be identified and the various stages of spermatogenesis evaluated. If spermatogenesis is incomplete, the stage at which it is blocked should be noted.

Degenerative changes and abnormal cells. Vacuolization, necrosis, or fragmentation of Sertoli and germ cells should be registered. Neoplastic cells typical of carcinoma in situ or invasive cancer and cancer metastases should be reported.

The changes in the testicular biopsy can be quantitated according to several systems (Johnsen, 1970; Skakkebaek and Heller, 1973; Makler and Abramovici, 1978; Sigg, 1979; Silber and Rodriguez-Rigau, 1981), which all show a good correlation with the sperm count.

Johnsen (1970) has devised a semiquantitative system on a scale of 1 to 10. Each seminiferous tubule is examined and given a score according to the following criteria:

10—If the germinal epithelium is multilayered around an open central lumen that contains numerous spermatozoa.

9—If the germinal epithelium appears multilayered but is slightly disorganized and shows sloughing into the central lumen, causing its obliteration. Spermatozoa are present and admixed to sloughed-off epithelium in the obliterated central lumen.

8—If the germinal epithelium is multilayered but fewer than 10 spermatozoa are present in the lumen.

7—If there are numerous spermatids but no spermatozoa (Fig. 2-7).

6—If there are no spermatozoa and less than 10 spermatids.

5—If there are only spermatocytes but no spermatids or spermatozoa (Fig. 2-8).

4—If there are no spermatozoa and spermatids and fewer than five spermatocytes.

3—If spermatogonia are the only germ cells present (Fig. 2-9).

2—If only Sertoli cells are present and no germ cells are visible (Fig. 2-10).

1—If no cells are inside the seminiferous tubule.

The sum of the scores assigned to each tubule is divided by the number of tubules counted, and a mean score is calculated. Typical examples illustrating Johnsen's system are shown in Figures 2-7 to 2-10.

In addition to seminiferous tubules, Johnsen (1970) mandates an evaluation of Leydig cells. The number of Leydig's cells is estimated, and a Leydig cell score (LS) is assigned on a scale of 1 to 6:

LS 1 indicates complete absence of Leydig cells.
LS 2 is a significant reduction.
LS 3 is an average number of Leydig cells.
LS 4 and LS 5 represent an increased number of Leydig cells.
LS 6 is nodular or diffuse hyperplasia of Leydig cells.

According to the scoring system of Johnsen (1970), the normal testis contains at least 60% of tubules with a score of 10, and less than 10% of tubules will have a score lower than 8. The mean score for the normal testis is 9.39

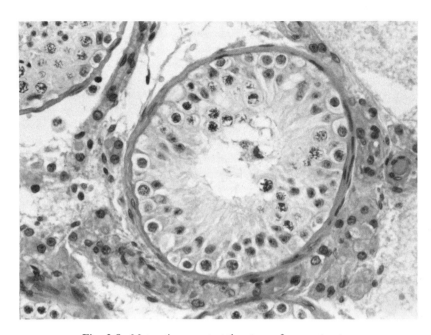

Fig. 2-8. Maturation arrest at the stage of spermatocytes.

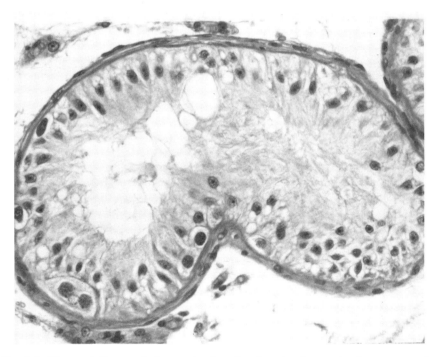

Fig. 2-9. The seminiferous tubule contains Sertoli cells and only occasional spermatogonia.

± 0.24. The mean score is decreased in conditions affecting spermatogenesis as reported by Johnsen (1970):

Oligozoospermia (less than 20 million sperm per milliliter): 5.32 + 2.13
Klinefelter syndrome: 1.25 ± 0.28
Pituitary hypogonadism: 3.95 ± 1.42
Sertoli-cell–only syndrome: 2.0 ± 0.03

Skakkebaek and Heller (1973) have attempted to quantify the spermatogenetic cells using the Sertoli cell numbers per tubule as a constant and expressing their results as a germ cell/Sertoli cell ratio. These authors have used biopsies fixed in Cleland's fixative, stained with iron hematoxylin, which made it possible to differentiate dark and pale type A spermatogonia from B spermatogonia; classify spermatocytes as preleptotene, leptotene, zygotene, and pachytene spermatocytes; and distinguish early and late spermatids. The total number of counted germ cells of

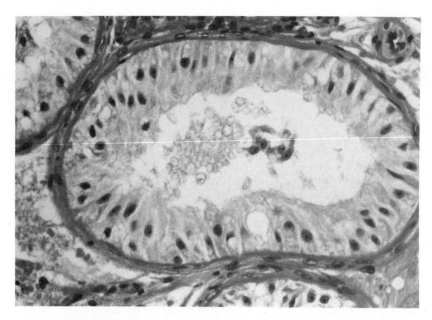

Fig. 2-10. The seminiferous tubule contains only Sertoli cells.

each type was divided by the total number of Sertoli cells in the same cross section of the tubule, and a Sertoli cell ratio (SCR) was calculated. In the normal testes the mean SCR for various cell types is as follows:

Spermatogonia A, dark	0.70
Spermatogonia A, light	0.79
Spermatogonia B	0.28
Spermatocytes, preleptotene	0.25
Spermatocytes, leptotene	0.22
Spermatocytes, zygotene and pachytene	1.96
Spermatids, early	3.05
Spermatids, late	2.14

The differences in the morphology of spermatogonia subtypes are not as apparent in Stieve's and Bouin's fixed tissue. Nevertheless, the ratio of three main forms of germ cells to Sertoli cells can be easily calculated in normal men. There are approximately 1.8 spermatogonia, 2 spermatocytes, and 5.2 spermatids per Sertoli cell per cross-sectioned tubule (Wheeler, 1991).

Makler and Abramovici (1978) designed an elaborate semiquantitative scoring system in which they took into account four parameters: the inner diameter of the tubules, the thickness of the basement membranes, the population of intratubular cells, and the degree of spermatogenic maturation. Each of these parameters was scored on a scale of 0 to 5, and results were added for a final score on a scale of 0 to 20.

The diameter of the tubules was scored as follows:

5—Normal tubules, 150 to 250 μm
4—Slightly reduced diameter, 75 to 100 μm
3—Moderately reduced diameter, 75 to 100 μm
2—Small tubules, 50 to 75 μm
1—Very small tubules, 25 to 50 μm
0—Almost obliterated tubules

The thickness of the tubular basement membrane was scored as follows:

5—Normal thickness, 3 μm
4—Slightly thickened, 3 to 5 μm
3—Moderately thickened, 5 to 7 μm
2—Severely thickened, 7 to 10 μm
1—Extremely thickened, 10 to 13 μm
0—Hyalinized

The cell populations were assessed by counting the number of cell layers in each cross-sectioned tubule and scored as follows:

5—More than four cell layers
4—Three to four cell layers
3—Two to three cell layers
2—One to two cell layers
1—One cell layer
0—No cells

The degree of spermatogenic maturation was scored as follows:

5—Maturation to spermatozoa
4—Maturation to spermatids
3—Maturation to secondary spermatocytes
2—Maturation to primary spermatocytes
1—Spermatogonia only
0—Sertoli cells only

Using this scoring system, Makler and Abramovici (1978) found that oligozoospermic men with a sperm count of 10 to 20 million sperm per milliliter have a score of approxi-

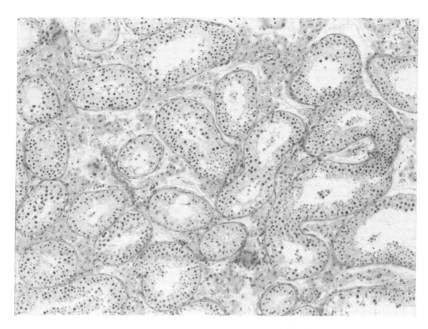

Fig. 2-11. Diffuse atrophy. All tubules show maturation arrest at the stage of round spermatids.

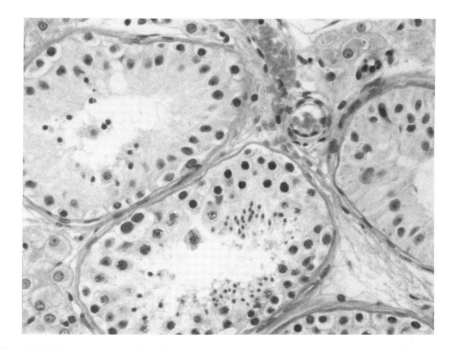

Fig. 2-12. Mixed atrophy. One tubule contains spermatozoa, the other a few round spermatids and the third only Sertoli cells.

mately 18 to 18.5. Men with a sperm count of 5 to 10 million sperm per milliliter had an average score of 12.5; those with a sperm count of 1 to 5 million sperm per milliliter had a mean score of 10.1; and those with less than 1 million had a mean score of 8.7. These authors conclude that in men with a sperm count over 12 million sperm per milliliter, the testicular biopsy provides little useful information and is warranted rarely if at all.

According to the system proposed by Sigg (1979), good results can be obtained by classifying the abnormal testicular findings into one of the following three groups: (1) diffuse atrophy, in which all the tubules show an approximately even degree of atrophy (Fig. 2-11); (2) focal atrophy, in which at least 5 cross-sectioned tubules show the same degree of atrophy; (3) mixed atrophy, in which adjacent tubules show varying degrees of atrophy (Fig. 2-12).

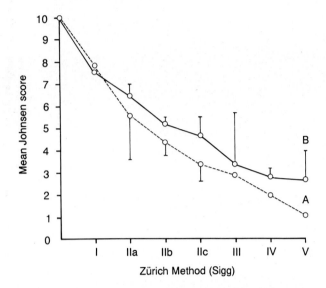

Fig. 2-13. The methods of Johnsen (1970) and Sigg (1979) yield comparable results, as shown by Mikuz et al. (1983). (Modified from Mikuz G, Schwarz C, Bartsch G. Der Pathologe 1983; 4:244, with permission.)

The degree of atrophy is estimated on a scale of I to V as follows:

I—Mild atrophy evidenced by spermatogenesis but a reduced number of spermatozoa (less than 10 per tubule)

II—Moderate tubular atrophy evidenced by (a) reduced thickness of germinal epithelium, (b) reduced diameter of seminiferous tubules, and (c) thickening of the basal membrane and lamina propria layers

IIa—Maturation arrest at the level of spermatids

IIb—Maturation arrest at the level of spermatocytes

IIc—Maturation arrest at the level of spermatogonia

III—Marked tubular atrophy recognized by (a) almost complete lack of germ cells, (b) markedly reduced diameter of tubules, (c) thickening of the basement membranes and lamina propria layers, and (d) occasional degenerative changes of Sertoli cells

IV—Sertoli-cell–only syndrome

V—Severe tubular atrophy with subtotal or total hyalinization and loss of intratubular cells

The evaluation of changes involving the seminiferous tubules is supplemented by observations pertaining to the (a) number and appearance of Leydig cells, (b) extent of interstitial fibrosis, (c) vascular changes, and (d) evidence of inflammation.

Mikuz et al. (1983) have applied the Zürich method of Sigg (1979) to their own material and compared it with the scoring system of Johnsen (1970). A good correlation was found between the two approaches (Fig. 2-13).

The quantitative methods for the evaluation of testicular biopsies are time-consuming and tedious. Alternative approaches based on simplified criteria have been recommended ranging from purely descriptive to semiquantitative assessments based on simplified criteria. Honoré (1979) uses four categories:

1. Suggestive of obstruction—a diagnosis applied to specimens whenever a discrepancy is found between the biopsy and sperm count
2. Hypospermatogenesis evidenced by incomplete maturation of spermatogenic cells
3. Sertoli cell–only syndrome
4. Testicular dysmorphogenesis related to chromosomal and developmental disorders.

Silber and Rodriguez-Rigau (1981) noted that an adequate assessment can be made by simply counting the number of round spermatids per tubule. The number of oval spermatids with dark, densely stained chromatin correlates roughly with the sperm count. In patients with more than 10 million sperm per milliliter, the tubule always contains more than 20 mature spermatids, whereas in patients without obstruction with less than 10 million sperm per milliliter, there were always less than 20 mature spermatids per tubule. Thus one can estimate spermatogenesis relatively quickly, expecting a high correlation with the sperm count.

Posttesticular causes of azoospermia and oligozoospermia

Azoospermia or severe oligozoospermia in the presence of normal testicular biopsy indicates either an obstruction of excretory ducts or retrograde ejaculation. In view of the fact that a vasogram might be indicated, some urologists prepare a touch preparation from the testicular sample to establish whether there are living spermatozoa in the testis (Dodson and Joshi, 1989). If there are no spermatozoa, a vasogram may be performed while the patient is still under generalized anesthesia to establish the site of obstruction or congenital aplasia. Other urologists defer additional treatment until a detailed analysis of the testicular biopsy is completed.

Hendry et al. (1990) have analyzed 37 patients with obstructive azoospermia and 80 patients with unilateral testicular obstruction. Their findings are summarized in Figure 2-14. In 176 (48%) cases, the obstruction was in the epididymis, 29% of which was in the head and 19% in the tail of the epididymis. Absent vas deferens was found in 86 (23%) cases, most of which were bilateral. Obstructed vas deferens was found in 40 (11%) cases and the obstruction of the ejaculatory duct in 14 (4%) cases. The etiology of these conditions varied. One can conclude that the obstruction of seminal excretory ducts could occur at many levels and that it may be caused by several pathogenetic mechanisms. Good reparative results can be obtained by microsurgery. In patients whose condition cannot be surgically corrected, epididymal sperm directly aspirated from the epididymis can be used for *in vitro* insemination (Silber et al., 1990).

Retrograde ejaculation is one of the more common

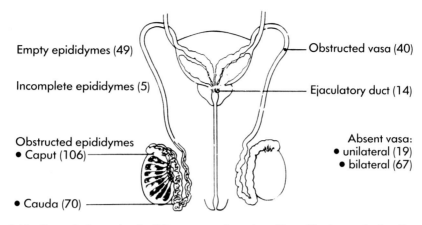

Fig. 2-14. Sites of obstruction in 370 azoospermic males. (From Hendry et al. Ann Roy Coll Surg Engl, 1990; 72:396, with permission.)

Table 2-4. Causes of retrograde ejaculation

Surgery	Retroperitoneal or intraperitoneal lymph node dissection
	Lumbar sympathectomy
	Prostate/bladder neck surgery
	Aortoiliac surgery
	Rectal surgery
Spinal cord injury	Posttraumatic paralysis
	Spinal cord surgery
	Spinal column surgery
Trauma of the bladder neck	
Neurologic diseases of the spinal cord	
	Multiple sclerosis
	Tabes dorsalis
	Poliomyelitis
	Viral encephalomyelitis
Diabetes mellitus	
Drugs	Alpha-adrenergic blocking agents
	Antihypertensive drugs
	Tranquilizers
Congenital anomalies of the bladder neck area	
Idiopathic	

Modified from Collins JP. In Baun J, Schill WB, Schwargstein Y (Eds). Treatment of Male Infertility. Berlin, Springer-Verlag; 1982, p. 179.)

Table 2-5. Pathophysiologic-etiologic classification of the principal causes of infertility in women

Hormonal disturbances	Hypothalamic release factors
	Pituitary hormones
	Ovarian hormonal secretion or response to stimulation
	Endometrial response
	Cervical response
Infection	Salpingitis
	Endometritis
	Cervicitis
Immune reactions	Autoimmune diseases
	Immune reaction to sperm
	Immune reactions to fetus and placenta
Congenital disorders	Gonadal dysgenesis
	Anomalies of the uterus
	Anomalies of the vagina and external genitalia
Idiopathic and poorly understood disorders	Endometriosis
	Metabolic disorders
	Habitual abortion

causes of low sperm count. The diagnosis of ejaculatory dysfunction should be suspected in men with oligoazoospermia, or azoospermia and a low ejaculatory volume (Dodson and Joshi, 1989). The diagnosis can be confirmed by examining the postejaculatory urine for spermatozoa. The most common causes of retrograde ejaculation are listed in Table 2-4.

WORK-UP OF THE FEMALE PATIENT

The work-up of the female should include the following:

1. Personal history
2. Reproductive and marital history
3. Physical examination
4. Gynecologic examination
5. If needed, special studies such as hormonal evaluation, laparoscopy, hysterosalpingography, and immunologic evaluation

On the basis of these data, the cause of infertility could be classified in one of the several categories listed in Table 2-5. A detailed discussion of the work-up of the woman is beyond the scope of this monograph. Clinical texts (Speroff et al., 1989; Seibel, 1990; Acosta et al., 1990; Yen and Jaffe, 1991) should be consulted for additional information. Nevertheless, as the pathologist plays an important role in evaluating the infertile couple, a brief summary of the clinician's task is presented to emphasize the team approach to all problems of infertility.

History

Past and present history should encompass information regarding the patient's general health status, past and present diseases, and whether such diseases have been treated medically or surgically. Previous abdominal surgery such as appendectomy should be noted. Adhesions after appendectomy are a documented risk factor for tubal infertility (Mueller et al., 1986). Many debilitating, chronic infectious, immune, and metabolic diseases are known to impair fertility. Temporal hair loss, supralabial hair growth, or excessive hirsutism and acne may reflect androgen excess. Galactorrhea may be a sign of hyperprolactinemia and pituitary lesions. Mood swings and easy fatigability, sweating, or changes in bowel habits may point to thyroid disturbances.

The patient should be asked about her eating habits because such questioning may reveal anorexia nervosa or bulimia. Dietary habits and recent weight loss or weight gain also could have an impact on reproductive function. Reasonable exercise is generally beneficial, but excessive strenuous exercise and athletic training may have profound effects on the menstrual cycle. Stress at work or in daily life may have similar effects.

Social history should encompass data about the workplace and habits such as smoking, alcohol consumption, or use of recreational drugs; all these may have adverse effects on reproduction (Verp, 1983). Intake of drugs, steroids, and other hormones should be scrutinized for potential side effects that may affect fertility.

Reproductive and marital history should include questions on prepubertal development, the onset of menarche, the regularity of the menstrual cycle, and the duration and amount of blood loss during menstruation. It should be recorded whether the patient has ever had spontaneous or induced abortions. Ectopic pregnancies, pelvic inflammatory disease, sexually transmitted disease, and pregnancies from previous marriages and their outcome should be documented. Specific questions should be asked about frequency of intercourse and sexual habits, contraception, and the duration of the effort to become pregnant. The salient points to be covered in the interview are listed in the box on the right.

Physical examination

A physical examination should take note of the patient's general health and nutritional status. Both obesity and extreme asthenia are associated with reproductive problems. Facial hirsutism and facial or body acne may be signs of androgen excess. The facial skin rash of systemic lupus erythematosus may signal an underlying autoimmune disorder. Exophthalmos and enlarged thyroid may be symptoms of Graves' disease. Tachycardia, sweaty palms, and overactivity may be other signs of hyperthyroidism. Excess body hair on the chest or abdomen or a male escutcheon can be indicative of virilization. Breast development should be assessed and the tissue palpated, including a

---

> **Important points to be covered in the history of the female partner of an infertile couple**
>
> 1. Duration of infertility (When did the couple decide to attempt pregnancy?)
> 2. Menstrual history—menarche, cycle length, regularity, duration of menses, and amount of menstrual bleeding
> 3. Previous contraception (IUD, oral contraceptives, diaphragm, spermicides, subcutaneous implantation devices, previous tubal sterilization)
> 4. Previous pregnancies, abortions (voluntary or spontaneous)
> 5. Coital frequency, timing, and techniques, including the use of lubricants
> 6. Current or previous medical conditions
> 7. Hormonal symptoms—galactorrhea, hirsutism, obesity, hyperactivity or hypoactivity
> 8. Sexually transmitted diseases or pelvic inflammatory disease
> 9. Previous surgical treatment, especially pelvic and gynecologic procedures
> 10. Medications, present and past
> 11. Social habits, recreational drugs, exposure to toxins in the environment or workplace
> 12. Family history of infertility or associated problems

---

gentle compression of nipples. If there is evidence of lactation, pituitary disorders, most notably prolactinemia (Koppelman et al., 1984), should be excluded with additional testing.

A gynecologic examination should record signs of inadequate development of the external or internal genital organs. Signs of masculinization, such as clitorimegaly, should be noted (Tagatz et al., 1979). During the vaginal examination one should pay special attention to infection and excess mucus. The shape of the cervix and its external os as well as the presence and amount of cervical mucus should be documented (Moghissi, 1987).

The size, position, and mobility of the uterus, fallopian tubes, and ovaries should be recorded. A rectovaginal examination should be performed to determine if there is tenderness or nodularity suggestive of endometriosis.

Special studies such as hormonal evaluation, endometrial biopsy, laparoscopy, hysterosalpingoscopy, and immunologic studies should be performed following the initial work-up, and basal body temperature should be charted over a 2-month period if abnormalities are disclosed.

Because disorders of ovulation account for at least 15% of all infertility problems, it is essential to establish whether the patient ovulates regularly. Indirect evidence of ovulation can be obtained by charting the basal body temperature. The patient is instructed on how to chart changes in basal body temperature for 2 months. Typically, an in-

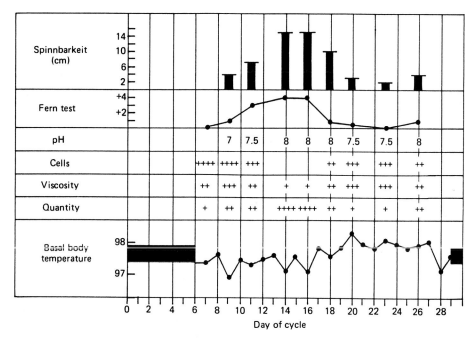

Fig. 2-15. Changes of basal body temperature and other physiologic parameters during the menstrual cycle. (From Goldfien A, Monroe SE. In Greenspan FS, Forsham PH. Basic and Clinical Endocrinology, 3rd ed. Norwalk, Appleton & Lange; 1986, and Maghissi K, Neuhaus OW. Am J Obstet Gynecol 1966; 96:91, with permission.)

crease in basal body temperature occurs 2 days after the preovulatory LH peak (Fig. 2-15).

However, basal body temperature provides only a rough estimate of menstrual cyclicity, and ovulation and the temperature surge actually correlate poorly with the hormonal changes of the periovulatory period and the precise time of ovum release (Quagliarello and Arny, 1986). Additional studies may be needed to determine the exact time of ovulation.

Cervical mucus changes during the menstrual cycle reflect the preovulatory rise in circulating estrogen. Under the influence of estrogen, the mucus becomes more copious, watery, thin, and clear. It shows an 8- to 10-cm stretchability *(spinnbarkeit)* and forms a typical fern pattern when smeared and dried on a microscope slide.

A system for scoring preovulatory cervical mucus on a scale of 0 to 3 has been devised by Moghissi (1987) (Table 2-6). It takes into account the amount of mucus, its viscosity, fern pattern formation, spinnbarkeit, and cellularity. Thick, opaque mucus with reduced stretchability and lack of fern pattern formation are associated with hormonal disturbances or cervical infection (Moghissi, 1987). However, the claims that poor-quality mucus reduces the chances for pregnancy have been disputed (Collins et al., 1984), and the value of cervical mucus examination remains controversial (Daly et al., 1989).

The examination of mucus is often combined with a postcoital sperm test. This test is performed several hours after coitus; the mucus is examined to determine the number of motile spermatozoa in the mucus. Minimal criteria

Table 2-6. Cervical mucus score for evaluation of preovulatory mucus

Amount	Spinnbarkeit
0 = 0	0 = < 1 cm
1 = 0.1 ml	1 = 1-4 cm
2 = 0.2 ml	2 = 5-8 cm
3 = 0.3 ml or more	3 = > 9 cm

Viscosity	Cellularity (white blood cells)
0 = Thick, highly viscous, premenstrual mucus	0 = >11 cells/hpf
1 = Intermediate type (viscous)	1 = 6–10 cells/hpf
2 = Mildly viscous	2 = 1–5 cells/hpf
3 = Normal midcycle mucus (preovulatory)	3 = 0 cells/hpf

Ferning
0 = No crystallization
1 = Atypical fern formation
2 = Primary and secondary stems
3 = Tertiary and quarternary stems

Modified from Moghissi KS. Obstet Gynecol Clin North Am 1987; 14:887, with permission.
hpf = high-power field.

for a positive test have not been accepted universally, and the predictive value of the test has been disputed (Griffith and Grimes, 1990).

If the basal body temperature charts reveal evidence of regular ovulation, special studies to exclude various cervi-

Table 2-7. Causes of anovulation

Cause	Mechanism	Condition
Hypothalamic	Idiopathic	Most common
	Functional	Rapid weight loss or gain, emotional stress
	Drug induced	Excessive exercise, opiates, alcohol
	Tumors	Craniopharyngioma, glioma, histiocytosis X
	Inflammation	Tuberculosis, sarcoidosis, viral encephalitis
Pituitary	Tumors	Prolactinoma, Cushing's syndrome
	Vascular	Hypopotuitarism
	Inflammation	Hypophysitis (tuberculosis, sarcoidosis)
Ovarian	Developmental	Gonadal dysgenesis, streak gonad (Turner's syndrome)
	Functional	Polycystic ovary, unresponsive ovary
	Iatrogenic	Chemotherapy, radiation
	Immune	Premature ovarian failure
	Idiopathic	Premature menopause (may be familial)
Metabolic	Functional	Hyperthyroidism, hypothyroidism, adrenal hyperfunction, diabetes mellitus

Modified from Pepperell et al. (1987) and Acosta et al. (1990).
Pregnancy, the most common cause of secondary amenorrhea, is not included.

cal, uterine, and oviductal anatomic causes of infertility should be performed depending on the leads from the initial studies.

Bacteriologic and serologic studies are indicated if there are signs of infection. A specimen of the discharge usually is obtained from the cervix. A speculum that has not been lubricated is inserted into the vagina. When the cervix is visualized, a swab is used to remove the exudate; even if there is no obvious lesion, the endocervix should be sampled. Sterile dacron swabs are used for sampling, and the specimens are sent for bacterial, chlamydial, and mycoplasma cultures. Thayer-Martin agar is used for culturing *Neisseria gonorrhoeae* (Kiviat et al., 1990); Anaswab tubes are used for anaerobes. Cycloheximide-treated McCoy cells in microtiter plates are used to culture *Chlamydia*. The *Chlamydia* Transwab system may be used as well (Zlatnik et al., 1990). Mycoplasma is cultured in beef heart infusion broth, which is available commercially as PPLO (pleuropneumonia-like organism) broth (Risi and Sanders, 1989). Alternative newer tests include direct immunofluorescence, enzyme immunoassay, and nucleic acid probes (Ridgway and Taylor-Robinson, 1991). Serum antibodies to *Chlamydia trachomatis* are valuable for the diagnosis of acute or chronic infection (Stacey et al., 1990).

Hormonal studies are essential in evaluating ovulatory disorders. Anovulation may result from hypothalamic, pituitary, ovarian, or metabolic disorders (Table 2-7). It is customary to distinguish primary amenorrhea from secondary amenorrhea, which is more common. According to Reindollar et al. (1986), the etiology of secondary amenorrhea is hypothalamic in 39% of cases (anovulation 28%, weight loss or anorexia 10%, hypothalamic suppression 10%, and hypothyroidism 1%); of pituitary origin secondary to prolactinomas in 7.5%; ovarian in 10.5%; and uterine in origin in 7%. The typical work-up of a patient with amenorrhea includes measurements of prolactin and TSH and a progestational challenge (Speroff et al., 1989).

Speroff et al. (1989) recommend screening for hypothyroidism in all women with amenorrhea, although hypothyroidism does not account for more than 3% to 5% of all cases. Amenorrhea secondary to hypothyroidism is not fully understood. In part, it is due to low levels of circulating thyroxin, which does not provide adequate negative feedback on hypothalamic secretion of thyrotropin-releasing hormone (TRH). Thyrotropin-releasing hormone stimulates pituitary TSH and prolactin-secreting cells. However, because TRH is increased only minimally in most amenorrheic women with hypothyroidism, other mechanisms must play a role as well.

Prolactin-secreting adenomas and microadenomas of the pituitary usually cause amenorrhea and galactorrhea and are easily identified and treated (Koppelman et al., 1984). Because the hypothalamus exerts an inhibitory influence on prolactin secretion, destructive lesions of the hypothalamus, brain surgery, or cranial irradiation may cause excessive prolactin secretion by disturbing this inhibitory axis. Dopamine is the presumed hypothalamic inhibitory substance, and all drugs interfering with production or release of dopamine have the potential to induce prolactinemia. Many drugs and hormones such as opiates, phenothiazines, and other neuroleptics (α-methyldopa, reserpine) and antihypertensive drugs may stimulate the secretion of prolactin. Estrogens, even in the small doses used for oral contraception, may stimulate prolactin secretion. Breast or thoracic surgery also may cause prolactinemia, theoretically via the stimulation of peripheral nerves that transmit signals similar to those produced by suckling. Finally, because prolactin is cleared through the kidneys, renal failure may be associated with hyperprolactinemia. The most important causes of hyperprolactinemia are listed in the box on p. 27.

Hormonal challenge with progesterone is used to assess central ovulatory mechanisms and the endogenous estrogen reserves and to exclude dysfunctional disturbances of

---

Causes of hyperprolactinemia

Hypothalamic

Tumors (glioma, craniopharyngioma, histiocytosis X)
Inflammation (encephalitis, sarcoidosis)
Functional, idiopathic

Pituitary

Prolactinoma, microscopic or macroscopic
Tumors of somatotropic cells
Destruction or transection of the stalk
Sheehan's syndrome
Empty sella syndrome

Thyroid

Hypothyroidism

Iatrogenic

Drugs (neurotropics, antihypertensives, anesthetics)
Hormones (estrogens, oral contraceptives, TRH)
Surgery (brain, thoracic, breast)
Irradiation of the hypothalamus

Renal failure

Table 2-8. Hormonal profiles of women with amenorrhea

Cause	LH	FSH	PRL	Estrogen	Response to progesterone stimulation
Hypothalamic					
Anatomic lesions	↓	↓	↓	↓	−
Dysfunctional	N	N	N	N	−
Stress	N	N	N	N	+
Anorexia	↓	↓	N	↓	−
Drug induced	N	N	N	N	+
Pituitary					
Tumor	↓	↓	↑ or ↓	↓	−
Destruction	↓	↓	↓	↓	−
Ovarian					
Failure	↑	↑	N	↓	−
Polycystic	N	N	N	N	+
Uterine	N	N	N	N	−

Modified from Davajan V, Kletzky OA. Secondary amenorrhea without galactorrhea or androgen excess. Mishell DR Jr, Davajan V, Lobo RA (Eds). In Infertility, Contraception, and Reproductive Endocrinology, 3rd ed. Boston, Blackwell Scientific, 1991; p 372, with permission. N, normal.

the endometrium. If the progesterone challenge does not produce uterine bleeding, insufficient estrogen production should be suspected, and the function of the hypothalamo-pituitary-ovarian axis and the uterus should be investigated further by measuring serum FSH and LH. Low levels of gonadotropins are indicative of central hypothalamic and pituitary lesions. Elevated levels of plasma LH and FSH point to ovarian insufficiency or unresponsiveness (Table 2-8).

Gonadotropin-releasing hormone and its analogues may be used to explore further the causes of anovulation or to induce ovulation (Conn and Crowley, 1991). Serum levels of testosterone and dehydroepiandrosterone sulfate (DHEA-S) (Hoffman et al., 1983) should be measured in women suspected of having polycystic ovary syndrome (Chang, 1984) or hormonally active adrenal lesions (Brodie and Wentz, 1987). Testosterone may be increased in polycystic ovary syndrome and related conditions of hypothalamo-pituitary-ovarian dysfunction. DHEA-S is, however, produced only by the adrenals and is a good marker of *adrenal* androgen production.

A pragmatic approach to women with amenorrhea is outlined in Algorithm 2-2.

Various immune mechanisms have been implicated in the pathogenesis of infertility of unknown origin (Haas, 1987), but in most cases their role remains poorly understood. Theoretically, immune mechanism accounting for female infertility could be classified as autoimmune or directed against male germ cells and seminal fluid components (Fig. 2-16).

In the ovary the targets of autoimmunity could be the oocyte or the follicular cells, ovarian stroma, secretory products of various cell compartments, and receptors for trophic hormones (Wilkins, 1990). Similarly, autoantibodies or sensitized T lymphocytes could be acting on tubal, endometrial, and cervical cells and their secretory products or surface receptors.

Heteroantibodies or cell-mediated immunity may be elicited by sperm and components of seminal fluid. Normal female genital organs contain immunoglobulins, which are in part derived from the circulation and in part locally synthesized (Haas and Beer, 1986). Thus antibodies to sperm can be detected in the cervical mucus or in the patient's serum. Serum antisperm antibodies are found in 5% or less of all couples with unexplained infertility (Coulam et al., 1988).

Antibodies to trophoblastic cells have been detected in patients with recurrent abortions who have lupuslike autoimmune disorders. Such patients may have high titers of lupus anticoagulant. Other autoimmune phenomena affecting the germ cells and the placenta have been reviewed recently by Tung and Lu (1991).

Reproductive immunity and the hypothetical protective role of maternal antibodies are poorly understood (Barratt et al., 1990). Nevertheless, it is quite possible that some recurrent abortions that cannot be explained otherwise are mediated by maternal antibodies or white blood cells in the genital tract. Asymptomatic cervicovaginal leukocytosis has been implicated as a cervical factor of infertility. The contribution of the immune system to infertility is intrigu-

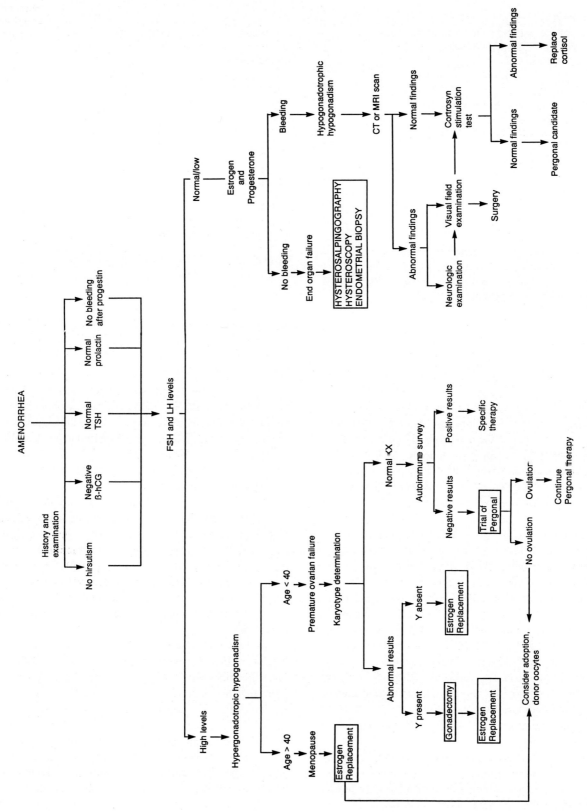

Algorithm 2-2. Evaluation of amenorrhea. (From DeCherney et al., 1988).

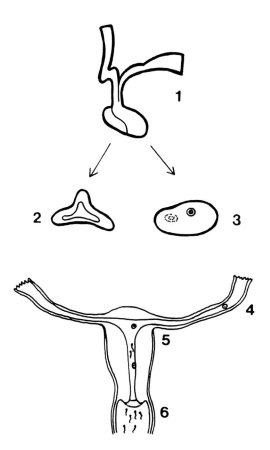

Fig. 2-16. Possible immune factors adversely affecting the female reproductive functions. *1.* Autoantibodies to the hormones of the hypothalamic-pituitary-adrenal-ovarian axis may cause a hormonal disbalance and anovulation. *2.* Pluriglandular immune diseases may affect the pituitary, the adrenals and the ovaries. *3.* Autoantibodies to ova, the zona pellucida, or the ovarian follicular cells cause early autoimmune ovarian failure. *4.* Various cytokines and mediators of inflammation, released in systemic immune disorders may affect the gamete transport through the tube or damage the XX gametes, the zygote, and the early embryo. *5.* Immune mechanisms may prevent intrauterine implantation or cause abortion. *6.* Antibodies to sperm may be cytotoxic or impede the sperm passage through the cervical mucus.

ing, but it is still poorly understood and needs further investigation.

Endoscopy and hysterosalpingography and sonography

Gynecologic endoscopy and radiologic contrast studies are used to visualize internal genital organs and attendant anomalies (Siegler, 1987). Hysteroscopy usually is performed on infertile women who have not responded to hormonal stimulation or who have suspected intrauterine lesions such as adhesions, submucosal myomas, adenomyosis, and polyps (Fayez et al., 1987). Metrorrhagia of unknown origin, prior intrauterine surgery, and a history of abortions are still other indications for hysteroscopy (March and Israel, 1976). Direct inspection of the uterine

cavity may be combined with biopsy and surgical or laser ablation of any lesions. Hysteroscopic biopsy based on direct visualization of lesions is more precise than a random sampling of endometrium (Gimpelson and Rappold, 1988). Hysteroscopy is contraindicated only in acute pelvic disease; in experienced hands it has few complications.

Hysterosalpingography is used to supplement hysteroscopic examination of the uterine cavity, and it is the method of choice for delineating uterine anomalies (Ben-Rafael et al., 1991) and tubal pathology. Direct visualization of intratubal lesions may be accomplished by salpingoscopy, which also allows sampling of tissues for histologic examination (Hershlag et al., 1991).

Salpingoscopic findings can be expressed semiquantitatively by using a scoring system established by Herschlag et al. (1991). This system takes into account five aspects of tubal morphology, i.e., patency of the tube, appearance of the epithelium, vascularity, adhesions, and extent of dilatation. Each category is scored on a scale of 1 to 3 for each tube. The maximal score is 30 (2×15) but additional 3 points can be assigned to lesions not included in the scoring system. The total score for normal tubes is 15; scores of 16 to 21 indicate mild changes, 27 to 27 moderate changes, and 28 to 33 severe changes.

Laparoscopy is an excellent approach for visualizing pelvic contents with minimal surgical risk to the patient. It is indicated in cases of suspected endometriosis, tubal disease, or pelvic adhesions and to assess the results of surgery. Tubal disease may be evaluated in terms of the extent and nature of adhesions, thickness of the tubal wall, and diameter of the hydrosalpinx (Boer-Meisel et al., 1986). A pelvic scoring system from 0 to 100 has been devised by Wu and Gocial (1988) by adding assigned scores for adhesion, salpingitis, and tubal occlusion. Adhesions are scored as:

0—None
1—Mild
2—Moderate
3—Severe
4—Extensive

Because the ovarian and tubal adhesions are considered to be most important, each score is multiplied by 2. Scores for other sites—uterus, bladder, intestine, and omentum—are added, with a maximum possible score of 48.

The salpingitis score is based on the assessment of the tubes bilaterally and then multiplied by 3 for a total not to exceed 24. The following criteria are used in this evaluation:

1—Mild salpingitis or hydrosalpinx. The tubes are edematous and hyperemic and the hydrosalpinx has a diameter of 0.5 to 1 cm.
2—Moderate salpingitis or hydrosalpinx. The tubes are fibrotic for less than half of their length, and the hydrosalpinx is 0.5 to 1 cm in diameter.

TABLE 1
THE AMERICAN FERTILITY SOCIETY CLASSIFICATION OF ADNEXAL ADHESIONS

Patient's Name _____ Date _____ Chart # _____

Age ____ G ____ P ____ Sp Ab ____ VTP ____ Ectopic ____ Infertile Yes ____ No ____

Other Significant History (i.e. surgery, infection, etc.) _____
_____

HSG _____ Sonography _____ Photography _____ Laparoscopy _____ Laparotomy _____

	ADHESIONS		<1/3 Enclosure	1/3 - 2/3 Enclosure	>2/3 Enclosure
OVARY	R	Filmy	1	2	4
		Dense	4	8	16
	L	Filmy	1	2	4
		Dense	4	8	16
TUBE	R	Filmy	1	2	4
		Dense	4*	8*	16
	L	Filmy	1	2	4
		Dense	4*	8*	16

* If the fimbriated end of the fallopian tube is completely enclosed, change the point assignment to 16.

Prognostic Classification for Adnexal Adhesions

	LEFT		RIGHT
A. Minimal	_____	0-5	_____
B. Mild	_____	6-10	_____
C. Moderate	_____	11-20	_____
D. Severe	_____	21-32	_____

Additional Findings: _____
_____
_____
_____
_____

Treatment (Surgical Procedures): _____
_____
_____
_____

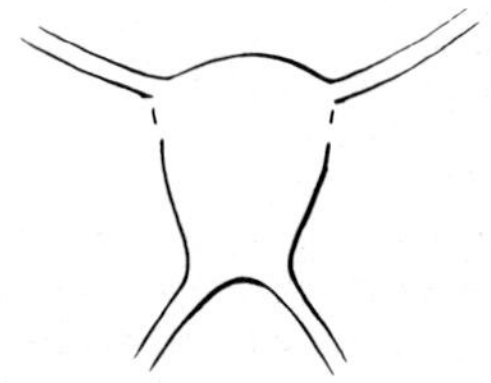

Prognosis for Conception & Subsequent Viable Infant**

_____ Excellent (> 75%)

_____ Good (50-75%)

_____ Fair (25%-50%)

_____ Poor (< 25%)

**Physician's judgment based upon adnexa with least amount of pathology.

Recommended Followup Treatment: _____
_____
_____

DRAWING

L   R

Property of
The American Fertility Society

For additional supply write to:
The American Fertility Society
2140 11th Avenue, South
Suite 200
Birmingham, Alabama 35205

Fig. 2-17. The American Fertility Society classification of adnexal adhesions. (Reproduced with permission.)

3—Severe salpingitis or hydrosalpinx. The tubes are fibrotic for more than half of their length, and the hydrosalpinx has a diameter of 1 to 2 cm.

4—Extensive salpingitis or hydrosalpinx. The tubes are rigid and fibrotic through their entire length and their lumen is obliterated. The hydrosalpinx has a diameter of greater than 2 cm.

The tubal occlusion score is derived by assigning 7 points for tubal constriction and 14 for complete occlusion (which is then multiplied by 2 for a maximum of 28). This pelvic scoring is inversely correlated with the reproductive potential of the patient. A similar classification and scoring system of adnexal adhesions has been developed by The American Fertility Society (Fig. 2-17).

Ultrasonography has been used extensively in the evaluation and treatment of infertility. Sonography is valuable for visualizing various congenital and acquired ovarian, tubal, and uterine lesions. The applications of ultrasonography in gynecology are too numerous to mention, and the reader is referred to specialized textbooks.

Serial sonography of the ovary is used routinely in assisted fertilization, especially when following preovulatory folliculogenesis and when harvesting ova for in vitro fertil-

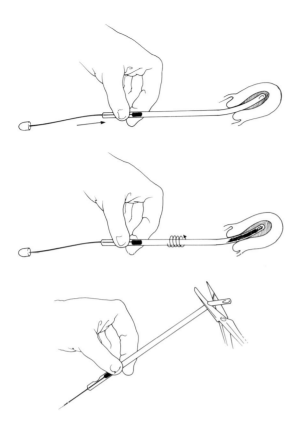

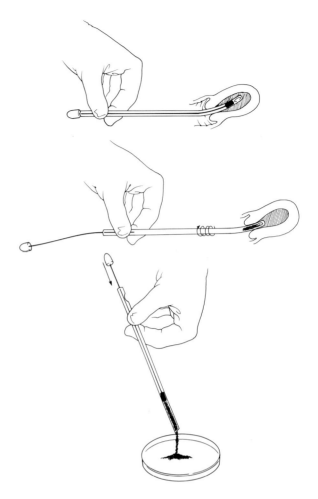

Fig. 2-18. Endometrial biopsy performed with Pipelle ©. (Courtesy of Unimar, Wilton, Connecticut. Redrawn and reproduced with permission.)

Indications for endometrial biopsy of infertile women

Irregular ovulation
Hormonal disturbances (luteal phase defect, hyperestrinism)
Endometritis
Uterine bleeding
Evaluation of hormonal treatment

---

ization (Daly et al., 1989). The use of various imaging techniques in the work-up of infertility problems in women has been comprehensively reviewed by Gutmann (1992).

Endometrial biopsy

Endometrial biopsy is commonly performed to assess possible ovarian and uterine causes of infertility. Luteal phase insufficiency, endometrial unresponsiveness to steroid hormones, endometritis, and endometrial hyperplasia are some of the most common findings that can be documented by tissue examination (Clement, 1991). Asherman's syndrome, marked by intrauterine adhesions that

may develop after endometrial curettage or uterine surgery, is often cured or ameliorated with careful cervical dilatation and uterine curettage (Schenker and Margalioth, 1982). Indications for endometrial biopsy in the work-up of infertile women are listed in the box at the left.

An adequate endometrial biopsy should provide enough tissue for the assessment of the endometrium but should not be performed too aggressively, to prevent traumatization of the uterus (Fig. 2-18). The fundal tissue is sampled with a special pipette aspirator or curet (Clement, 1991) that does not require cervical dilatation. Because the superficial layer, the functionalis, reflects most accurately the functional status of the endometrium, it should be included in the specimen. The basalis layer and the mucosa of the lower uterine segment and endocervix respond less to hormonal stimulation and thus provide less insight into potential abnormality. Fragments of endometrial polyps are sometimes included, but these should not be taken into consideration for hormonal evaluation of the endometrium.

The biopsy should be submitted with adequate clinical information, including data pertinent to the fertility work-up. The patient's age, date of the last menstrual period, suspected cause of infertility, and history of treatment, especially all hormonal therapies, should be listed. All special requests should be stated clearly.

An endometrial biopsy specimen should be fixed immediately in one of the standard histologic fixatives. Buffered formalin and Bouin's fixative are used most commonly. Each of these fixatives has its advantages and disadvantages (Buckley and Fox, 1989), but essentially comparable results are obtained. The tissue is then embedded in paraffin and sectioned at 5 to 8 μm; hematoxylin and eosin staining is routinely performed, and usually there is no need for special stains or special processing of the tissue. Frozen sections and electron microscopy are of limited value and are not used in the evaluation of endometrial biopsies. Immunohistochemistry has been used as an investigative approach. It remains to be seen whether immunohistochemical demonstration of complement and immunoglobulins (Bartosik et al., 1987), epidermal growth factor receptor (Damjanov et al., 1986), or progesterone and estrogen receptors (Garcia et al., 1988) is of clinical significance. Additional details about endometrial biopsies and their histopathologic interpretation can be found in monographs by Hendrickson and Kempson (1980), Dallenbach-Hellweg (1987), and Buckley and Fox (1989).

The pathologist interpreting the endometrial biopsy must answer several critical questions before providing the report to the clinician (Hendrickson and Kempson, 1980; Keel and Webster, 1990). It is essential to assert whether:

1. The specimen is obtained properly and submitted in adequately preserved form. It is important to ascertain that the biopsy contains enough *endometrial* tissue, not just blood or mucus; that the tissue is submitted in standard histologic fixatives; and that the specimens have not desiccated because they were not fixed immediately or become distorted from extended time in a saline solution. Hysteroscopic biopsy may be affected by the high-molecular-weight dextran used for visualization of the uterine cavity during hysteroscopy, but this usually does not interfere with the histologic interpretation.
2. The uterus is adequately sampled. It is essential to obtain fundal mucosa, which should include functionalis and a strip of surface endometrium (the "capsule"). Dating of early secretory phase is made on the basis of the appearance of the stratum spongiosum, whereas the surface stratum compactum becomes important for the evaluation of the endometrium from day 23 to the end of an ideal 28-day cycle.
3. The endometrium can be classified histologically as normal proliferative, secretory, menstrual, gestational, or abnormal. If the endometrium is classified as normal, it should be dated as corresponding to a specific phase of the menstrual cycle. If the endometrium is abnormal, the specific pathologic diagnosis of atrophy, hyperplasia, neoplasia, or inflammation should be assigned.
4. There is evidence of placental tissue or fetal parts,

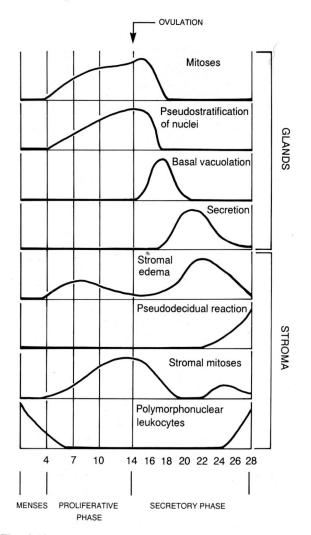

Fig. 2-19. Criteria for histologic dating of the endometrium. (Modified from Noyes RW et al. Fertil Steril 1950; 1:3, with permission.)

intrauterine or extrauterine pregnancy, or hormonal treatment. It should be kept in mind that pregnancy is the most common cause of amenorrhea in women of reproductive age. Data on hormonal therapies and methods of contraception should be provided by the clinician to the pathologist. Without these data there is a risk of misinterpreting the histologic findings.

Histologic dating of the endometrium is based on the principles and criteria developed by Noyes et al. (1950), which are summarized in Figure 2-19. This widely used system is imprecise (Li et al., 1987; Gibson et al., 1991) primarily because of interobserver variability, which accounts for approximately two thirds of all errors (Gibson et al., 1991). Duplicate readings by the same evaluator have proved to be inconsistent in 27% of cases. Regional differences between segments of uterine mucosa accounted for 8% of errors in dating (Gibson et al., 1991). Thus many pathologists prefer to date the endometrium only as proliferative or secretory and subdivide each phase into early,

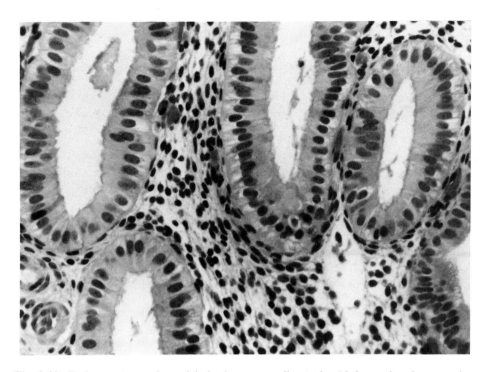

Fig. 2-20. Early secretory endometrial glands corresponding to day 16 show subnuclear vacuoles.

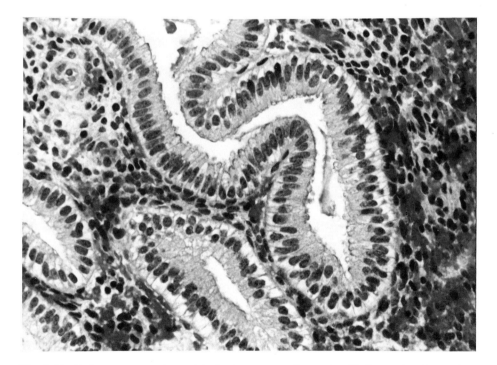

Fig. 2-21. Early secretory endometrial glands corresponding to day 18 show subnuclear and supranuclear vacuoles.

midterm, and late. The morphologic features of normal endometrium are illustrated in Figures 2-20 to 2-27 and described subsequently.

Proliferative endometrium. The glands are straight and narrow and lined by cuboidal cells with a high nucle-

ocytoplasmic ratio in the early proliferative phase. In a later proliferative phase, the glands are coiled and lined by cylindrical cells that have more cytoplasm. The nuclei are plump and elongated, have coarse chromatin, and are arranged in a pseudostratified manner. Mitoses are promi-

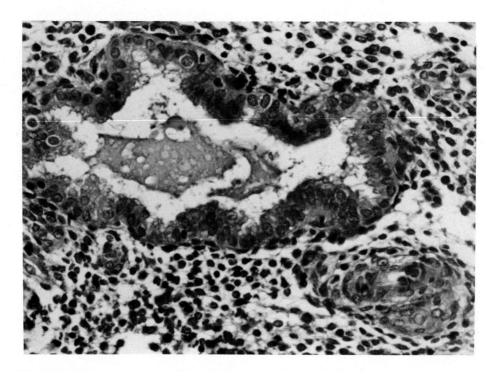

Fig. 2-22. Midsecretory endometrial glands corresponding to day 20 show ragged luminal borders and contain inspissated secretory material.

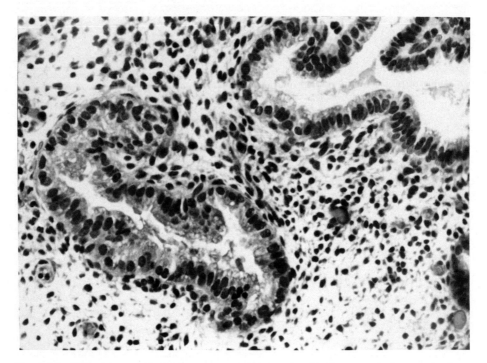

Fig. 2-23. Midsecretory endometrium corresponding to day 21 shows marked stromal edema. Stromal cells appear as "naked nuclei." The grandular luminal lining appears ragged, and secretory material is in the lumen.

nent. The stroma is dense, uniform, and composed of spindle-shaped cells with elongated, plump nuclei. The ratio of glands to stroma (G:S) is approximately 1. Midproliferative stroma shows varying degrees of edema, which is not seen in the early proliferative phase.

Interval endometrium. This term is used by Hendrickson and Kempson (1980) to denote the transition from the proliferative to secretory endometrium during the first 36 hours after ovulation. Coiled glands of late proliferative phase predominate. Scattered glands with subnu-

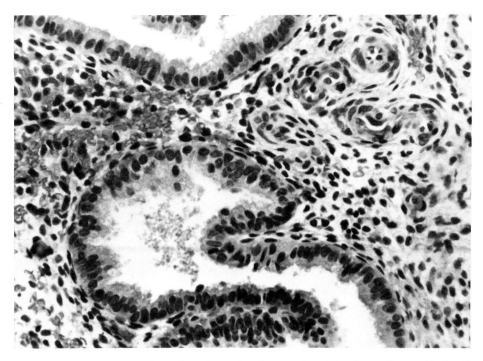

Fig. 2-24. Late secretory endometrium shows dorminent periarteriolar sheets of predecidual cells and secretory exhaustion of the glands.

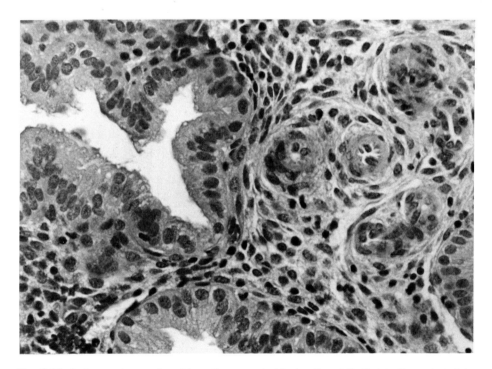

Fig. 2-25. Late secretory endometrium shows predecidual cells not limited to the periarteriolar areas only. Scattered lymphocytes are seen in the stroma. Glands show secretory exhaustion.

clear vacuolization are found but account for less than 50% of all glands. The stroma consists of spindle-shaped cells with plump, elongated nuclei, and the G:S is 1.

Secretory endometrium. The endometrium can be dated as early secretory, midsecretory, and late secretory

(Hendrickson and Kempson, 1980) or as corresponding to days 16 to 28 of an ideal 28-day cycle (Noyes et al., 1950; Noyes and Haman, 1953; Noyes, 1956).

In early secretory phase (days 16 to 19), the endometrial glands show subnuclear vacuolization, whereas the

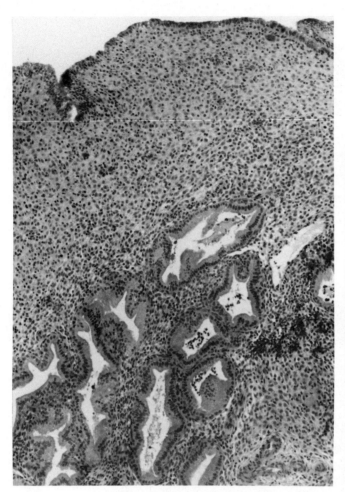

Fig. 2-26. Late secretory premenstrual endometrium shows a solid sheet of decidua in the stratum compactum.

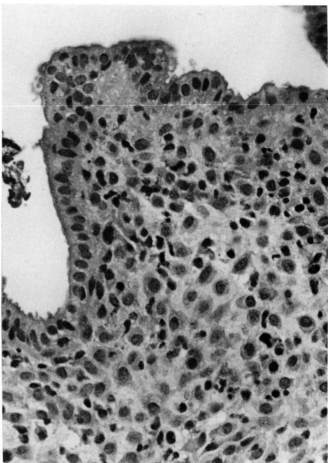

Fig. 2-27. Detail of the decidualized stroma and glandular epithelium of late secretory endometrium.

stroma has retained features of proliferative endometrium (Figs. 2-20 and 2-21).

In midsecretory phase (days 20 to 23), the glandular lumina contain secretory material and are lined by nonvacuolated cells. The stroma is composed of spindle cells and appears edematous (Figs. 2-22 and 2-23).

Late secretory endometrium (days 24 to 28) shows predeciduation of the stroma, which begins around the spiral arteries and gradually involves the entire functionalis, resulting in a superficial compact layer. Premenstrual endometrium is infiltrated by leukocytes and shows signs of focal cell necrosis and hemorrhage (Figs 2-24 to 2-27).

Day-to-day timing of the secretory endometrium using the criteria of Noyes et al. (1950) is based on the assessment of the morphology of glands and stroma. If this system is used, it is recommended to use a 2-day span and relate the date to days 16 to 28 of the idealized normal cycle (Keel and Webster, 1990).

The secretory endometrium shows the following features:

Day 16—Glands are coiled and show pseudostratified alignment of nuclei with subnuclear vacuoles. Mitoses of glandular and stromal cells are seen.

Day 17—Glands show subnuclear and some supranuclear vacuoles. Nuclei become somewhat but not completely aligned. Mitoses still are present in glands and stroma.

Day 18—Glands show prominent subnuclear and supranuclear vacuoles. Luminal surface vacuoles appear. Nuclei are linear and are located in the midportion of the clear cytoplasm. Rare mitoses are seen in glands and stroma.

Day 19—Intraluminal secretory material appears. The cytoplasm of glandular cells no longer contains discrete vacuoles, and the cells appear empty. There are no mitoses.

Day 20—Glandular secretions peak. The glands have ragged luminal borders and are filled with intraluminal mucus, which may show signs of inspissation.

Day 21—There is prominent stromal edema. The stro-

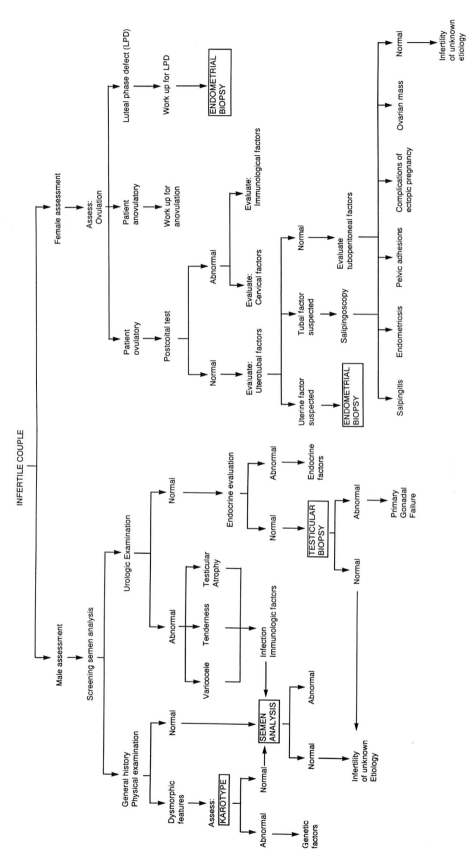

Algorithm 2-3. Evaluation of the infertile couple. (From DeCherney et al., 1988.)

mal cells show little cytoplasm and appear as "naked" nuclei. The glands are filled with inspissated mucous material.

Day 22—Stromal edema reaches its peak. There are numerous naked stromal nuclei. The glands contain an inspissated mucous. Occasional stromal mitoses are seen.

Day 23—Signs of deciduation appear around spiral arteries, which are surrounded by cuffs of predecidual cells. Predecidual cells are derived from stromal cells that proliferate and acquire more cytoplasm. Typically, they have less condensed nuclei. The glands show secretory exhaustion and are lined by cuboidal epithelium.

Day 24—The glands are secretorily exhausted and show ragged luminal borders. There are prominent periarteriolar sheets of predecidual cells. Stromal mitoses are prominent.

Day 25—Predecidual cells form sheets in the compacta and are not limited to the periarteriolar sheets. The glands contain inspissated material. Lymphocytes and occasional neutrophils appear in the stroma.

Day 26—Widespread decidualization of stromal cells is seen at a distance from periarteriolar sheets outside of the compacta. A prominent influx of neutrophils occurs.

Day 27—A solid sheet of decidua forms in the stratum compactum. The glands contain inspissated material. The stroma is infiltrated with neutrophils.

Day 28—Foci of hemorrhage and necrosis are seen. The nuclei of stromal and glandular cells show clumping of the chromatin, and the endometrial glands appear ruptured. Prominent infiltrates of neutrophils are admixed with red blood cells.

Menstrual epithelium is marked by the fragmentation of glands, clumping of stromal nuclei, hemorrhage, and edema of the stroma. At the end of the menstrual phase, regeneration of the endometrial gland and stroma begins from the basalis layer.

CLINICAL EVALUATION OF THE INFERTILE COUPLE

The clinical approach to the evaluation of the infertile couple could follow several standardized protocols discussed in detail in textbooks on reproductive medicine (Seibel, 1990; Lipshultz and Howards, 1991). A typical work-up of the infertile couple is outlined in Algorithm 2-3.

REFERENCES

Acosta AA, Swanson RJ, Ackerman SB, Kruger TF, van Zyl JA, Menkveld R: Human Spermatozoa in Assisted Reproduction. Baltimore, Williams & Wilkins, 1990.

Adeghe J-H A, Cohen J, Sawers SR: Relationship between local and systemic antibodies to sperm, and evaluation of immunobead test for sperm surface antibodies. Acta Eur Fertil 1986; 17:99.

Afzelius BA: Genetical and ultrastructural aspects of the immotile-cilia syndrome. Am J Hum Genet 1981; 33:852.

Ali JI, Grimes EM: Sperm morphology: Unstained and stained smears in fertile and infertile men. Arch Androl 1989; 22:191.

Amann RP: Can the fertility potential of a seminal sample be predicted accurately? J Androl 1989; 10:89.

Ayodeji O, Baker HWG: Is there a specific abnormality of sperm morphology in men with varicoceles? Fertil Steril 1986; 45:839.

Baccetti B, Burrini AG, Collodel G, Magnano AR, Piomboni P, Renieri T, Sensini C: Morphogeneis of decapitated and decaudated sperm defect in two brothers. Gamete Res 1989; 23:181.

Badenoch DF, Evans PR, Gray A, Evans SJW: Sperm morphological analysis: Comparison of two methods in human semen. Br J Urol 1990; 65:294.

Baker ER: Menstrual dysfunction and hormonal status in athletic women: A review. Fertil Steril 1981; 36:691.

Baker HWG, Burger HG, deKretser DM, et al: A study of the endocrine manifestations of hepatic cirrhosis. J Med 1976; 177:145.

Barratt CLR, Bolton AE, Cooke ID: Functional significance of white blood cells in the male and female reproductive tract. Hum Reprod 1990; 5:639.

Bartosik D, Damjanov I, Viscarello RR, Riley JA: Immunoproteins in the endometrium: Clinical correlates of the presence of complement fractions C3 and C4. Am J Obstet Gynecol 1987; 156:11.

Bartsch G, Frank S, Marberger H, Mikuz G: Testicular torsion: Late results with special regard to fertility and endocrine function. J Urol 1980; 124:375.

Ben-Rafael Z, Seidman DS, Recabi K, Bider D, Mashiach S: Uterine anomalies. A retrospective matched-control study. J Reprod Med 1991; 36:723.

Blacklock NJ, Beavis JP: The response of prostatic fluid pH in inflammation. Br J Urol 1974; 46:537.

Blackwell RE, Chang RJ: Report of the national symposium on the clinical management of prolactin-related reproductive disorders. Fertil Steril 1986; 45:607.

Boer-Meisel M, te Velde ER, Habbema JDF, Kardaun JWPF: Predicting the pregnancy outcome in patients treated for hydrosalpinx: A prospective study. Fertil Steril 1986; 45:23.

Bonde JPE: Subfertility in relation to welding. A case reference study among male welders. Dan Med Bull 1990; 37:105.

Bostofte E, Serup J, Rebbe H: Interrelations among the characteristics of human semen, and a new system for classification of male fertility. Fertil Steril 1984; 41:95.

Bostofte E, Serup J, Rebbe H: The clinical value of morphological rating of human spermatozoa. Int J Fertil 1985; 30:31.

Brodie BL, Wentz AC: Late onset congenital adrenal hyperplasia: A gynecologist's perspective. Fertil Steril 1987; 48:175.

Bronson RA, Cooper GW, Rosenfeld DL: Sperm antibodies: Their role in infertility. Fertil Steril 1984; 42:171.

Buckley CH, Fox H: Biopsy Pathology of Endometrium. New York, Raven Press, 1989.

Burger H, deKretser DM: The Testis. New York, Raven Press, 1989.

Casano R, Orlando C, Caldini AL, Barni T, Natali A, Serio M: Simultaneous measurement of seminal L-carnitine, 1-4-glucosidase, and glycerylphosphorylcholine in azoospermic and oligozoospermic patients. Fertil Steril 1987; 47:324.

Chang RJ: Ovarian steroid secretion in polycystic ovarian disease. Semin Reprod Endocrinol 1984; 2:244.

Charny CW: Testicular biopsy. Its value in male sterility. JAMA 1940; 115:1429.

Clarke G: An improved immunobead test procedure for detecting sperm antibodies in serum. Am J Reprod Immunol 1987; 13:1.

Clement PB: Pathology of gamete and zygote transport: Cervical, endometrial, myometrial, and tubal factors of infertility. In Pathology of Reproductive Failure, edited by Kraus FT, Damjanov I, Kaufman N. Baltimore, Williams & Wilkins, 1991, p 140.

Clifton DK, Bremmer WJ: The effect of testicular x-irradiation on spermatogenesis in man. A comparison with the mouse. J Androl 1983; 4:387.

Close CE, Roberts PL, Berger RE: Cigarettes, alcohol and marijuana are related to pyospermia in infertile men. J Urol 1990; 144:900.

Coburn M, Wheeler T, Lipshultz LI: Testicular biopsy. Its use and limitations. Urol Clin North Am 1987; 14:587.

Cockett ATK, Takihara H, Cosentino MJ: The varicocele. Fertil Steril 1984; 41:5.

Cohen J, Malter H, Wright G, Kort H, Massey J, Mitchell D: Partial zona dissection of human oocytes when failure of zona pellucida penetration is anticipated. Hum Reprod 1989; 4:435.

Collins JA, So Y, Wilson EH, Wrixon W, Casper RF: The postcoital test as a predictor of pregnancy among 355 infertile couples. Fertil Steril 1984; 41:703.

Collins JP: Retrograde ejaculation. In Baun J, Schill WB, Schwargstein Y (Eds): Treatment of Male Infertility. Berlin, Springer, 1982, p. 179.

Conn PM, Crowley WF Jr: Gonadotropin-releasing hormone and its analogues. N Engl J Med 1991; 324:93.

Coulam CB, Moore SB, O'Fallon W: Investigating unexplained infertility. Am J Obstet Gynecol 1988; 158:1374.

Dallenbach-Hellweg G: Histopathology of the Endometrium, 3rd ed. New York, Springer, 1987.

Daly DC, Reuter K, Cohen S, Mastroianni J: Follicle size by ultrasound versus cervical mucus quality: Normal and abnormal pattern in spontaneous cycles. Fertil Steril 1989; 51:598.

Daly DC, Soto-Albors C, Walters C, Ying Y, Riddick DH: Ultrasonographic assessment of luteinized unruptured follicle syndrome in unexplained infertility. Fertil Steril 1985; 43:62.

Damjanov I, Mildner B, Knowles BB: Immunohistochemical localization of the epidermal growth factor receptor in normal human tissues. Lab Invest 1986; 55:588.

DeCherney AH: Decision Making in Infertility. Philadelphia, BC Decker; 1988.

DeVere White R (Ed): Aspects of Male Infertility. Baltimore, Williams & Wilkins, 1982.

Dodson MG: Transvaginal Ultrasound. New York, Churchill Livingstone, 1991.

Dodson MC, Joshi PN: Male factor infertility and the gynecologist. Am J Gynecol Health 1989; 3:175.

Dubin L, Amelar RD: Etiologic factors in 1294 consecutive cases of male infertility. Fertil Steril 1971; 22:469.

Elias AN, Valenta LJ, Domurat ES: Male hypogonadism due to nontumorous hyperestrogenism. J Androl 1990; 11:485.

Eliasson R: Standards for investigation of human semen. Andrologia 1971; 3:49.

Eliasson R: Supravital staining of human spermatozoa. Fertil Steril 1977; 28:1257.

Evans HJ, Fletcher J, Torrance M, Hargreave TB: Sperm abnormalities and cigarette smoking. Lancet 1981; 1:627.

Fayez JA, Mutie G, Schneider PJ: The diagnostic value of hysterosalpingography and hysteroscopy in infertility investigation. Am J Obstet Gynecol 1987; 156:558.

Fossa SD, Aass N, Kaalhus O: Radiotherapy for testicular seminoma stage I: Treatment results and long-term post-irradiation morbidity in 365 patients. Int J Radiat Oncol Biol Phys 1989; 16:383.

Fowler JE, Kessler R: Genital tract infections. In Infertility in the Male, edited by Lipshultz LI, Howards SS. New York, Churchill Livingstone, 1990, p 283.

Freund M: Standards for the rating of human sperm morphology: A cooperative study. Int J Fertil 1966; 11:97.

Garcia E, Bouchard P, de Brux J, et al: Use of immunocytochemistry of progesterone and estrogen receptors for endometrial dating. J Clin Endocrinol Metab 1988; 67:80.

Gavaler JS, Van Thiel DH: Gonadal dysfunction and inadequate sexual performance in alcoholic cirrhotic men. Gastroenterology 1988; 95:1680.

Gibson M, Badger GJ, Byrn F, Lee KR, Korson R, Trainer TD: Error in histologic dating of secretory endometrium: Variance component analysis. Fertil Steril 1991; 56:242.

Gimpelson RJ, Rappold HO: A comparative study between panoramic hysteroscopy with direct biopsies and dilatation and curettage. A review of 276 cases. Am J Obstet Gynecol 1988; 158:489.

Glass AR, Swerdloff RS, Bray GA, Dahms WT, Atkinson RL: Low serum testosterone and sex-hormone-binding-globulin in massively obese men. J Clin Endocrinol Metab 1977; 45:1211.

Glezerman M, Bernstein D, Zakut C, Misgav N, Insler V: Polyzoospermia: A definite pathologic entity. Fertil Steril 1982; 38:605.

Gomez F, de la Cueva R, Wauters JP, Lemarchand-Beraud T: Endocrine abnormalities in patients undergoing long-term hemodialysis. Am J Med 1980; 68:522.

Gonen Y, Casper RF, Jacobson W, Blankier J: Endometrial thickness and growth during ovarian stimulation: A possible predictor of implantation in vitro fertilization. Fertil Steril 1989; 52:446.

Griffith CS, Grimes DA: The validity of the postcoital test. Am J Obstet Gynecol 1990; 162:615.

Guerin J-F, Ben Ali H, Cottinet D, Rollet J: Seminal alpha-glucosidase activity as a marker of epididymal pathology in nonazoospermic men consulting for infertility. J Androl 1990; 11:240.

Gutmann JN: Imaging in the evaluation of female infertility. J Reprod Med 1992; 37:54.

Haas GG: Immunologic infertility. Obstet Gynecol Clin North Am 1987; 14:1069.

Haas GG, Beer AE: Immunologic influences on reproductive biology: Sperm gametogenesis and maturation in the male and female genital tracts. Fertil Steril 1986; 46:753.

Hadžiselimović F (Ed): Cryptorchidism. Management and Implications. Berlin, Springer-Verlag, 1983.

Hammen R: Studies on Impaired Fertility in Man with Special Reference to the Male. Copenhagen-London, Munksgaard and Milford, 1944.

Hammond MG: Evaluation of the infertile couple. Obstet Gynecol Clin North Am 1987; 14:821.

Handelsman DJ, Conway AJ, Boylan LM, Turtle JR: Young's syndrome. Obstructive azoospermia and chronic sinopulmonary infections. N Engl J Med 1984; 310:3.

Hansen PV, Trykker H, Helkjaer PE, Andersen J: Testicular function in patients with testicular cancer treated with orchiectomy alone or orchiectomy and cisplatin-based chemotherapy. J Natl Cancer Inst 1989; 81:1246.

Heller CB, Clermont Y: Kinetics of the germinal epithelium in men. Recent Prog Horn Res 1964; 20:545.

Hendrickson MR, Kempson RL: Surgical Pathology of the Uterine Corpus. Philadelphia, WB Saunders, 1980.

Hendry WF, Levison DA, Parkinson MC, Parslow JM, Royle MG: Testicular obstruction: Clinicopathologic studies. Ann Roy Coll Surg Engl 1990; 72:396.

Hershlag A, Seifer DB, Carcangiu ML, Patton DL, Diamond MP, DeCherney AH: Salpingoscopy: Light microscopic and electron microscopic correlation. Obstet Gynecol 1991; 77:399.

Hjort T, Linnet L, Skakkebaek NE: Testicular biopsy: Indications and complications. Eur J Pediatr 1982; 138:23.

Ho PC, Poon ILM, Chan SYW, Wang C: Intrauterine insemination is not useful in oligoasthenospermia. Fertil Steril 1989; 5:582.

Hoffman D, Love K, Lobo RA: The prevalence and significance of elevated DHEA-S levels in anovulatory women. Fertil Steril 1983; 39:404.

Homonnai ZT, Pax G, Kraicer PF: A retrospective diagnostic study of fifty cases of vas deferens agenesis. Andrologia 1978; 10:410.

Honoré LH: Testicular biopsy for infertility: A review of sixty-eight cases with simplified histologic classification. Int J Fertil 1979; 24:49.

Howe G, Westhoff C, Vessey M, Yeates D: Effects of age, cigarette smoking and other factors on fertility: Findings in a large prospective study. BMJ 1985; 290:1697.

Huszar G, Vigue L, Corrales M: Sperm creatine kinase activity in fertile and infertile oligospermic men. J Androl 1990; 11:40.

James WH: Secular trend in reported sperm counts. Andrologia 1980; 12:381.

Jensen RT, Collen MJ, Pandol SJ: Cimetidine-induced impotence and breast changes in patients with gastric hypersecretory states. N Engl J Med 1983; 308:883.

Johnsen SG: Testicular biopsy score count-method for registration of spermatogenesis in human testes: Normal values and results in 335 hypogonadal males. Hormones 1970; 1:2.

Johnson L, Petty CS, Neaves WB: The relationship of biopsy evaluations and testicular measurements to over-all daily sperm production in human testes. Fertil Steril 1980; 34:36.

Kandeel FR, Swerdloff RS: Role of temperature in regulation of spermatogenesis and the use of heating as a method for contraception. Fertil Steril 1988; 49:1.

Katz DF, Diel L, Overstreet JW: Differences in the movement of morphologically normal and abnormal human seminal spermatozoa. Biol Reprod 1982; 26:566.

Keel BA, Webster BW: CRC handbook of the laboratory diagnosis and treatment of infertility. Boca Raton, Florida, CRC Press, 1990.

Kennedy WP, Kaminski JM, Vander Ven H, Jeyendran RS, Reid DS, Blackwell J, Bielfeld P, Zaneveld LJD: Simple clinical assay to evaluate acrosin assay in human spermatozoa. J Androl 1989; 10:221.

Kiviat NB, Paavonen JA, Wolner-Hanssen P et al: Histopathology of endocervical infection caused by Chlamydia, simplex virus, Trichomonas vaginalis, and Neisseria gonorrhoeae. Hum Pathol 1990; 21:831.

Klaiber EL, Broverman DM, Pokoly TB: Interrelationships of cigarette smoking, testicular varicoceles, and seminal fluid indices. Fertil Steril 1987; 47:481.

Knuth UA, Yeung C-H, Nieschlag E: Computerized semen analysis: Objective measurement of semen characteristics is biased by subjective parameter setting. Fertil Steril 1987; 48:118.

Koppelman MCS, Jaffe MJ, Rieth KG, Caruso RC, Loriaux DL: Hyperprolactinemia, amenorrhea, and galactorrhea: A retrospective assessment of twenty-five cases. Ann Intern Med 1984; 100:115.

Krause W: Long-term variations of seminal parameters. Andrologia 1984; 16:175.

Kruger TF, Acosta AA, Simmons KF, Swanson RJ, Matta JF, Oehninger S: Predictive value of abnormal sperm morphology in in vitro fertilization. Fertil Steril 1988; 49:112.

Kruger TF, Menkveld R, Stander FSH, Lombard CJ, van der Merwe JP, van Zyl JA, Smith K: Sperm morphologic features as a prognostic factor in vitro fertilization. Fertil Steril 1986; 46:1118.

Leung AKC: Polyorchidism. Am Fam Physician 1988; 38:153.

Levine RJ, Mathew RM, Chenault CB et al: Differences in the quality of semen in outdoor workers during summer and winter. N Engl J Med 1990; 321:12.

Li T-C, Rogers AW, Lenton EA, Dockery P, Cooke ID: A comparison between two methods of chronological dating of human endometrial biopsies during the luteal phase, and their correlation with histological dating. Fertil Steril 1987; 48:928.

Lincoln GA: Seasonal aspects of testicular function. In The Testis, edited by Burger H, deKretser DM. New York, Raven Press, 1989, pp 225–302.

Lipshultz LI, Howards SS (Eds): Infertility in the Male, ed 2. St Louis, Mosby–Year Book, 1990.

Lipson LG: Treatment of hypertension in diabetic men: Problems with sexual dysfunction. Am J Cardiol 1984; 53:46a.

Ludwig G, Frick J: Spermatology. Atlas and Manual. Berlin, Springer-Verlag, 1990.

MacLeod J: Effect of chicken pox and of pneumonia on semen quality. Fertil Steril 1951; 2:523.

MacLeod J: Human seminal cytology as a sensitive indicator of the germinal epithelium. Int J Fertil 1964; 9:281.

MacLeod J, Gold RZ: The male factor in fertility and infertility. VI. Semen quality and certain other factors in relation to ease of conception. Fertil Steril 1953; 4:10.

Magid MS, Cash KL, Goldstein M: The testicular biopsy in the evaluation of infertility. Semin Urol 1990; 8:51.

Mahmood T, Templeton TA: Prevalence and genesis of endometriosis. Hum Reprod 1991; 6:544.

Makler A, Abramovici H: The correlation between sperm count and testicular biopsy using a new scoring system. Int J Fertil 1978; 23:300.

Makler A, Tatcher M, Mohilever J: Sperm semi-autoanalysis by a combination of multiple exposure photography (MEP) and computer techniques. Int J Fertil 1980; 25:62.

Males JL, Townsend JL, Schneider RA: Hypogonadotropic hypogonadism with anosmia-Kallmann's syndrome. A disorder of olfactory and hypothalamic function. Arch Intern Med 1973; 131:501.

March CM, Israel R: Intrauterine adhesions secondary to elective abortion: Hysteroscopic diagnosis and management. Obstet Gynecol 1976; 48:422.

Menkveld R, Kruger TF: Basic semen analysis. In Human Spermatozoa in Assisted Reproduction, edited by Acosta AA, Swanson RJ, Ackerman SB, Kruger TF, van Zyl JA, Menkveld R. Baltimore, Williams & Wilkins, 1990, p 68.

Menkveld R, Stander FSH, Kotze TJVW, Kruger TF, van Zyl JA: The evaluation of morphological characteristics of human spermatozoa according to stricter criteria. Hum Reprod 1990; 5:586.

Merce LT, Andrino R, Barco MJ, de la Fuente F: Cyclic changes of the functional ovarian compartments: Echographic assessment. Acta Obstet Gynecol Scand 1990; 69:327.

Mettler L: Cervical factors in infertility. Curr Opin Obstet Gynecol 1990; 2:193.

Mikuz G, Schwarz C, Bartsch G: Wert der semiquantitativen morphologischen Beurteilung von Hodenbiopsien bei Fertilitätstörungen des Mannes. Pathologe 1983; 4:244.

Mishell DR Jr, Davajan V, Lobo RA: Infertility, Contraception and Reproductive Endocrinology, 3rd ed. Boston, Blackwell Scientific, 1991.

Moghissi KS: Cervical and uterine factors in infertility. Obstet Gynecol Clin North Am 1987; 14:887.

Mortensen JT: Risk for reduced sperm quality among metal workers, with special reference to welders. Scand J Environ Health 1988; 14:27.

Mortimer D: The male factor in infertility. Part I. Semen analysis. Probl Obstet Gynecol Fertil 1985; 8:3.

Mortimer ST, Mortimer D: Kinematics of human spermatozoa incubated under capacitating conditions. J Androl 1990; 11:195.

Mueller BA, Daling JR, Moore DE, Weiss NS, Spadoni LR, Stadel BV, Sooules MR: Appendectomy and the risk of tubal infertility. N Engl J Med 1986; 315:1506.

Nagler HM, White RD: The effect of testicular torsion on the contralateral testis. J Urol 1982; 128:1343.

Nilsson S, Edvinsson A, Milsson B: Improvement of semen and pregnancy rate after ligation and division of the internal spermatic vein: Fact or fiction? Br J Urol 1979; 51:591.

Nistal M, Paniagua R: Infertility in adult males with retractile testes. Fertil Steril 1984; 41:395.

Noyes RW: Normal phases of the endometrium. In The Uterus, edited by Norris HJ, Hertig AT. Baltimore, Williams & Wilkins, 1973, p 110.

Noyes RW, Haman JO: Accuracy of endometrial dating. Fertil Steril 1953; 4:504.

Noyes RW, Hertig AT, Rock J: Dating the endometrial biopsy. Fertil Steril 1950; 1:3

Osser S, Gennser G, Liedholm P, Ranstam J: Variation in semen parameters in fertile men. Arch Androl 1983; 10:127.

Papić Z, Katona G, Škrabalo Z: The cytologic identification and quantification of testicular cell subtypes. Reproducibility and relation to histologic findings in the diagnosis of male infertility. Acta Cytol 1988; 32:697.

Pepperell RJ, Hudson B, Wood C (Eds): The Infertile Couple, 2nd ed. London, Butterworth, 1987.

Pesce CM: Testicular biopsy in the evaluation of male fertility. Semin Diagn Pathol 1987; 4:264.

Poland ML, Moghissi KS, Giblin PT, Ager JW, Olson JM: Variation of semen measure within normal men. Fertil Steril 1985; 44:396.

Posinovec J: The necessity for bilateral biopsy in oligo and azoospermia. Int J Fertil 1976; 21:189.

Pryor JP: Evaluation of the infertile patient. In Aspects of Male Infertility, edited by DeVere White R. Baltimore, Williams & Wilkins, 1982, p 186.

Pryor JP: Seminal analysis. Clin Obstet Gynecol 1981; 8:571.

Quagliarello J, Arny M: Inaccuracy of basal body temperature charts in predicting urinary luteinizing hormone surges. Fertil Steril 1986; 45:334.

Reindollar RH, Novak M, Tho Spt, McDonough PG: Adult-onset amenorrhea: A study of 262 patients. Am J Obstet Gynecol 1986; 155:531.

Ridgway GL, Taylor-Robinson D: Current problems in microbiology: 1. Chlamydial infections: Which laboratory test? J Clin Pathol 1991; 44:1.

Risi GF, Sanders CV: The genital mycoplasmas. Obstet Gynecol Clin North Am 1989; 16:611.

Rivkees SA, Crawford JD: The relationship of gonadal activity and chemotherapy-induced gonadal damage. JAMA 1988; 259:2123.

Schenker JG, Margalioth EJ: Intrauterine adhesions: An updated appraisal. Fertil Steril 1982; 37:593.

Schilsky RL, Lewis BJ, Sherins RJ, Young RC: Gonadal dysfunction in patients receiving chemotherapy for cancer. Ann Intern Med 1980; 93:109.

Schlappack OK, Kratzik C, Schmidt W, Spona J, Schuster E: Response of the seminiferous epithelium to scattered radiation in seminoma patients. Cancer 1988; 62:1487.

Schlegel PN, Chang TSK, Marshall FF: Antibiotics: Potential hazards to male fertility. Fertil Steril 1991; 55:235.

Schwartz D, Laplanche A, Jouannet P, David G: Within subject variability of human semen in regard to sperm count, volume, total number of spermatozoa and length of abstinence. J Reprod Fertil 1979; 57:391.

Scott LS: Mumps and male fertility. Br J Urol 1960; 32:183.

Segal S, Yaffe H, Laufer N, Ben-David M: Male hyperprolactinemia: Effects on fertility. Fertil Steril 1979; 32:556.

Seibel MM: Infertility. A Comprehensive Text. Norwalk, CT, Appleton & Lange, 1990.

Siegler AM: Gynecologic endoscopy in infertility. Obstet Gynecol Clin North Am 1987; 14:1015.

Sigg C: Klassifizierung tubulärer Hodenatrophien bei Sterilitätsabklärungen. Bedeutung der sogenannten bunten Atrophie. Schweiz Med Wochenschr 1979; 109:1284.

Siimes MA, Routonen J: Small testicles with impaired production of sperm in adult male survivors of childhood malignancies. Cancer 1990; 65:1303.

Silber SJ, Ord T, Balmaceda J, Patrizio P, Asch RH: Congenital absence of the vas deferens. The fertilizing capacity of human epididymal sperm. N Engl J Med 1990; 323:1799.

Silber SJ, Rodriguez-Rigau LJ: Quantitative analysis of testicular biopsy: Determination of partial obstruction and production of sperm count after surgery for obstruction. Fertil Steril 1981; 36:480.

Simon A, Younis J, Lewin A, Bartoov B, Schenker JG, Laufer N: The correlation between sperm cell morphology and fertilization after zona pellucida slitting in subfertile males. Fertil Steril 1991; 56:325.

Singer R, Sagir M, Barnett M, Segenreich E, Allalouf D, Landau B, Servadio C: Motility, vitality and percentages of morphologically abnormal forms of human spermatozoa in relation to sperm counts. Andrologia 1980; 12:92.

Skakkebaek NE: Carcinoma in situ of the testis: Frequency and relationship to invasive germ cell tumors in infertile men. Histopathology 1978; 2:157.

Skakkebaek NE, Heller CG: Quantification of human seminiferous epithelium. III. Histological studies in 21 fertile men with normal chromosomal complements. J Reprod Fertil 1973; 32:179.

Smith CG, Asch RH: Drug abuse and reproduction. Fertil Steril 1987; 48:355.

Smithwick EB, Young LG: Solid phase indirect immunogold localization of human sperm antigens reacting with antisperm antibodies in human sera. J Androl 1990; 11:246.

Spark RF: The Infertile Male. The Clinician's Guide to Diagnosis and Treatment. New York, Plenum, 1988.

Speroff L, Glass RH, Kass NG: Clinical Gynecologic Endocrinology and Infertility. Baltimore, Williams & Wilkins, 1989.

Stacey C, Munday P, Thomas B, Gilchrist C, Taylor-Robinson D, Beard R: Chlamydia trachomatis in the fallopian tubes of women without laparoscopic evidence of salpingitis. Lancet 1990; 336:960.

Stillman RJ, Rosenberg MJ, Sachs BP: Smoking and reproduction. Fertil Steril 1986; 46:545.

Swerdloff RS, Overstreet JW, Sokol RZ, Rajfer J: Infertility in the male. UCLA conference. Ann Intern Med 1985; 103:906.

Tagatz GE, Kopher RA, Nagel TC, Okagaki T: The clitoral index: A bioassay of androgenic stimulation. Obstet Gynecol 1979; 54:562.

Tjoa WS, Smolensky MH, Hoi BP, Steinberger E, Smith KD: Circannual rhythm in human sperm count revealed by serially independent sampling. Fertil Steril 1982; 38:454.

Toovey S, Hudson E, Hendry WF, Levi AJ: Sulphasalazine and male infertility: Reversibility and possible mechanism. Gut 1981; 22:452.

Tung KSK, Lu CY: Immunologic basis of reproductive failure. In Pathology of Reproductive Failure, edited by Kraus FT, Damjanov I, Kaufman N. Baltimore, Williams & Wilkins, 1991, p 308.

Van Thiel DH, Gavalet JS, Smith WI, Swendolyn P: Hypothalamic-pituitary-gonadal dysfunction in men using cimetidine. N Engl J Med 1979; 300:1012.

Verp MS: Environmental causes of ovarian failure. Semin Reprod Endocrinol 1983; 1:101.

Vogt HJ, Heller WD, Borelli S: Sperm quality of healthy smokers, exsmokers, and never-smokers. Fertil Steril 1986; 45:106.

Wah RM, Anderson DJ, Hill JA: Asymptomatic cervicovaginal leukocytosis in infertile women. Fertil Steril 1990; 54:445.

Weinberg CR: Infertility and the use of illicit drugs. Epidemiology 1990; 1:189.

Weinberg U, Kraemer FB, Kammerman S: Coexistence of primary endocrine deficiencies: A unique case of male hypergonadism associated with hypoparathyroidism, hypodrenocorticism, and hypothyroidism. Am J Med Sci 1976; 272:215.

Wentz AC, Herbert CM III, Maxon WS, Hill GA, Pittaway DE: Cycle of conception endometrial biopsy. Fertil Steril 1986; 46:196.

Werner CA: Mumps orchitis and testicular atrophy. Ann Intern Med 1950; 32:1066.

Wheeler JE: Histology of the fertile and infertile testis. In Pathology of Reproductive Failure, edited by Kraus FT, Damjanov I, Kaufman N. Baltimore, Williams & Wilkins, 1991, p 56.

Whorton, D, Krauss RM, Marshall S, Milby TH: Infertility in male pesticide workers. Lancet 1977; 2:1259.

Wilkins TJ: Receptor autoimmunity in endocrine disorders. N Engl J Med 1990; 323:1318.

Williamson RA, Koehler JK, Smith WD, Stenchever MA: Ultrastructural sperm tail defects associated with sperm immotility. Fertil Steril 1984; 41:103.

Winfield AC, Wentz AC: Diagnostic Imaging in Infertility, 2nd ed. Baltimore, Williams & Wilkins, 1992.

Wong TW, Strauss FH II, Jones TM, Warner NE: Pathological aspects of the infertile testes. Urol Clin North Am 1978; 5:503.

World Health Organization: Laboratory Manual for the Examination of Human Semen and Semen-Cervical Mucus Interaction. Cambridge, UK, Cambridge University Press, 1987.

World Health Organization Task Force on Methods for Regulation of Male Fertility: Contraceptive efficacy of testosterone-induced azoospermia in normal men. Lancet 1990; 336:955.

Wu CH, Gocial B: A pelvic scoring system for infertility surgery. Int J Fertil 1988; 33:341.

Yen SSC, Joffe RB: Reproductive Endocrinology: Physiology; Pathophysiology and Clinical Management, ed 3. Philadelphia, WB Saunders, 1991.

Ying S-Y: Inhibins activins and follistatins: Gonadal proteins modulating the secretion of follicle-stimulating hormone. Endocr Rev 1988; 9:267.

Zamboni L: Sperm ultrastructural pathology and infertility. In Pathology of infertility. Clinical Correlations in the Male and Female, edited by Gondos B, Riddick DH. New York, Thieme, 1987, p 353.

Zamboni L: Clinical relevance of evaluation of sperm and ova. In Pathology of Reproductive Failure, edited by Kraus FT, Damjanov I, Kaufman N. Baltimore, Williams & Wilkins, 1991, p 10.

Zaneveld LJD, Jeyendran RS: Modern assessment of semen for diagnostic purposes. Semin Reprod Endocrinol 1988; 6:323.

Zaneveld LJD, Polakoski LK: Collection and the physical examination of the ejaculate. In Techniques of Human Andrology, edited by Hafez E. Amsterdam, Elsevier, 1977, p 147.

Zlatnik FJ, Gellhaus TM, Benda JA, Koontz FP, Burmeister LF: Histologic chorioamnionitis, microbial infection, and prematurity. Obstet Gynecol 1990; 76:355.

Chapter 3

DISORDERS OF SEXUAL DIFFERENTIATION AND DEVELOPMENT

NORMAL DEVELOPMENT

Sexual differentiation is determined by a series of sequential processes involving primary genetic and secondary hormonal determinants of maleness and femaleness. These distinct stepwise events include:

1. Determination of genetic sex
2. Differentiation of the gonads
3. Development of extragonadal reproductive organs and male and female characteristics
4. Establishment of the function of reproductive organs
5. Establishment of psychological gender

In most instances development of the genetic sex corresponds to the development of secondary sexual characteristics and the psychological gender, but in a considerable number of cases some discordance evolves, leading to various forms of hermaphroditism, intersexuality, bisexuality, and homosexuality. The consequences may be anatomic, functional, psychological, or any combination of these, resulting in major, minor, or subliminal forms of reproductive dysfunction and infertility.

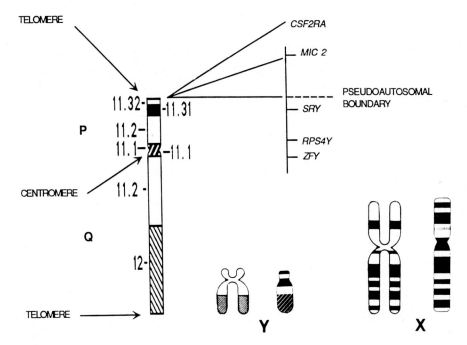

Fig. 3-1. Diagram of sex chromosomes. The enlarged Y chromosome shows the location of sex determining gene region; SRY-sex determining. (Courtesy P. Goodfellow).

Chromosomal sex

Chromosomal sex is determined by the X and Y chromosomes at the time of fertilization (Fig. 3-1). Individuals with two X chromosomes become females, and those with XY become males primarily through the action of sex chromosomes on germ cells that have migrated from the yolk sac into the undifferentiated gonadal primordium (Austin and Edwards, 1981). It became evident that the Y chromosome has the most important role in directing the undifferentiated gonad to become a testis when it was noted that a fetus with only one X chromosome will form ovaries and acquire a female phenotype and those carrying a Y chromosome, irrespective of the number of X chromosomes, become male (McLaren, 1990b and 1991b). The genetic determinant of maleness responsible for the formation of testes was named testis determining factor (TDF) in humans and testis determining Y gene (Tdy) in mice. Although there is compelling evidence that the critical TDF of men and mice is located on the Y chromosome, it is not known whether the development of testes depends on one or several genes that could be acting coordinately or under the dictate of one principal regulator (Goodfellow and Lovell-Badge, 1991).

The TDF has been named SRY (sex-determining region on chromosome Y) in humans and Sry in mice (McLaren, 1991b). Human SRY is located in the Y-specific region on the short arm of the Y chromosome below the pseudoautosomal pairing region. The genes in the pseudoautosomal region pair with the X chromosome and participate in the homologous recombination of the genes on the homolo-

gous sex chromosome (Ellis, 1991). The genes of the Y-specific region, including the SRY, do not cross over normally and are inherited in a patrilinear manner. Koopman et al. (1991) have constructed transgenic mice by inserting Sry or SRY into the germ line and have shown that transgenic female mice carrying the mouse Sry develop testes. These experiments prove that the murine 14-kilobase sequence of genomic DNA carries the determinant of maleness. The action of Sry requires, however, an interaction with other genes and the mutation of these regulatory or effector genes could affect the final expression of Sry. It also appears that Sry is sensitive to positional effects exerted by other genes on the sex chromosomes as evidenced by the fact that not all transgenic mice carrying Sry develop testes (Koopman et al., 1991). Furthermore, female mice carrying human SRY did not develop testes. Thus it is not known whether Sry and SRY are equivalent to one another and whether SRY is indeed the human testis determinant (McLaren, 1991b).

Data most strongly implicating SRY as the human TDF were derived from the study of two sex-reversed XY daughters, with a mutation in the SRY region that was not detectable in their father (Berta et al., 1990; Jäger et al., 1990). Because the testes did not develop in these two offspring with the mutated SRY, it was concluded that the normal SRY sequence is essential for testiculogenesis. Sensitivity to positional influences and the poorly understood interaction of SRY with other genes could account for some clinical observations such as the development of male gonads in XX individuals lacking SRY (Palmer et al., 1989) and the development of female gonads in XY females with intact SRY (Berta et al., 1990; Jäger et al., 1990). Positional effects could account for the fact that female mice transgenic for SRY did not develop testes (Koopman et al., 1991).

In contrast to the progress made toward understanding of testis determining genes, very little is known about the ovary determining genes. Eicher and Washburn (1983) have proposed that the ovary determining genes are located on the autosomes and that they interact with the Y chromosomal genes. In XX individuals the ovary determining genes have no competition, and as a result of their action, ovaries are formed. In XY individuals the Y chromosome is activated before the ovary determining genes on the autosome influence female differentiation, thus ensuring the development of testes. However, if the ovary determining genes are activated before Y chromosomal gene activation, as postulated for sex-reversed mice, an ovary or ovotestis will develop even in the presence of the Y chromosome because the ovary determining genes have already *primed* the undifferentiated gonad. This hypothesis needs to be corroborated, and the putative human ovary determining genes remain to be identified.

Gonadal sex

Gonadal sex determination and the development of gonads and genital organs have been reviewed extensively (Austin and Edwards, 1981; McLaren, 1991a). Mammalian gonads develop from several cell lineages, which include primordial germ cells, coelomic epithelium lining the genital ridge, mesenchymal cells of the urogenital ridge, and the mesonephric structures (Byskov, 1986). Germ cells originate in the yolk sac and migrate along the midline of the embryo into the genital ridges, which appear as protuberances on the posterior wall of the coelomic cavity anteromedial to the mesonephric ridges and adrenals. Genital ridges consist of mesenchymal cells, mesonephric tubules, and a two- to three-layer-thick coelomic epithelium covering their free surface (Fig. 3-2). During the first 6 weeks of development, the genital ridge is in an undifferentiated bipotential state; development may proceed in the direction of either testes or ovary. Initial induction occurs as a result of the interaction between gonocytes and supporting sex cord cells (McLaren, 1991a). Subsequent development of fetal gonads and internal and external genital organs is then under the influence of sex hormones and the müllerian-inhibiting substance (MIS) also known as antimüllerian hormone (AMH) nonsteroidal glycoprotein. The functions of this were reviewed by Josso et al. in 1991.

The exact role of germ cells in gonadogenesis is not fully understood. Ovaries do not develop without germ cells, indicating that these cells are critical for the development of the female gonad (Merchant, 1975). The morphogenesis of testes may proceed without germ cells, as evi-

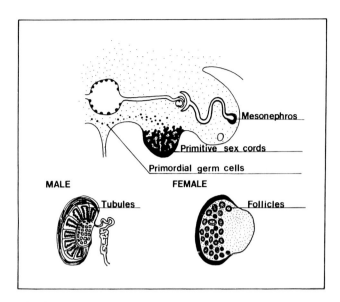

Fig. 3-2. Schematic presentation of the development of the genital ridges. Seminiferous tubule form within the male gonad and follicles form in female gonads. (Modified from Grumbach MM. In Wilson JD, Foster DW (Eds). Williams Textbook of Endocrinology, 8th ed. Philadelphia, WB Saunders, 1992, with permission.)

denced by relatively unimpeded tubulogenesis in male mice that are genetically sterile and lack gonocytes (Merchant, 1975). Fetal Sertoli cells can differentiate even without gonocytes but, at least in experimental animals, complete maturation of Sertoli cells is impeded in the absence of spermatogenesis (McLaren, 1991a).

Fetal Sertoli cells secrete AMH, the function of which is to mediate the involution of the müllerian duct in the male. However, as murine fetal Sertoli cells continue synthesizing AMH throughout an entire gestation and still in the early postnatal period, it has been proposed that AMH might have additional functions in development of the testis (McLaren, 1990a). AMH may act as inhibitor of meiosis of germ cells in the testis, which at least in the mouse testis begins coincidentally with the decreased expression of the AMH gene in the postnatal Sertoli cells (Munsterberg and Lovell-Badge, 1991). Hence it was proposed that the AMH is toxic to meiotic cells in testis, and that the function of AMH in the fetal testes is to eliminate any germ cell that has entered meiosis precociously.

Early in development and at high concentration, AMH is toxic to fetal ovarian oocytes (Vigier et al., 1989). Female germ cells enter meiosis early in the fetal gonad. If AMH is toxic for meiotic cells, female gonocytes would be affected adversely. However, because the female fetus does not synthesize AMH under normal circumstances, there is no danger that fetal oocytes entering meiosis will be damaged. In adult female mice, AMH is synthesized by granulosa cells, presumably exerting meiosis-inhibitory effects on the intrafollicular oocytes. Once released from the follicle and from the presumptive inhibitory influence of AMH, oocytes reenter meiosis, which is completed at the

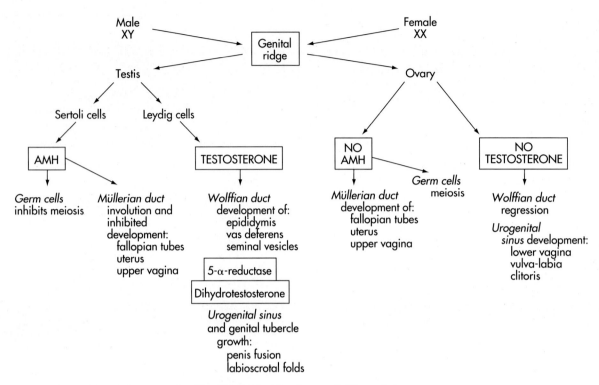

Algorithm 3-1. Female sexual differentiation.

time of fertilization. Fetal testes synthesize and secrete testosterone (Serra et al., 1970), which is essential for the development of male gonad, virilization of the urogenital sinus, wolffian ducts, and the urogenital tubercle (George and Wilson, 1988). Jost and his collaborators have shown that male rabbit fetuses castrated in utero develop female genital organs; in addition fetal testes implanted next to the fetal ovary stimulated local regression of müllerian ducts and the development of the wolffian duct (Jost, 1972). One could conclude that local secretion of testosterone by the fetal testis is essential for the morphogenesis of internal genital organs.

Genital sex

Phenotypic sex is assigned to an individual on the basis of the typical male or female features of the external and internal genital organs. Secondary sexual characteristics develop at puberty under the influence of sex hormones produced by the testis or the ovary.

Internal genital organs develop from müllerian and wolffian ducts and the urogenital sinus; the external genital organs develop from the genital tubercle (Algorithm 3-1). These primordia are present in both the female and male fetus before the eighth week of intrauterine development (Wilson et al., 1981). Under the influence of AMH, the müllerian ducts involute in the male fetus by the tenth

week. In the female fetus, whose gonads do not secrete AMH, the müllerian ducts form the fallopian tubes, uterus, and upper portion of the vagina (George and Wilson, 1988) (Fig. 3-3). In the male fetus, the mesonephric (wolffian) ducts give rise to the epididymis, vas deferens, and seminal vesicles. Full development of male genital ducts occurs only under the influence of male sex hormones.

Androgenic sex hormones are essential for the masculinization of both internal and external genitalia. Androgens are synthesized initially by fetal Leydig cells and the adrenal cortex under the influence of human chorionic gonadotropin (hCG), fetal adrenocorticotropic hormone (ACTH), and gonadotropins. Fetal testosterone levels and the number of Leydig cells peak at 15 to 17 weeks (Lee et al., 1980). Thereafter, sex hormone levels drop and Leydig cells decrease in number. Female fetuses derive androgens from adrenals. Adrenal disturbances such as 21-hydroxylase deficiency are characterized by overproduction of androgens and subsequent virilization of external genital organs (White et al., 1987); however, the wolffian ducts do not differentiate into male genital ducts, indicating that the development of the wolffian system in the male occurs only in the presence of the testes. Likewise, in genotypic males with ambiguous external genitalia, the epididymis, ductus deferens, and seminal vesicles develop

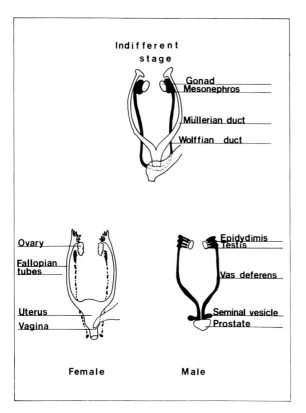

Fig. 3-3. The regression of müllerian ducts in the male is regulated by the AMH derived from fetal Sertoli cells (redrawn from Wilson et al. Science 1981; 211:1278, with permission, © 1981 AAAS).

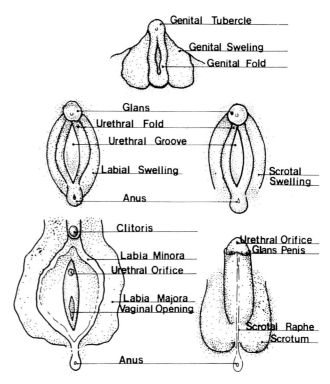

Fig. 3-4. The external genital organs develop from the genital tubercle and the urogenital sinus. Androgens are needed for the virilization of external genital. (Modified from Spaulding, 1921; and Grumbach and Conte, 1992).

only if the testes are present. If the testis develops only unilaterally, genital ducts develop from the wolffian ducts ipsilaterally from saturation of the developmental fields with testicular androgens presumably through direct diffusion (Grumbach and Conte, 1992). Apparently, the virilization of the external genitalia requires smaller amounts of androgens than the male genital ducts, which form only if local androgen concentrations are sufficiently high. This oversaturation of developmental fields with androgens occurs in males through direct diffusion from the ipsilateral testis.

It appears that virilization of the wolffian ducts is mediated by testosterone, whereas virilization of the urogenital sinus and formation of external genitalia are under the influence of dihydrotestosterone, which is formed peripherally from testosterone through the action of 5-α-reductase. The critical role of 5-α-reductase in the virilization of external genitalia is best illustrated in male pseudohermaphrodites caused by 5-α-reductase deficiency. Although these patients have testes and male wolffian duct derivatives, the external genitalia are female (Peterson et al., 1977). Although testes of the patients produce testosterone, the hormone is not converted into dehydrotestosterone, which is essential for the virilization of the external genitalia. Hence, the gonadal tubercle and urogenital sinus do not

form penis and scrotum but give rise to female external genitalia.

External genital organs develop primarily from the genital tubercle, with a contribution from the lower part of the urogenital sinus (Fig. 3-4). In the female fetus the müllerian ducts establish contact with the urogenital sinus, forming the uterovaginal plate (Bulmer, 1957). The proliferation of cells in the uterovaginal plate separates the cervix from the vulva. Lengthening of the vaginal primordium occurs, followed by central cavitation and formation of the vaginal lumen. The remaining portion of the urogenital sinus remains open and gives rise to the vulva.

In the male, epithelial buds proliferate from the upper urogenital sinus to form the prostate; the lower part forms the urethra. In contrast to the vulvar portion of the urogenital sinus, which remains open, the lower part of the male urogenital sinus closes and is incorporated into the protruding genital swellings to form the penile urethra.

Differentiation of the urogenital tubercle giving rise to the penis in males and clitoris in females occurs at different rates. The growth of the urogenital tubercle is under the influence of fetal androgens.

Because the genital tubercle of the female fetus has essentially the same number of androgen receptors per cell as the cells of the male genital anlage, the presence or absence of hormonal influences during this sensitive period of organogenesis is a critical determinant of normal development (George and Wilson, 1988). Male fetal deficiency of androgens can, for example, result in micropenis (Lee et al., 1980). Virilization of female external genital organs occurs when the female fetus is exposed to excess androgens, such as in the adrenogenital syndrome due to 11-β-hydroxylase deficiency (Zachmann et al., 1983).

The effects of estrogens on phenotypic differentiation of female genital organs are less understood. It is also not known whether an estrogen excess could inhibit the normal development of male genitalia. Abnormalities induced by diethylstilbestrol, an analogue of estrogen, have been documented in both females and males exposed in utero (Herbst and Bern, 1981).

Sexual maturation

Sexual maturation occurs at the time of puberty (reviewed comprehensively by Speroff et al., 1989). It involves activations of the hypothalamo-pituitary-gonadal axis and results in the final differentiation of the gonads, genital organs, and acquisition of secondary sexual characteristics. From infancy to prepuberty the hypothalamus is extremely sensitive to negative feedback inhibition, which maintains the secretion of gonadotropin-releasing hormone (Gn-RH) at very low levels (Speroff et al., 1989). Endogenous inhibition of the hypothalamus also contributes to maintaining hypothalamic inactivity, but this mechanism is poorly understood.

At puberty these inhibitory influences wane, and a pulsatile Gn-RH secretion is instituted, resulting in the initiation of gametogenesis. The pattern of FSH and LH secretion in response to Gn-RH changes and gradually assumes the pattern typical of adulthood.

In the female, landmark events are *thelarche,* evidenced by breast budding, and *pubarche,* marked by pubic and axillary hair growth. Hair growth in the pubic and axillary regions occurs under the influence of adrenal androgens, the secretion of which is independent of gonadotropins, ACTH, and prolactin. Hence it is also called *adrenarche.* Growth spurts, mediated by the effect of estrogens on long bones, occur in a crescendo-decrescendo manner, the peak occurring at 12 years for girls and 14 for boys. *Menarche* typically occurs after the peak growth rate.

The onset of puberty is influenced genetically and socially. Among others, these exogenous influences include living conditions (urban-rural, high altitude or sea level, geographic latitude), nutritional status, and body weight. Strenuous physical activity, chronic disease, or chemotherapy may delay puberty.

A general trend toward earlier menarche has been recorded in the nineteenth and early twentieth centuries in all Western countries, but in the United States the biologic optimum apparently has been reached and the mean age of girls entering menarche has stabilized at 12.8 years. Inter-

estingly, black females generally enter puberty earlier than white females. Males mature somewhat slower than females, with *spermarche* occurring typically 6 to 12 months later in life than menarche in females.

Psychosocial gender

Final gender identity is the end result of gonadal development, differentiation of genitalia, acquisition of male or female sexual characteristics, imprinting of the fetal brain, and social sex assignment and rearing. Psychosocial gender is thus in part nature and in part nurture. The reproductive function of such individuals will vary over a broad range from minor deviation from the norm to severe impairment, requiring various forms of psychosocial, medical, or surgical interventions.

Human sexual behavior has been graded on a seven-point scale by Kinsey et al. (1948), who recognized that this aspect of sexuality simply cannot be discussed in terms of heterosexual and homosexual orientation. The issues pertaining to psychosocial and biologic aspects of homosexuality remain controversial and poorly understood. Recent claims that there are anatomic differences between the hypothalamic nuclei of heterosexual and homosexual have fueled the controversy even more (LeVay, 1991). These studies and others (reviewed by Gorski, 1991), although inconclusive, have defined a sexual dimorphism of the human brain and have focused on the hypothalamus (interstitial nuclei of hypothalamus 3) as one of the most important anatomic sites regulating human sexuality. The exact mechanisms of brain imprinting and the acquisition of male or female sexual orientation are poorly understood in the human (for review, see Gorski, 1991).

Fetal and neonatal rat brains may be imprinted under the influence of sex hormones. The brain of rats shows sexual dimorphism, most prominently in the sexually dimorphic nucleus of the preoptic area (SDN-POA). This nucleus is approximately five times larger in males than in females. Administration of testosterone to female fetuses or newborn pups increases the size of the SDN-POA, indicating that the development of this structure is directly influenced by androgenic hormones. Administration of antiestrogens inhibits the growth and development of the SDN-POA and is associated with defeminization, albeit without evidence of masculinization. Hence it appears that in rodents both estrogens and androgens act on the developing brain and contribute to its sexual dimorphism. The human equivalent of rodent SDN-POA has been described, but there still is controversy regarding the exact location of this area and whether these hypothalamic nuclei show sexual dimorphism (Gorski, 1991).

Swaab and Hoffman (1988) quantitatively studied the hypothalamic nuclei of male homosexuals, transsexuals, and male and female heterosexuals. They found that the SDN-POA of homosexuals did not differ from that of heterosexual males, whereas in the male transsexuals the number of neurons in the nucleus was in the range for heterosexual females. Psychosocial development in intersexes provides additional arguments for understanding the sexual differentiation of the brain. Excessive prenatal exposure to androgens, as it occurs in congenital adrenal hyperplasia, causes virilization of the external genitalia but does not change the heterosexual orientation of affected females. Genotypic males with testicular feminization have female external organs and well-developed breasts and are raised as and behave like females. The effect of social influences cannot be excluded, but the deficiency of androgen receptors in these people is more likely to have a major determinant influence. On the other hand, genetic males with 5-α-reductase deficiency have a urogenital sinus instead of a vagina and female external genitalia organs and are raised in early life as females. These individuals change their gender identity at the time of puberty (Imperato-McGinley et al., 1987) presumably in part because of the imprinting of the brain with male hormones during prenatal life.

Psychosocial gender development or assignment, or both, may result in *gender dysphoria,* a term used to denote discomfort with one's anatomic or assigned sex (Brown, 1990). Gender dysphoria includes various conditions such as transvestism and transsexualism. The endocrinology of transsexualism has been reviewed by Gooren (1990), and the medical implications of it were discussed in an editorial in *Lancet* (1991).

Disorders of erotic arousal, such as dislocation of arousal imagery from the "normal" heterosexual or intrusion of extraneous imagery such as fetishism, are grouped under the term *paraphilia* (Money, 1984). These include homosexuality, fetishism, exhibitionism, necrophilia, coprophilia, and a wide range of similar disorders. None of these aberrations is linked thus far to an organic or hormonal cause.

The contributions of nature and nurture closely intertwine with one another and cannot be readily distinguished. Nevertheless, the genetic factors are of paramount influence, as illustrated in the study of homosexuality in twins and adoptive brothers (Bailey and Pillard, 1991). According to this study 52% of monozygotic twins, 22% of dizygotic twins, and 11% of adoptive brothers were homosexual. Although such data favor the genetic basis of homosexuality, this entire area of inquiry is in great flux and remains controversial.

Clinical determination of sex

Clinical investigations of sexual differentiation and development include laboratory studies, gynecologic and andrologic examination, and, if needed, psychological evaluation (Grumbach and Conte, 1992). Chromosomal sex is established on the basis of cytogenetic studies. Gonadal sex can be determined by examining the external and internal genital organs, supplemented by biopsy if needed. Functional maturation and competence of the hypothala-

---

Genetic anomalies of sexual differentiation, gonadogenesis, and genital organ development

A. Sex chromosome abnormalities
 1. Klinefelter's syndrome and its variants
 2. Gonadal dysgenesis
   Turner's syndrome
   Pure gonadal dysgenesis
   Mixed gonadal dysgenesis
 3. True hermaphroditism
B. Single gene defects
 1. Adrenogenital syndromes
   21-hydroxylase deficiency
   11-β-hydroxylase deficiency
   3-β-hydroxysteroid dehydrogenase deficiency
   17-α-hydoxylase deficiency
   17,20-lyase deficiency
   Cholesterol desmolase deficiency
   17-β-hydroxysteroid oxidoreductase deficiency
 2. Androgen insensitivity
   Androgen receptor deficiency
   5-α-reductase deficiency
 3. Antimüllerian hormone deficiency
C. Congenital syndromes associated with gonadal abnormalities

---

mo-pituitary-gonadal axis may necessitate hormonal studies.

ABNORMALITIES OF SEXUAL DIFFERENTIATION

Abnormalities of sexual differentiation, gonadogenesis, and the development of external genital organs and secondary sexual characteristics can be classified as consequences of:

1. Sex chromosomal defects
2. Autosomal single gene defects
3. Idiopathic developmental birth defects
4. Prenatal hormonal effects
5. These disorders are listed in the box above and in general correspond to conditions that have been classified traditionally as disorders of gonadal differentiation, female pseudohermaphroditism, male pseudohermaphroditism, and unclassified forms of abnormal sexual development (Grumbach and Conte, 1992).

Sex chromosome abnormalities

As discussed in the first part of this chapter, the sex chromosomes play a crucial role in determining the development of gonads and indirectly the external genitalia. Without the Y chromosome the fetus will develop into a female. In the fetus that has a Y chromosome, the external genitalia will be male unless there is androgen resistance.

Table 3-1. Sex chromosome abnormalities in 34,910 liveborn children in Århus during a 13-year period 1969-1974 and 1980-1988

Sex chromosome abnormalities	Liveborn	Rate per 1000	Rate total
Klinefelter's syndrome	30		
47,XXY	20		
46,XY/47,XXY	7	1.68	1/596
46,XX (male)	2		
48,XXYY	1		
XYY syndrome	20		
47,XYY	18	1.12	1/894
46,XY,47,XYY	2		
Triple X syndrome (47,XXX)	17	1.00	1/1002
Turner's syndrome	8		
45,X	1		
45,X/46,XX	2		
45,X/47,XXX	1		
45,X/46,X,r(X)	1		
45,X/46,X,inv(X)	1	0.47	1/2130
45,X/46,X,i(Xq)/ 47,X,i(Xq),i(Xq)	1		
45,Xinv(9)/ 46,XX,inv(9)	1		
Others	3		
45,X/46,XY (male)	1		
46,XX/47,XX,del(Yq) (female)	1	0.09	1/11,637
46,XX/46,XY (female)	1		
TOTAL	78	2.23	1/448

From Nielsen and Wohlert. Birth Defects 1991; 26(4):211, © March of Dimes Foundation, with permission

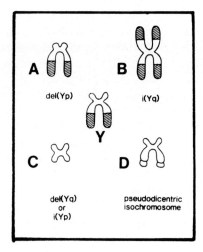

Fig. 3-5. Structurally abnormal Y chromosomes. *Y,* Normal chromosome. *A,* Isochromosome for the long arm. *B,* Deletion of the long arm or isochromosome for the short arm. *D,* Pseudodicentric isochromosome for the short arm also containing two copies of the proximal part of the long arm. (Modified from de la Chapelle A. In Emery AEH, Rimoin DL (Eds). Principles and Practice of Medical Genetics, 2nd ed. Edinburgh, Churchill Livingstone, 1990, with permission).

Table 3-2. Characteristics of patients with Klinefelter's syndrome*

Feature	Karyotype	
	47, XXY (%)	Mosaics 46, XY/ 47, XXY (%)
Testicular histopathology	100	94
Testicular size decreased	99	73
Azoospermia	93	50
Increased gonadotropins	75	33
Decreased testosterone	79	33
Decreased facial hair	77	64
Decreased axial hair	49	46
Gynecomastia	55	33
Decreased length of penis	41	21
Decreased sexual function	68	56

Modified from Gordon et al. Arch Intern Med 1972; 130:726, © 1972, American Medical Association, by permission.
*Data are based on the study of 519 47,XXY and 51 46,XY/47,XXY mosaic patients.

However, if the karyotype of an XY individual contains additional X chromosomes, these will interfere with normal male development and the affected individual will show features of Klinefelter's syndrome. Sex chromosome abnormalities occur at a rate of approximately 2.5 per 1000 newborns (Table 3-1).

Klinefelter's syndrome. Klinefelter's syndrome is a form of male hypogonadism associated with sex chromosome abnormalities that include at least two X chromosomes and one Y chromosome (de la Chapelle, 1990). Three forms of Klinefelter's syndrome can be diagnosed cytogenetically:

1. Classic
2. Variant
3. Mosaics

The classic form is associated with the 47, XXY karyotype. Variant forms are marked by supernumerary sex chromosomes 48, XXXY, 48, XXYY, 49, XXXXY, and 49, XXXYY karyotypes or structurally abnormal chromosomes such as 47, XX, i (Xq) Y, 47, XX, inv Y (p+q−); or 47, XX (q−) Y (Fig. 3-5). Some 46, XX males also present with hypogonadism and are included under this heading. Mosaics have one normal male or female line and one or more sex chromosome trisomic lines (e.g., XY/

XXY or XX/XXY) or two chromosomally abnormal lines (e.g., 47, XXY/48, XXXY).

Incidence. Klinefelter's syndrome is the most common chromosomal disorder associated with infertility and affects approximately 1 in 500 to 1 in 1000 phenotypic males (Philip et al., 1976; de la Chapelle, 1990). Approximately 80% to 90% of these patients have the classic form, and 10% to 15% have mosaicism. The variant forms are rare and account for 1% to 5% of all cases. Among azoospermic men, approximately 10% to 13% have Klinefelter's syndrome (Chandley, 1979). In mental institutions for the chronically ill, approximately 15% of the

Table 3-3. Hormonal findings in infertile men

	N	Mean testis volume (ml)	Testosterone (nmol/l)	LH (U/l)	Testosterone/ LH ratio	FSH (Bioactive)	FSH (Immunoreactive)	FSH Bioactive/ immunoreactive ratio
Fertile	23	18.74 ± 0.8	16.5 ± 1.4	3.3 ± 0.9	6.3 ± 0.9	6.2 ± 0.3	4.1 ± 0.4	1.8 ± 0.2
XXY	11	2.4 ± 0.5	10.6 ± 1.2	22.1 ± 3.1	0.6 ± 0.1	24.1 ± 6.0	26.9 ± 3.0	0.9 ± 0.2
Azoospermia	15	9.6 ± 1.5	14.0 ± 1.0	6.5 ± 1.2	3.6 ± 0.6	25.1 ± 4.3	22.2 ± 4.0	1.2 ± 0.1
Cryptorchidism	36	10.8 ± 0.7	15.8 ± 1.2	5.9 ± 0.6	3.8 ± 0.5	12.5 ± 1.4	14.6 ± 1.6	0.9 ± 0.1
Oligospermia (<5 million)	50	12.2 ± 0.7	15.5 ± 1.0	5.8 ± 0.7	4.1 ± 0.4	11.9 ± 1.2	11.2 ± 1.0	1.1 ± 0.1
Oligospermia (<20 million)	45	15.0 ± 0.8	16.7 ± 1.1	4.9 ± 1.1	5.9 ± 0.6	8.9 ± 1.5	8.0 ± 1.1	1.2 ± 0.1

Modified from Jockenhovel et al. Acta Endocrinol 1989; 121:902, with permission.

residents have a Klinefelter's syndrome karyotype (Pecile and Filippi, 1991).

Clinical findings. In the original description of Klinefelter et al. (1942), the syndrome was delineated as consisting of gynecomastia, small, firm testes, and high urinary follicle-stimulating hormone (FSH). Characteristic hypoandrogenism and low levels of serum testosterone were recognized only later (Klinefelter, 1973). Subsequently, it was discovered that serum testosterone concentrations varied and were either mildly, moderately, or severely below normal values for males. The degree of virilization or eunuchoidism reflected endogenous androgen production and thus varied over a wide range (Hsueh et al., 1978). The increasing degree of disability encountered in patients with an additional X or Y chromosome probably can be ascribed to a dosage effect of genes that are homologous on the X and Y chromosomes and escape X inactivation (Ferguson-Smith, 1991).

Clinical features of the syndrome have been reviewed by Schwartz and Root (1991). The most common symptoms include delayed puberty and incomplete masculinization, eunuchoid habitus, lack of body hair, female escutcheon, and gynecomastia (Table 3-2). Most patients are taller than average but not to the extent as initially thought—177.4 cm for patients versus 173.5 cm for controls in the study quoted by de la Chapelle (1990). Symptoms are expressed variably, and the only constant findings are microorchidism and azoospermia. Testes measure on average less than 2 cm in length in comparison with normal testes, which are 3.5 to 4.5 cm long. A small penis is seen in one fourth of all cases (Smith and Rodriguez-Rigau, 1989) and occasionally may be associated with hypospadias. Intellectual capacity of patients with classic Klinefelter's syndrome is within normal range or slightly lower than in their sibs (Netley, 1981). These patients show reduced achievement in reading, spelling, and arithmetic and may have some impairment of expressive and receptive language skills (Graham et al., 1988). The patients with variant syndromes seem to show more pronounced psychosocial deviations (Grumbach and Conte, 1992). The psychosocial orientation of most patients, irrespective of the karyotype, is male.

Patients with cytogenetically diagnosed variant or mo-

saic forms of Klinefelter's syndrome have essentially the same features as those with the classic form of the syndrome. Nevertheless, some argue that it is important to distinguish various subtypes (Grammatico et al., 1990). Patients with the 48, XXYY karyotype tend to be taller, whereas the 46, XY/47, XXY mosaics have higher levels of testosterone in the serum and thus appear more masculinized. Those with the 48, XXXY karyotype resemble the classic form of the syndrome. Those with 48, XXXY or 49, XXXXY have extremely small, "pea-sized" testes and micropenis (de la Chapelle, 1990; Grumbach and Conte, 1992). Mental retardation is most pronounced in the 48, XXYY individuals (Grammatico et al., 1990).

One in 25 patients with Klinefelter's syndrome has a 46, XX karyotype (de la Chapelle, 1981). Phenotypically, 46, XX males show all the features of Klinefelter's syndrome, and the only differences are that they are generally not as tall and have a normal intelligence (de la Chapelle, 1990). In most instances the X chromosome of XX males carries the TDF of the Y chromosome translocated to the X chromosome (Andersson et al., 1986) because of an abnormal terminal X-Y interchange (Petit et al., 1987). The nature of the defect, however, remains enigmatic, especially in some familial cases that show no detectable Y chromosome fragments in their karyotype (Abbas et al., 1990). Some of these familial XXs are true hermaphrodites, indicating that the pathogenesis of the two conditions may be interrelated and caused by an autosomal or pseudoautosomal mechanism based on the activity of genes outside of the TDF of the Y chromosome.

Hormonal findings. Postpubertal patients typically show elevated serum levels of FSH and luteinizing hormone (LH) in the range comparable to that of infertile men who have surgically corrected cryptorchidism (Giagulli and Vermeulen, 1988). This elevation of serum gonadotropins apparently is related to testicular abnormalities and the inability of the Leydig cells to respond appropriately to hypothalamic stimulation that occurs at puberty. As one would expect, the prepubertal levels of FSH and LH are within normal limits (Ratcliffe, 1982), but become elevated after puberty (Jockenhovel et al., 1989; Table 3-3). Since the Leydig cells do not respond adequately to gonadotropic stimulation at the time of puberty or later with a

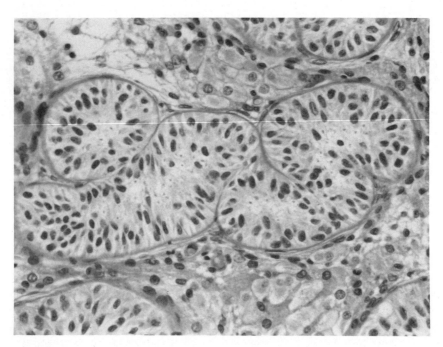

Fig. 3-6. Histologic findings in the testis of a prepubertal patient with Klinefelter's syndrome. The tubules do not contain identifiable germ cells.

therapeutic injection of Gn-RH, serum levels of testosterone are considerably lower than normal in most patients. Wang et al. (1975) reported, nevertheless, that 43% of patients in their series had serum levels in the low normal range, which again points out the heterogeneity of the testicular defects. Serum estradiol may be elevated (Wang et al., 1975). However, as this is not typical of all patients, it was proposed that gynecomastia and other signs of incomplete virilization are not direct consequences of hyperestrinism but rather of a higher than normal estradiol to testosterone ratio (Grumbach and Conte, 1992).

Pathologic findings. Typical histologic features of Klinefelter's syndrome in the postpubertal or adult testis are tubular atrophy with hyalinization, aspermatogenesis, interstitial fibrosis, and prominence of Leydig cells. Scattered germ cells and residual signs of spermatogenesis may be found focally. Spermatogenesis is usually abortive, and viable spermatozoa are rarely found. This is the usual case in mosaics as well, although they occasionally are fertile (Court-Brown et al., 1964). As a rule, most patients with Klinefelter's syndrome are azoospermic and suffer from irreversible sterility.

The lack of spermatogenic cells in the tubules can be traced to prepubertal development during which the testicular tubules appear smaller than those in normal age-matched controls (Ferguson-Smith, 1959). In these prepubertal testes only 20% of the tubules contain spermatogonia in normal numbers in contrast to normal testes, which have germ cells in at least 80% of the tubules (Fig. 3-6).

In postpubertal testes the hypoplastic tubules can be recognized by their smooth contours. Normal seminiferous tubules become invested with elastic tissue at the time of puberty; however, in Klinefelter's syndrome the tubules lack elastic tissue, indicating that they have not undergone pubertal development (Rutgers and Scully, 1987). With progressive atrophy the tubular basement membrane becomes corrugated and frayed and surrounded by multilayered concentric rings of fibrous interstitial tissue. Germ cells disappear, and the lumen of most tubules contains only Sertoli cells. Finally, the tubules depleted of cells undergo hyalinization, collapse, and transform into hyaline masses without a central lumen (Fig. 3-7).

Interstitial spaces contain increased amounts of fibrous tissue and aggregates or even nodules of Leydig cells. Aggregates of Leydig cells may give a false impression of hyperplasia but volumetric analysis has shown that the total number of Leydig cells is not increased (Ahmad et al., 1971). By electron microscopy these Leydig cells contain fewer Charcot crystals and more paracrystalline inclusions and megamitochondria (Sigg and Hedinger, 1984; Soderstrom, 1984). It is not obvious whether these changes are reactive or degenerative or whether they reflect an endogenous insufficiency or inability of Leydig cells to respond to gonadotropic stimulation or just nonspecific ultrastructural changes unrelated to the basic pathogenetic mechanisms of Klinefelter's syndrome.

Gonadal dysgenesis. *Gonadal dysgenesis* is a term that encompasses a gamut of gonadal developmental anomalies associated with X-chromosome monosomy (45,X) and related disorders in which fragments of the

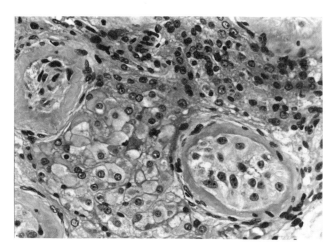

Fig. 3-7. The testis of an adult patient with Klinefelter's syndrome. There is tubular atrophy and basement membrane thickening. Tubules containing Sertoli cells are surrounded with prominent Leydig cells.

Table 3-4. Karyotypes associated with Turner's syndrome

Karyotype	Description	Incidence (%)
45,X	Monosomy X	58
46,Xi (Xq)	Isochromosome of long arm of X	16
45,X/46,XX	Mosaic	9
45,X/46,XY	Mosaic	6
45,X/47,XXX	Mosaic	1
46,XXp−	Deletion of short arm of X	2.5
46,XXq−	Deletion of long arm of X	2.5
46,X,r(X)	Ring X	2.5
46,Xi(Xp)	Isochromosome of short arm of X	Rare
46,X t(X,autosome)	Translocation	Rare
46,X, ter rea (X,X)	Terminal rearrangement	Rare

Data on incidence are modified from Lippe, 1991.

other X or Y chromosome are preserved in the karyotype. Although the gonads and genital organs may vary in appearance from almost normal female to almost normal male in most instances, this syndrome is associated with predominantly female genital organs and rudimentary ovaries forming streak gonads. Two clinically distinct subtypes of gonadal dysgenesis can be identified as Turner's syndrome and pure gonadal dysgenesis.

Turner's syndrome. The term *Turner's syndrome* is used to denote gonadal dysgenesis associated with the clinical stigmata described by Turner in 1938 as streak ovaries, stunted growth, webbing of the neck, cubitus valgus, and chromosomal abnormalities involving the sex chromosomes, most often monosomy X (45, X karyotype).

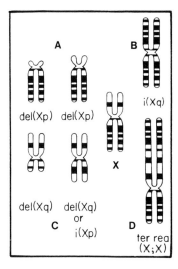

Fig. 3-8. Chromosomal abnormalities in Turner's syndrome. *X*, Normal chromosome *A*, Deletion of most of the short arm. *B*, Isochromosome of long arm. *C*, Probably interstitial deletion of the middle portion of the short arm, deletion of the long arm at band q22. This abnormality is difficult to distinguish from an isochromosome for the short arm. *D*, Short arm end-to-end terminal rearrangement. (Modified from de la Chapelle A. In Emery AEH, Rimoin DL (Eds). Principles and Practice of Medical Genetics, 2nd ed. Edinburgh, Churchill Livingstone, 1990, by permission).

Incidence. Turner's syndrome is diagnosed in 1 of every 2500 to 3500 females (Hook and Warburton, 1983; de la Chapelle, 1990) and thus is approximately five times less common than Klinefelter's syndrome. Among the spontaneously aborted fetuses, approximately 10% have the 45, X karyotype, indicating that monosomy X is one of the most common chromosomal abnormalities. Because it is associated with high fetal mortality, only a small fraction of affected conceptuses are viable and survive to term.

There is no consensus on the prevalence of various chromosomal genotypes in Turner's syndrome (Ferguson-Smith, 1965; Palmer and Reichmann, 1976; Hook and Warburton, 1983; Hall and Gilchrist, 1990). Such surveys are difficult to perform. The technical problems in identifying structurally abnormal sex chromosomes and uncertainty pertaining to the definition of mosaicism confound the issues even more (de la Chapelle, 1990). Overall, it appears that the 45, X karyotype accounts for 50% to 60% of cases (Table 3-4), whereas others show mosaicism, structurally abnormal or fragmented X and Y chromosomes, or both numerical and structural chromosomal defects (Fig. 3-8). In 45 X individuals the X chromosome is of maternal origin in approximately 75% of cases (Hassold et al., 1988). The structurally abnormal chromosomes are mostly paternal.

Clinical features. The multisystemic symptoms of Turner's syndrome have been reviewed on several occasions (Ferguson-Smith, 1965; Palmer and Reichmann, 1976; Simpson, 1976; Hall and Gilchrist, 1990; Rosenfeld

Table 3-5. Estimated incidence of somatic features of patients with Turner's syndrome

	Feature	Incidence (%)
Skeletal	Short stature	100
	Abnormal upper to lower segment ratio	90
	Short neck	40–80
	Cubitus valgus	30–75
	Genu valgus	30–40
	Short metacarpals	35–65
	High-arched palate	35–50
	Micrognathia	30–60
	Shield chest with widely spaced nipples	50–75
Gonadal	Streak gonad	75–95
	Gonadoblastoma	3
Skin and subcutis	Webbed neck	20–65
	Low posterior hair line	40–80
	Edema of hands and feet	21–70
	Nail dysplasia or hypoplasia	10–70
	Pigmented nevi	25–60
Cardiovascular	Congenital defects	20–50
	Renal or renovascular	25–60
Other	Thyroiditis	35
	Ear or hearing problems	45–70
	Carbohydrate intolerance	40

The range of incidence for each feature has been extrapolated from data in Simpson, 1975; Hall and Gilchrist, 1990; and Lippe, 1991.

and Grumbach, 1990; Lippe, 1991). After the original report of Turner, who listed short stature, sexual infantilism, webbing of the neck, low posterior hair line, and cubitus valgus as the typical features, it became obvious that only gonadal dysgenesis and short stature are invariably present in all patients (Lippe, 1991). All other symptoms and a long list of subsequently identified pathologic findings (Table 3-5) are found less predictably. The interconnectedness of symptoms is not fully understood, and for the time being it is not possible to discern whether these symptoms all reflect a single basic defect; whether they are consequences of an abnormality in a pleiotropic gene complex; or whether they all relate to abnormal gonadogenesis. Disordered mesenchymal tissue growth could definitely account for many if not most of the anomalies (Lippe, 1990), but it remains to be proven whether this functional defect is causally related to the chromosomal changes.

The cardinal symptoms of Turner's syndrome are listed in Table 3-5. Short stature is found in essentially all patients with the 45, X karyotype (Fig. 3-9). Mosaics and those with an additional fragment of the X chromosome may be somewhat taller. Height ranges from 122 to 152 cm (Hall and Gilchrist, 1990) with a mean of 143 cm (Lyon et al., 1985). Abnormal growth may even be noticed during intrauterine life; at birth, children with Turner's syndrome are an average 2.8 cm below the normal

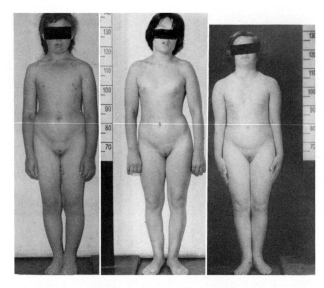

Fig. 3-9. Three patients with Turner's syndrome. The patients are 17-18 years old and are 132-143 cm tall. (From Drobnjak, 1974).

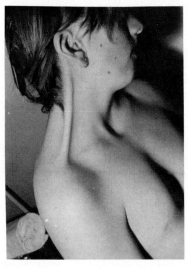

Fig. 3-10. Webbed neck in a patient with Turner's syndrome. (From Drobnjak, 1974).

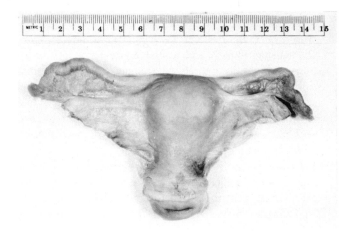

Fig. 3-11. The uterus and streak gonads in Turner's syndrome.

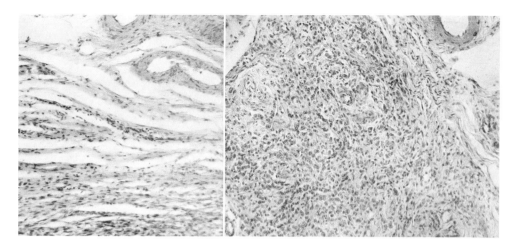

Fig. 3-12. The streak gonads are composed of fibrous tissue which may show signs of luteinization.

mean (Hall and Gilchrist, 1990). Patients with Turner's syndrome grow more slowly during the prepubertal period and fail to have a pubertal growth spurt (Ranke et al., 1983 and 1987). Failure of body growth along the longitudinal axis accounts for the abnormal upper to lower body proportions (Massa et al., 1990) and the relatively broad thorax, which contributes to the illusory wide spacing of the nipples (Lippe, 1991). A short neck and the valgus deformities of the cubital and knee joints, scoliosis, and short metacarpal bones are common skeletal abnormalities. Typical facial features include a triangular face, downslanting palpebral fissures, epicanthal folds, and ptosis (Hall and Gilchrist, 1990). Micrognathia, a small mandible with widely spaced rami, high-arched palate, and radiologic abnormalities of the base of the skull are additional manifestations of abnormal bone growth.

A webbed neck (Fig. 3-10) is found in only 25% to 50% of all patients (Ferguson-Smith, 1965; Lippe, 1991). The anomaly is probably related to lymphatic obstruction, which causes nuchal hygroma of 45, X fetuses and most likely edema of the dorsum of the hands and nail deformities found in one fifth of all patients (Lippe, 1991). It is possible that defective formation of lymphatic vessels is causally related to congenital defects of the aortic arch and other cardiac anomalies (Clark, 1984; Larco et al., 1988). Cardiovascular abnormalities, such as coarctation of the aorta and bicuspid aortic valves, are present in 20% to 30% of cases (Hall and Gilchrist, 1990). Renal malformations, which include structural and positional abnormalities (Lippe, 1980), are pathogenetically unrelated to cardiac anomalies but contribute to circulatory disturbances and cardiovascular morbidity.

Turner's syndrome is associated with a predilection to autoimmune disorders, most prominent of which are thyroiditis and hypothyroidism (Hall and Gilchrist, 1990). Disturbances of carbohydrate metabolism have been detected in some patients, but the pathogenesis and significance of these remain undetermined (Lippe, 1991).

Psychosocial problems are relatively common (Hall and Gilchrist, 1990). These include maladjustment, poor self-perception, and mild cognitive defects pertaining to conceptualization of spatial relations and numerical aptitude (Hall and Gilchrist, 1990). Intelligence quotients are in the normal range.

Hormonal changes. As a result of gonadal dysgenesis and abortive folliculogenesis, most patients have hypoestrinism and do not show signs of cyclic estrogen-progesterone secretion typical of normal postpubertal females. Pituitary gonadotropin levels are elevated as a result of inadequate feedback inhibition. Response to Gn-RH, which is used to assess the hypothalamo-pituitary-gonadal axis, is exaggerated. These pituitary and hypothalamic disorders, however, have no clinical implications (Lippe, 1991).

Estrogen replacement therapy administered cyclically with progesterone has been used routinely (Lippe, 1991). Estrogen replacement also is used for preparing the uterus for donor oocyte transfer, which has enabled several patients with Turner's syndrome to become pregnant and maintain the pregnancy to term (Navot et al., 1986; Serhal and Craft, 1989). Although the benefits of estrogen replacement exceed the usual risks and adverse reactions are relatively uncommon, the risk for endometrial adenocarcinoma should not be neglected (Krishnamurthy et al., 1977; Louka et al., 1978).

Gonadal pathology. External and internal genital organs are female albeit often hypoplastic. In place of normal ovaries patients with Turner's syndrome have dysgenetic gonads that appear as fibrous streaks. The streak gonads are located in the mesosalpinx; their longitudinal axis is parallel with the fallopian tube (Fig. 3-11).

Histologically, streak gonads are composed of elongated connective tissue cells and collagenous intercellular substance resembling ovarian stroma (Fig. 3-12). The hilar and stromal cells may be luteinized and there may be signs of hyperthecosis (Scully, 1991). Mesonephric duct remnants may be seen scattered randomly outside the hilar

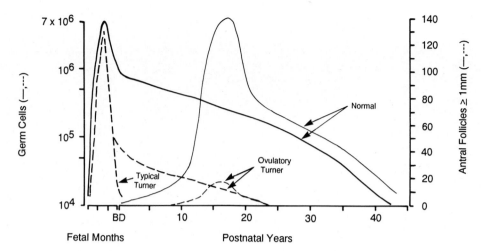

Fig. 3-13. In most Turner's syndrome patients the oocytes are lost at an accelerated rate. However in some cases the ovaries retain oocytes until early adulthood. Such patients can become pregnant. (Redrawn from Rosenfield and Grumbach Turner's Syndrome. New York, Marcel Dekker, 1990, with permission).

area. Typically, there is no evidence of folliculogenesis; oocytes are not seen in most postpubertal patients. Corpora lutea or albicantia also are not evident.

It generally has been held that approximately 10% of all patients with Turner's syndrome experience puberty and menstruate (Ferguson-Smith, 1965), although this may be an underestimate (Massa et al., 1990). Eight percent of patients with a 45 X karyotype and 21% of those with 45 X/46 XX karyotype experience puberty and menstruate (Ferguson-Smith, 1965). Theoretically, these patients are fertile, and one could anticipate that their gonads contain graafian follicles and viable oocytes, albeit in smaller numbers than in age-matched controls. Most of the pregnancies recorded were in Turner's syndrome patients with mosaicism (Singh et al., 1980), although at least 19 cases of pregnancy are documented in 45, X patients (reviewed by Kaneko et al., 1990).

A small number of patients (2% to 6%) with phenotypic features of Turner's syndrome have a Y chromosome or a fragment of the Y chromosome (Lippe, 1991). These patients are at risk for developing tumors from germ cells residing in their gonads. Most of the tumors diagnosed in these patients were gonadoblastomas.

The pathogenesis of gonadal dysgenesis is not understood, although it is apparent that it begins before birth. Until the third month of pregnancy the gonads of 45, X fetuses are indistinguishable from those in normal age-matched controls (Singh and Carr, 1966). Coincidental with the onset of primordial folliculogenesis, the gonads of 45, X fetuses begin losing oocytes considerably faster than those of normal females. This continuously accelerated loss continues until at term many but not all gonads will contain only a fraction of the normal oocyte contingent or none at all. The histologic picture may vary considerably (Carr et al., 1968), reflecting to some extent the variable nature of Turner's syndrome and in part the nature of the underlying chromosomal anomalies. A small number of patients will retain enough oocytes until puberty, when they may ovulate and feasibly even become pregnant.

This hypothetical model of oocyte loss constructed by Rosenfeld (Fig. 3-13) explains why some patients with Turner's syndrome become pregnant. However, because these ovulating patients with Turner's syndrome have from the beginning a smaller number of available oocytes than normal women, depletion of oocytes occurs earlier and typically these women become anovulatory by the age of 25 years. The reasons for the accelerated atresia of oocytes in the gonads of patients with Turner's syndrome are not understood, although one could speculate that both X chromosomes are needed for the adequate survival of female germ cells in the gonad (Ferguson-Smith, 1991). The fact that an additional fragment of the second X chromosome may improve the survival of oocytes and that mosaics have more oocytes in the gonad than 45, X patients is consistent with this hypothesis.

Pure gonadal dysgenesis. Gonadal dysgenesis occurs in many forms; it may be associated with chromosomal anomalies; and it may present in various clinical forms. This complex issue has been extensively reviewed in textbooks of endocrinology (Conte and Grumbach, 1989; Grumbach and Conte, 1992).

For practical purposes and for simplicity, pure gonadal dysgenesis is defined here as dysgenesis of gonads in phenotypic females who show signs of sexual infantilism but are of normal height and do not show any other stigmata of Turner's syndrome (de la Chapelle, 1990). Individuals with these phenotypic features may have a 46, XY or 46, XX karyotype or are mosaics and show structurally abnormal X or Y chromosomes. However, because the diagnosis of mosaicism requires extensive tissue sampling and is often difficult to exclude, it is arguable that some cases reported as nonmosaics are indeed misdiagnosed mosaics. The same argument applies to chromosomal structural abnormalities and translocations, which may remain undetected by standard chromosomal techniques. Hence, this discussion is limited to the classic form of pure gonadal dysgenesis and with the understanding that numerous aberrations may occur and that this entity represents a spectrum of disorders that cannot be entirely separated from one another (Grumbach and Conte, 1992).

Incidence and pathogenesis. Because the criteria for diagnosing pure gonadal dysgenesis vary and because some studies are based only on chromosomal surveys whereas others take into consideration clinical features, it is impossible to determine the precise incidence of this condition. Karyotype 46, XY with a female phenotype cannot be equated with pure gonadal dysgenesis since some patients will have features of Turner's syndrome (Affara et al., 1987; Disteche et al., 1986). Simpson (1976) studied women with primary amenorrhea and recorded pure gonadal dysgenesis in 16% of cases. Among the 75 individuals with 45, X/46, XY mosaicism diagnosed prenatally, only one had female external genitalia (Chang et al., 1990), indicating that most of these mosaics will not have developed into females with pure gonadal dysgenesis. Familial aggregates have been reported (Pallister and Opitz, 1979; Kraus et al., 1987).

A small deletion of the short arm of chromosome Y has been detected in some 46, XY females (Disteche et al., 1986). Longer deletion of Yp may result in shortened growth and the development of Turner's stigmata (Ferguson-Smith, 1991). Several 46, XY females were found to have mutations in the SRY locus (Berta et al., 1990; Jäger et al., 1990), which suggests that the lack of testicular development in these individuals is a consequence of the loss of TDF of the Y chromosome. However, in 80% of XY patients tested, no mutation of SRY could be found, suggesting that other sequences must be involved (Ferguson-Smith, 1991).

Interstitial deletions of the X chromosome also have been described, and these may account for the vertical transmission in some familial cases (Bernstein et al., 1980; Kraus et al., 1987).

Clinical findings. Patients with pure gonadal dysgenesis develop as females (Fig. 3-14). External genitalia are female, although occasional clitorimegaly may be encountered (Conte and Grumbach, 1989). Puberty is delayed, and infertility is a typical presenting complaint in patients then diagnosed with gonadal dysgenesis. Signs of hypoestrinism dominate in later years. Patients who have not had gonadectomy are at an increased risk for developing gonadal neoplasia, especially those who have a Y chromosome (Savage and Lowe, 1990).

Gonadal dysgenesis may occur in a familial form, which seems to be inherited as an X-linked trait (Espiner

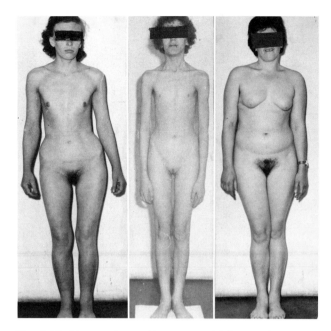

Fig. 3-14. Three patients with pure gonadal dysgenesis. Two patients to the left appear to have small breasts. The third patient was treated with estrogens and has well developed breasts. (From Drobnjak, 1974).

et al., 1970; German et al., 1978). Gonadal dysgenesis's may be a component of certain rare congenital syndromes, such as Perrault's syndrome, which is marked by sensorineural deafness (Pallister and Opitz, 1979); camptomelic dwarfism, which comprises numerous congenital anomalies (Hall and Spranger, 1980); Drash's syndrome, which includes parenchymal renal disease and a tendency for development of Wilms tumors (Eddy and Mauer, 1985); and Frasier's syndrome, which is marked by childhood renal failure (Moorthy et al., 1987).

Hormonal findings. Most patients have low serum estrogen and elevated serum gonadotropin levels. Hormonally, pure gonadal dysgenesis is thus indistinguishable from Turner's syndrome. Some patients show mild virilization and evidence of increased androgen secretion.

Pathologic findings. Both gonads appear as symmetric fibrous streaks located in the mesosalpinx and are essentially indistinguishable from those in patients with Turner's syndrome. Histologically, most gonadal streaks consist of elongated nondescript connective tissue cells (Fig. 3-15) reminiscent of ovarian stroma (Sohval, 1965). Sometimes it is possible to distinguish a cortical zone, which is composed of dense wavy stroma, from medullary tissue, which is composed of loose stroma (Berkovitz et al., 1991). The hilar area contains rete ovarii and hilar, luteinized cells. Scattered clusters of granulosa cells, distinctly differentiated ovarian cortical stroma, and occasional primordial follicles may be encountered (Cussen and MacMahon, 1979; Bernstein et al., 1980; Berkovitz et al., 1991).

Gonadoblastomas are found in 30% of XY patients (de

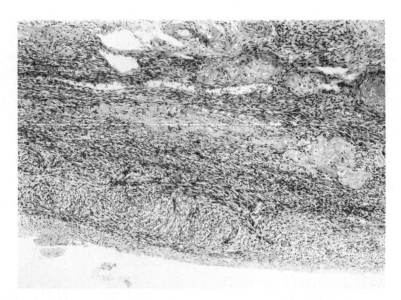

Fig. 3-15. Streak gonads of mixed gonadal dysgenesis are composed of nondescript connective tissue stroma.

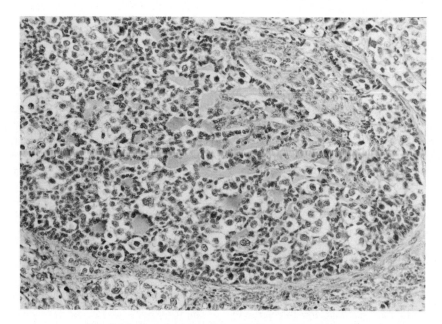

Fig. 3-16. Gonadoblastoma in mixed gonadal dysgenesis.

la Chapelle, 1990). These are either microscopic, especially if diagnosed early (Damjanov and Klauber, 1980), or macroscopic (Scully, 1970). Approximately 40% of tumors are bilateral (Mackay et al., 1974).

Gonadoblastoma is currently considered a potentially malignant lesion corresponding to a malignancy in situ (Scully, 1991). It is composed of primitive germ cells surrounded by sex cord derivatives equivalent to fetal or adult granulosa or Sertoli cells (Fig. 3-16). Sex cord cells secrete basement membrane material, which is deposited either in the form of extracellular membranes, which delimit groups of cells from the remainder of the gonadal stroma,

or in the form of discrete hyaline globules amid nests of germ cell–sex cord cell aggregates. The hyaline globules frequently undergo calcification.

Most invasive germ cell tumors originating in gonadoblastomas have the histologic features of seminoma-dysgerminoma (Scully, 1970; Hart and Burkons, 1979). Other germ cell tumors are less common. Histologically, they present as mixed germ cell tumors, teratocarcinomas, choriocarcinomas, and yolk sac carcinomas and do not differ from equivalent tumors in the normal male or female gonads (Hart and Burkons, 1979; Muzsnai and Feinberg, 1980; Savage and Lowe, 1990). Gonadoblastomas and seminomas have an excellent prognosis. Other germ cell tumors of dysgenetic gonads have a less favorable prognosis.

Mixed gonadal dysgenesis. Mixed gonadal dysgenesis denotes asymmetric development of gonads in individuals with sex chromosome abnormalities and usually ambiguous external genitalia (Scully, 1991). Most often, one of the gonads is a fibrous streak and the other a testis or streak testis; or there are bilateral streak testes. A uterus typically is present, and at least one fallopian tube has developed. The testis most often is located in the labioscrotal folds, which are usually asymmetric. The testes also may be intraabdominal or within the inguinal canal.

Incidence and pathogenesis. Mixed gonadal dysgenesis is the second most common cause of sexual ambiguity (Scully, 1991). There are, however, no reliable epidemiologic data on the true incidence of this condition. Approximately two thirds of patients have 45, X/46, XY mosaicism (Zah et al., 1975), a chromosomal anomaly found in 15 per 100,000 neonates (Hamerton et al., 1975). However, most 45, X/46, XY mosaics appear to be male, at least during the fetal and neonatal periods (Chang et al., 1990). Furthermore, 6% of these mosaics have Turner's stigmata and are clinically treated for Turner's syndrome (Lippe, 1991). Thus any prediction of the real incidence of mixed gonadal dysgenesis based on extrapolation from chromosomal survey data would be inaccurate. The issue is complicated further by the fact that many patients have an apparently normal 46, XY karyotype (Scully, 1991). Some of these patients probably have undetected mosaicism, whereas others have structurally abnormal chromosomes or mutated loci on the sex chromosomes (Ferguson-Smith, 1991).

Asymmetric development of gonads in mosaic individuals reflects the segregation of X and Y chromosome cell lineages. On the side that contains 46, XY cells the gonad will develop into a testis, which will in turn inhibit the development of ipsilateral müllerian ducts. Accordingly, on the side with a functional testis, the fallopian tube will not develop and the uterus may appear deformed, unicornuate, or hypoplastic. The gonad populated by 45 X cells will constitutively develop into an ovary, and the müllerian ducts will form the fallopian tube, uterus, and upper vagina. However, because the germ cells on that side contain only one X chromosome, they are less viable and, for the most part, mostly undergo atresia, which leads to the formation of the streak gonad in a manner analogous to gonadogenesis in Turner's syndrome. External genitalia develop asymmetrically, which prevents the fusion of labioscrotal folds. The clitoris is usually slightly enlarged, or a diminutive penis may develop, accounting for the fact that one third of all 45, X/46, XY individuals are raised as males (Ferguson-Smith, 1991).

Under the heading of mixed gonadal dysgenesis it is customary to include patients with dysgenetic male pseudohermaphroditism (Robboy et al., 1982; Rajfer and

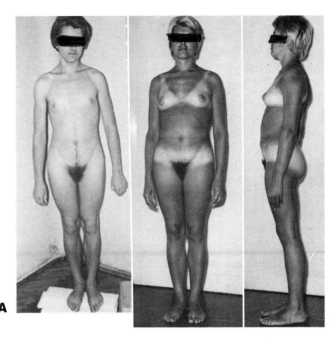

A   **B,C**

Fig. 3-17. Mixed gonadal dysgenesis. **A,** Untreated patient on the left appears to be female, but shows signs of virilization. **B, C,** Following the removal of the testis and the dysgenetic gonad and estrogen treatment breasts developed. (From Drobnjak, 1974).

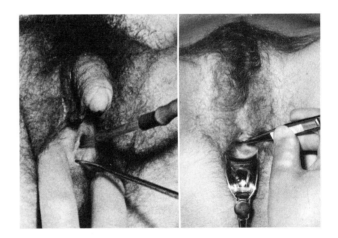

Fig. 3-18. Mixed gonadal dysgenesis. External genitalia of the same patient, at the initial presentation and after the amputation of the hypoplastic penis. (From Drobnjak, 1974).

Walsh, 1981), although this may be a distinct entity. These patients have cryptorchid bilateral dysgenetic testes, persistent müllerian structures, and inadequate virilization of external genitalia. Most patients are mosaics with a 45, X/46, XY karyotype.

Clinical findings. The clinical picture is highly variable depending on the extent of masculinization of the external genitalia and the social assignment of sex in infancy. Two thirds of those affected are raised as females (Yeh et al., 1975), although many have signs of virilization (Figs. 3-17 and 3-18). The definitive diagnosis is usually based on laparoscopic or operative exploration of internal genital organs and chromosomal and hormonal studies. Puberty and sexual maturation do not occur, and the patients are essentially infertile.

Hormonal findings. Serum levels of estrogens are low, and the levels of androgens are variable depending on the amount of testicular tissue. The capacity of the patient to produce testosterone can be tested with chorionic gonadotropin stimulation, which will provide also an estimate of functional testicular tissue in the male gonad (Conte and Grumbach, 1989).

It is of interest that estrogens may be derived from gonadoblastomas in the gonadal streak (Yeh et al., 1975). Hormonal substitution therapy routinely is given, and it includes either estrogen/progesterone or androgen replacement depending on the assigned gender of the patient (Conte and Grumbach, 1989).

Pathologic findings. The gonadal streak histologically is similar to gonadal streaks in pure gonadal dysgenesis or Turner's syndrome, although they often contain more poorly developed tubules than the former (Scully, 1991). In infants the streak gonad may contain numerous primordial or primary follicles and thus resemble a true ovary. However, with time, most of these germ cells disappear, but a significant number may survive. The streak gonad may also contain histologic foci of gonadoblastoma or even grossly visible tumorous gonadoblastomas. The germ cells in the gonadal streak and in gonadoblastomas have a strong tendency toward malignant neoplastic transformation and give rise to malignant tumors at a higher rate than in pure gonadal dysgenesis.

The testes that develop in patients with mixed gonadal dysgenesis may resemble normal testes except for a decreased number of germ cells and an occasional admixture of ovarian-like stroma (Scully, 1991). The tubules may be racemose, irregularly shaped, and focally devoid of basement membrane (Berkovitz et al., 1991). Often it is possible to distinguish an outer cortical portion from the more centrally located tubules, although the tunica albuginea is in most cases focally absent (Berkovitz et al., 1991). The superficial cortex may resemble ovarian stroma with gradual transition into testicular tissue, which consists of widely spaced seminiferous tubules occasionally lacking a limiting basement membrane. On the other hand, the centrally located tubules appear more normal, although even here the stroma appears edematous. Germ cells are present in most patients. Leydig cells are scattered or in small groups, but spermatids and spermatozoa are not seen (Wallace and Levine, 1990).

The admixture of ovarian stroma and testicular tubules may occur in several patterns: at random; in a gradient from superficial, where the tissue is more ovarian-like toward central, where the tissue consists of tubules only; and finally, in patches with areas composed only of ovarian stroma and areas composed only of seminiferous tubules, each sharply demarcated from the other.

Gonadoblastomas and malignant invasive germ cell tumors may develop in the gonadal streak and the testicular tissue, as stated. Intratubular carcinoma in situ may precede invasive germ cell tumors (Wallace and Levine, 1990). Because the testis secretes androgens, it is recommended to leave the descended testes in situ in male patients. These patients should, however, be under constant medical supervision, and if a tumor develops, gonadectomy should be performed immediately. Streak gonads usually are removed surgically for prophylaxis soon after the diagnosis is established.

Hermaphroditism. True hermaphroditism is a disturbance of gonadal differentiation and is characterized by the simultaneous presence of both male and female gonads in the same individual. The gonads may develop into bilateral ovotestes or alternatively a testis on one side and an ovary on the other (Scully, 1991). This diagnosis should be made only if ovarian and testicular tissue are unequivocally demonstrated on histologic examination and the diagnosis of mixed gonadal dysgenesis has been ruled out (Grumbach and Conte, 1992). Occasionally, it may be difficult to distinguish hermaphroditism from mixed gonadal dysgenesis which could have testicular tissue on one side and a streak gonad contralaterally. These tissues may contain, especially in children, a considerable number of oocytes, thus imparting the false impression of a functional ovary. It is important, therefore, not to misdiagnose the status of an ovary on the basis of a few scattered oocytes.

Incidence and pathogenesis. Hermaphroditism is rare, with less than 400 fully documented cases in the literature (Jones et al., 1965; van Niekerk, 1976; Berkovitz et al., 1982). Of the karyotypes 60% are 46, XY, 12% are 46, XY, and 13% are mosaics with a 46, XX/46 XY karyotype (van Niekerk and Retief, 1981). Familial cases are also described (Armendares et al., 1975; Skordis et al., 1987; Abbas et al., 1989).

As discussed by Grumbach and Conte (1992), true hermaphroditism may result from sex chromosome mosaicism, based on meiotic or mitotic errors; double fertilization of a binucleated ovum with two sperms, one containing an X and the other a Y chromosome (Gartler et al., 1962); translocation of the Y chromosome or its fragments to an autosome or the X chromosome; or, finally, mutation of autosomal genes in loci that are involved in gonadogenesis. True hermaphrodites with a 46, XX karyotype may carry Y-specific sequences (Palmer et al., 1989; Jäger et al., 1990). However, a high percentage of cases do not have a detectable SRY (Ferguson-Smith, 1991). In familial cases of true hermaphroditism described by Skordis et al. (1987) and Abbas et al. (1989) there was no evidence of SRY. In these families the 46, XX karyotype was associated with either hermaphroditism, sterile hypogonadic males, or normal females, suggesting that SRY is not the only TDF and that another X-linked determinant may be operational.

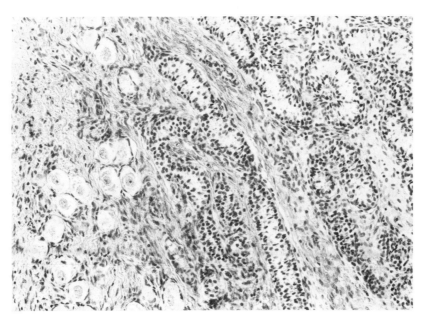

Fig. 3-19. Ovotestis.

Clinical findings. The clinical picture may be highly variable. Most patients are raised as males. The height of most patients is in the normal female range. They have ambiguous genitalia, hypospadias, a vaginal pouch, and variably developed uteri and fallopian tubes (Ferguson-Smith, 1991). Three types are recognized (Grumbach and Conte, 1992):

1. Unilateral—Testis on one side and ovary on the other
2. Bilateral—Both testis and ovary, usually fused into an ovotestis on both sides
3. Unilateral—The ovotestis on one side and a testis or an ovary on the other

The testis will inhibit the development of müllerian ducts into fallopian tubes and a uterus. However, these structures regularly develop on the side of the ovary. Ovotestes induce very little virilization (Ferguson-Smith, 1991). Most cases with bilateral hermaphroditism have a uterus and fallopian tubes. Ovotestes in these cases are typically located in the mesosalpinx. Virilization and breast development occur at puberty, and menses occurs in about half of patients (Grumbach and Conte, 1991). Pregnancy was recorded in several patients (Kim et al., 1973; Talerman et al., 1990).

Hormonal findings. Most patients have hypogonadism, but the hormonal profile obviously may be quite variable.

Gonadal pathology. In most cases, the ovary and the testis forming the ovotestis are fused into a single structure; nevertheless, they are sharply demarcated from each other (Scully, 1991). In a minority of cases, testes appear as hilar inclusions of the ovary. In the ovary or the ovarian portion of the ovotestis, there are numerous follicles with viable oocytes (Fig. 3-19). As a consequence of ovulation, after puberty corpora lutea and albicantia are apparent.

The testicular part of the ovotestis consists of hypoplastic seminiferous tubules, which are often devoid of germ cells and frequently are hyalinized. Testes that are located in the inguinal canal or the labioscrotal folds contain better preserved seminiferous tubules; scrotal testes may even show signs of spermatogenesis (Scully, 1991).

Ovotestes and the male or female gonad of true hermaphrodites are at an increased risk for neoplasia, but the extent of this risk cannot be ascertained because of the rarity of cases and especially the rarity of those who did not have gonadectomy in childhood. Gonadoblastomas and dysgerminomas have been described (Schwartz et al., 1980; Talerman et al., 1990).

Sex chromosome abnormalities without gonadal changes

Several numerical chromosomal abnormalities such as additional copies of X chromosome in females and additional copies of Y chromosome in males are relatively common. Some of these karyotypes are associated with mental retardation but no endocrine or reproductive problems. Current evidence indicates that the karyotypes 47,XXX, 48,XXXX, 49,XXXXX, or 47,XXY and 48,XYYY are not associated with gonadal abnormalities. Most of these patients have normal gonads and external genitalia (Grumbach and Conte, 1992).

ADRENOGENITAL SYNDROMES

Congenital defects involving genes that encode the enzymes mediating the biosynthesis of steroid hormones result in distinct syndromes (reviewed by White et al., 1987; Miller, 1991). All these syndromes are characterized by a

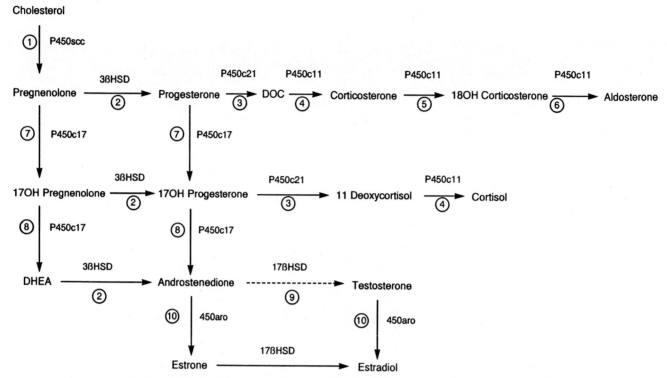

Fig. 3-20. Principal pathways of steroidogenesis. ① Mitochondrial cytochrome P450scc converts cholesterol to pregnenolone by 20-α-hydroxylation, 22-hydroxylation, and scission of the c20-22 carbon bond (formerly known as *20,22 desmolase*). ② 3-β-Hydroxysteriod dehydogenase (3-βHSD), a non-P450 enzyme bound to the endoplasmic reticulum, catalyzes both 3-βHSD and $\triangle^5 \rightarrow \triangle^4$ isomerase activities. ③ P450c21 in the endoplasmic reticulum catalyzes 21-hydroxylation of progesterone to DOC and of 17-hydroxyprogesterone to 11-deoxycortisol. ④ ⑤ and ⑥, Mitochondrial P450c11 catalyzes three reactions: 11-β-hydroxylase ④, 18-hydroxylase ⑤, and 18-methyl oxidase ⑥, thus converting DOC to aldosterone and 11-deoxycortisol to cortisol. ⑦ and ⑧: P450c17 in the endoplasmic reticulum mediates both 17-α-hydroxydase ⑦ and 17,20 lyase ⑧ activities for both $\triangle^5$ substrates (pregnenolone and 17-hydroxypregnenolone) and $\triangle^4$ substrates (progesterone and 17-hydroxyprogesterone). ⑨ and ⑩, 17-β-hydroxysteriod dehydrogenase (17-βHSD), also known as 17 ketosteroid reductase, is a non-P450 enzyme of the endoplasmic reticulum that converts androstenedione to testosterone ⑨; it may then be converted to estradiol by P450aro (⑩), another P450 enzyme in the endoplasmic reticulum. P450aro can convert androstenedione to estrone (10) which is converted to estradiol by 17-βHSD ⑨. The reactions ⑨ and ⑩ are found primarily in the gonads. (Modified from Miller WL. Endocrinol Metab Clin N Am, 1991; 20:721, with permission).

metabolic block in steroid hormone synthesis (Fig. 3-20), lack of cortisol, and accumulation of intermediate steroids, which shift hormone synthesis into an irregular pathway with compensatory overproduction of ACTH and secondary, albeit congenital adrenal hyperplasia (CAH). Hyperandrogenism is common and can cause fetal virilization of external genitalia in females as well as other signs of hyperandrogenism in postnatal life, including hirsutism, deep voice, and musculoskeletal development typical of males. Males are also affected, although, in most instances, they show normal genital development. Symptoms in the male include hyperandrogenism and early virilization or hypoandrogenism that characterizes some forms of adrenogenital syndrome such as 17-hydroxylase deficiency, which usually becomes evident only at puberty. Other common metabolic disturbances found in males and fe-

males relate to abnormal metabolism of mineralocorticoids and glucocorticoids.

Adrenogenital syndromes may be divided into three categories that affect:

1. Adrenal cortex only, such as 21-hydroxylase and 11-β-hydroxylase deficiencies
2. Adrenals and gonads
3. Testes, primarily biosynthesis of steroids in the testes, such as 17,20-desmolase and 17-β-hydroxysteroid oxidoreductase deficiencies.

The salient features of various adrenogenital syndromes are listed in Table 3-6.

Deficiency of 21-hydroxylase

Deficiency of 21-hydroxylase is the most common form of CAH, accounting for almost 90% of all cases of con-

Table 3-6. Defects of adrenal steroidogenesis

Deficiency	Syndrome	Genitalia		Postnatal Virilization	Salt Metabolism	Increased Steroids	Decreased Steroids	Chromosome	Incidence
		Female	Male						
Cholesterol des-molase (P450 scc)		F	A	No	Salt-wasting	None	All	15	Rare
3β-Hydroxy-steroid dehy-drogenase	Classic	A	A	Yes	±Salt-wasting	DHEA,17-OH-pregnenolone	Aldo, cortisol, T	1	Rare
	Nonclassic	F	M	Yes	Normal	DHEA, 17-OH-pregnenolone	—		Frequent
17-α-Hydro-xylase (P450 c17)	—	F	A	No	Hypertension	DOC, cortico-sterone	Cortisol, T	10	Rare
17,20-Lyase (P450 c17)	—	F	A	No	Normal	—	DHEA, T, an-drostenedione	10	Rare
21-Hydroxylase (P450 c21)	Salt-wasting	A	M	Yes	Salt-wasting (70%)	17-OHP, an-drostenedione	Aldo, cortisol	6p	1:10,000
	Simple viril-izing	A	M	Yes	Normal	17-OHP, an-drostenedione	Cortisol	6p	1:10,000
	Nonclassic	F	M	Yes	Normal	17-OHP, an-drostenedione	—	6p	1:100
11-Hydro-xylase (P450 c11)	Classic	A	M	Yes	Hypertension	DOC, 11-deoxy cortisol	Cortisol, ±aldo	8q	1:100,000
	Nonclassic	F	M	Yes	Normal	11-deoxy-cortisol, ±DOC	—	8q	Frequent
Corticosterone methyl oxi-dase II (P450 c11)	—	F	M	No	Salt-wasting	18-OH-corticosterone	Aldo	8q	Rare

Adapted from information appearing in *The New England Journal of Medicine*, White PC, New MI, Dupont B, Congenital adrenal hyperplasia. 1987; 316:1519, with permission.
DHEA = dehydroepiandrosterone; DOC = deoxycorticosterone; 17-OHP = 17-hydroxyprogesterone; and T = testosterone; Aldo = aldosterone.
Genitalia are F = female; M = male; A = ambigous

genital adrenogenital syndrome (Pang et al., 1988; Thilen and Larsson, 1990). The metabolic block causes a deficiency of cortisol and aldosterone, with increased levels of 17-hydroxyprogesterone and androgens. The gene for 21-hydroxylase has been localized to the short arm of chromosome 6 (Fig. 3-21) in close proximity to the HLA locus (Strachan, 1990). Mutations, deletions, and conversions in this locus on chromosome 6 lead to an enzyme deficiency that may be severe, moderate, or mild (Speiser and New, 1987).

The classic form of 21-hydroxylase deficiency affects 1 in approximately 10,000 newborns (Pang et al., 1988; Thilen and Larsson, 1990). About 70% of these infants have deficiency of both cortisol and aldosterone, and therefore, the disease presents as the salt-losing form of CAH. A late onset form of this disease has been identified as the most common autosomal recessive human inborn error of metabolism, affecting 1 in 100 individuals, and as many as 1 in 30 Askenazi Jews (Brody and Wentz, 1987; Pang et al., 1988). The mild form of 21-hydroxylase deficiency does not cause genital abnormalities and may present at the time of puberty with hirsutism and mild virilization (Azziz and Zacur, 1989).

Clinical findings. Increased fetal androgen production causes virilization of the external genitalia in females but has few obvious consequences in males. Females are born with an enlarged clitoris, fused labioscrotal folds, and a phallic urethra that develops from the closed urogenital sinus. The internal female reproductive organs are normal. Male infants may have a slightly enlarged penis, but the diagnosis is rarely made on physical examination alone. Salt loss causes dehydration, which typically is the most common finding that suggests the diagnosis. Excess androgen production affects bone growth in males and females, and therefore, most children show advanced bone age. Epiphyses tend to close earlier, which accounts for the

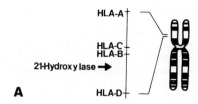

CLINICAL SPECTRUM OF HLA-LINKED STEROID 21-HYDROXYLASE DEFICIENCY

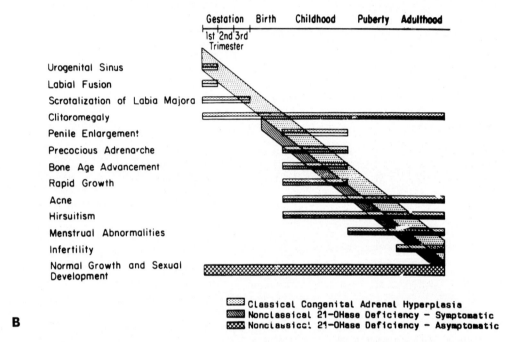

Fig. 3-21. A, Deficiency of 21-hydroxylase is linked to structural abnormalities of chromosome 6. B, Clinical spectrum of 21-hydroxylase deficiency. (From New MI et al. In Stanbury JB et al. The Metabolic Basis of Inherited Disease, 5th ed. New York, McGraw-Hill, with permission).

short stature of affected individuals. Clitorimegaly or macrogenitosomia, premature appearance of sexual hair, acne, and adult body odor typically are found in older children. Adult females may show signs of virilization (Fig. 3-22) or present with polycystic ovaries, menstrual irregularities, and infertility (White et al., 1987). Spermatogenesis may be depressed, accounting for the infertility in males (Wischusen et al., 1981).

The late-onset so-called nonclassic form of 21-hydroxylase deficiency presents with menstrual irregularities or infertility (Birnbaum and Rose, 1984). Approximately 5% to 9% of adult women with hirsutism and other signs of hyperandrogenism have this metabolic disorder (McLaughlin et al., 1990).

Hormonal findings. Clinical symptoms are caused by an androgen excess released from the adrenals. Because the enzyme deficiency prevents the production of cortisol, which normally provides the inhibitory feedback signal to the pituitary and is the principal regulator of ACTH, blood levels of ACTH are also elevated. ACTH stimulates the adrenal cortex to synthesize progesterone, which cannot be

converted to cortisol beyond the 21-hydroxylase-mediated step. Hence 17-hydroxyprogesterone accumulates and is released into the blood. This is accompanied by an increased urinary excretion of pregnanetriol, which is its main degradation product (White et al., 1987). Facilitated androgen synthesis raises blood androgen levels. Aldosterone synthesis is inhibited in 70% of cases, and the blood levels of this mineralocorticoid can be slightly or significantly below normal level. However, renin always is elevated and the renin/aldosterone ratio is increased. The ACTH stimulation test, which is used to confirm the diagnosis, causes a rise of blood 17-hydroxyprogesterone that is higher than in normal controls.

Pathologic findings. Fetal and neonatal adrenal glands show bilateral cortical hyperplasia with prominent convolutions, which on cross sectioning impart a cerebriform appearance (Fig. 3-23). Focal or diffuse nodularity occurs commonly in older patients. Hyperplastic cortex is composed predominantly of lipid-depleted eosinophilic cells and scattered cells with clear cytoplasm. Ultrastructurally, these cells appear well differentiated and contain abundant

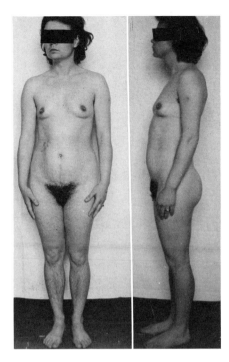

Fig. 3-22. Adrenogenital syndrome. The patient has small breasts, abdominal striae and hirsutism. (From Drobnjak, 1974).

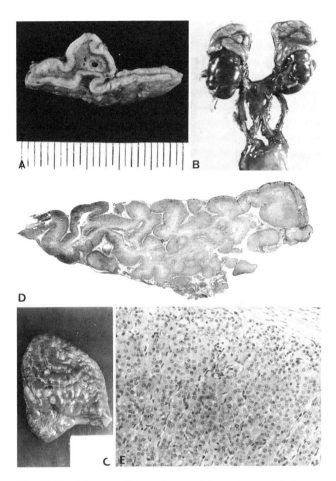

Fig. 3-23. Adrenogenital syndrome. Enlarged convoluted adrenal glands were found at the autopsy of this child. (From Nistal M and Paniagua R. Testicular Epididymal Pathology. New York, Thieme-Stratton, 1984, with permission).

amounts of smooth and rough endoplasmic reticulum with well-developed Golgi apparatus and numerous mitochondria with tubular cristae. Lipid droplets and lipofuscin are present in variable amounts. Electron microscopy features are typical of steroid-secreting cells but do not allow a distinction between normal and hyperplastic or neoplastic cells. Furthermore, it is not possible morphologically to determine to which zone of the adrenal cortex the hyperplastic cells correspond (Tannenbaum, 1973).

Males with 21-hydroxylase deficiency and CAH may develop adrenal rest tumors of the testes (Burke et al., 1973). These tumors present as paratesticular nodules, which may be multiple or even bilateral (Cunnah et al., 1989). Adrenal rest tumors of the testis may decrease in size upon dexamethasone treatment, but some appear to be nonsuppressible (Newell et al., 1977). Histologically, these tumors are composed of cells that are indistinguishable from Leydig cells. Sometimes it is difficult to differentiate adrenal rest tumors from Leydig cell tumors even with the most sophisticated techniques of molecular biology (Solish et al., 1989).

Deficiency of 11-β-hydroxylase

Deficiency of 11-ß-hydroxylase is the second most common form of CAH diagnosed in infants and it accounts for 5% to 8% of all neonatal cases (White et al., 1987). In addition to the classic neonatal form, a nonclassic form, characterized by mild biochemical abnormalities, has been noted in adults (Cathelineau et al., 1980). The classic form

affects 1 in 100,000 newborns (Zachmann et al., 1983). The disorder is more common in Jews of Moroccan origin, in whom it occurs at a rate of 1 in 5000 (Rösler et al., 1992). The gene is located on chromosome 8. This enzyme deficiency blocks the formation of cortisol and aldosterone and leads to the accumulation of 11-deoxycortisol and deoxycorticosterone and their conversion into androgens. The disease presents with signs of congenital virilization in girls. Hypertension is found in 70% of patients, presumably because deoxycorticosterone acts as a mineralocorticoid. The nonclassic form has no major influence on the development of genitalia, and even in adults it presents with few symptoms. The disorder is diagnosed on the basis of biochemical abnormalities.

Hormonal studies show elevated blood levels of 11-deoxycortisol and deoxycorticosterone, androstenedione, testosterone, and ACTH. Urinary 17-ketosteroids are elevated, whereas 18-hydroxylated steroids are decreased (White et al., 1987). Plasma renin and aldosterone are low. In the nonclassic form the biochemical abnormalities may be minimal and appear only after ACTH stimulation.

Deficiency of 3-β-hydroxysteroid dehydrogenase

This enzyme deficiency occurs in a classic neonatal form, which is rare, and as a more common nonclassic late-onset disease, which may be more prevalent than the mild form of 21-hydroxylase deficiency (Zerah et al., 1991). The gene-encoding 3-β-hydroxysteroid dehydrogenase has been mapped to chromosome 1 (Zerah et al., 1991). However, since there are several isoenzymes, it is possible that they are encoded by several genes.

Activity of 3-β-hydroxysteroid dehydrogenase can be demonstrated in the adrenals and gonads. Deficiency of 3-β-hydroxysteroid dehydrogenase affects the synthesis of all steroids. The classic form is marked by salt wasting and genital ambiguity in both males and females. Although the adrenal glands and gonads accumulate dehydroepiandrosterone, the conversion of this weak androgen into the more potent androstenedione and testosterone is ineffective. Dehydroepiandrosterone will suffice to produce virilization of external genitalia in females but results in suboptimal virilization of male genitalia. Female infants show clitorimegaly usually without posterior labial fusion. There is considerable phenotypic variation. Children have early growth of axillary and pubic hair and develop signs that are indistinguishable from those of idiopathic precocious pubarche. The late-onset disease may present with hirsutism, menstrual irregularities, and infertility. Other symptoms usually assigned to polycystic ovaries are also described in certain women. This may be related to the existence of isoenzymes that are expressed differently in the ovary and the adrenal. It has been hypothesized that partial deficiency affects the ovary differently than the adrenals.

It is estimated that the mild 3-β-hydroxysteroid dehydrogenase deficiency accounts for at least 15% of all cases of hyperandrogenism in adult women (Zerah et al., 1991). Hormonal studies show elevated blood levels of 17-hydroxypregnenolone and dehydroepiandrosterone. The diagnosis is confirmed by demonstrating raised ratios of B ring ($\triangle^5$) to A ring ($\triangle^4$) steroids.

Deficiency of 17-α-hydroxylase/17,20-lyase

This deficiency is marked by an inborn error involving P450c17, which catalyzes both the 17-α-hydroxylase and 17,20-lyase reaction (reviewed by Yanase et al., 1991). The disease is rare, and Yanase et al. (1991) found approximately 100 cases reported thus far.

The enzyme P450c17 is encoded by a gene on chromosome 10. The block in steroid synthesis results in a deficiency of glucocorticoids and sex hormones, but the mineralocorticoids are not affected. Male infants are shown to have defective virilization and later prove to be infertile. Females appear normal but have amenorrhea at puberty or show sexual infantilism.

Pathologic findings. The adrenals show diffuse hyperplasia, nodular hyperplasia, or both. These lesions are composed of compact eosinophilic or clear cells. Myelo-lipoma has been described in two cases (for review, see Yanase et al., 1991).

Testes occasionally are removed because of their ectopic position. Histologically, the testes show tubular atrophy and little or no spermatogenesis. Leydig cells may be hyperplastic. A single case of Sertoli cell adenoma was reported in one patient. Ovaries are often grossly polycystic and contain a high number of atretic follicles and few graafian follicles.

Deficiency of cholesterol desmolase

Deficiency of cholesterol desmolase results in severe inhibition of the entire steroidogenic metabolism (Degenhart, 1984). The condition is marked by lipoid adrenal hyperplasia and is usually lethal in childhood. Owing to the inhibition of androgen synthesis, male infants are born incompletely virilized. The adrenal glands are enlarged and have a nodular cortex composed of lipid-filled cells and extracellular deposits of cholesterol crystals.

Deficiency of 17-β-hydroxysteroid oxidoreductase (17-ketosteroid reductase)

The deficiency of 17-β-hydroxysteroid oxidoreductase, an enzyme reversibly catalyzing the oxidoreduction of androstenedione to testosterone, estrone to estradiol, and dehydroepiandrosterone to $\triangle^5$, androstenediol, causes male pseudohermaphroditism (Grumbach and Conte, 1992). Despite the ubiquitous distribution of the enzyme, the defect primarily affects the gonads (Imperato-McGinley et al., 1979; Rösler and Kohn, 1983). Most other symptoms are secondary and can be related to a deficiency of testosterone production in fetal testes.

Male children affected by this disease are born with ambiguous genitalia. They may be raised as males or females. The external genitalia are female with a blind vaginal pouch. Testes are usually inguinal, and wolffian duct derivatives are well developed. Müllerian duct derivatives atrophy during fetal life and are not seen at birth. At puberty, virilization ensues, marked by a growing phallus, male body hair distribution, and voice changes. Gynecomastia may develop depending on the ratio of estrogens to androgens (Imperato-McGinley et al., 1979, 1987).

Hormonally, puberty is marked by increased blood levels of androstenedione and estrone and low levels of testosterone, dehydrostenedione, and estrone, which cannot be formed because of the enzyme deficiency.

Individuals reared as males are typically treated surgically and with testosterone to achieve complete masculinization, whereas castration and estrogen therapy are given to those raised as females. Testosterone does not restore fertility.

Histologically, the testes show persistent hypoplasia and atrophy seminiferous tubules. These changes persist even after corrective surgery. Deficiency of 17-β-hydroxysteroid oxidoreductase may concur with 5-α-reductase deficiency and affect members of the same family (Imperato-McGinley et al., 1987). The genes for 5-α-reductase and 17-β-hydroxysteroid oxidoreductase segregate separately within the kindred and are apparently unrelated to each other.

Deficiency of 17-β-hydroxysteroid oxidoreductase does not interfere with the development of female genital organs. However, it has been suggested that some patients with the polycystic ovary syndrome have a deficiency of this enzyme (Toscano et al., 1990).

ANDROGEN INSENSITIVITY

Peripheral resistance to androgens occurs as a result of two basic defects: androgen receptor deficiency and deficiency of 5-α-reductase, an enzyme that plays a crucial role in the activation of testosterone (Griffin, 1992).

Androgen receptor deficiency

Androgen receptor deficiency is a genetic disorder marked by a resistance to androgens. Because the gene for the androgen receptor resides on the X chromosome, the syndrome is inherited as a sex-linked trait affecting males only. Females are carriers but show no clinical symptoms.

Pathogenesis. Androgen receptor is a nuclear protein that belongs to the family of steroid receptors. It is encoded by a gene located on the long arm of the X chromosome (Brown et al., 1989). Without the receptor, testosterone and its more bioactive derivative, 5-α-dihydrotestosterone, cannot activate genes in the target cells; thus, these androgens have little or no effect on tissues dependent on the male sex hormone.

Androgen receptor deficiency affects the development of external genital organs in the fetus, sexual maturation at puberty, and the regulation of gonadotropin secretion in adult life. Ineffective virilization of the fetal genital tubercle and the urogenital sinus leads to the external genital organs assuming a constitutively female appearance. The vagina develops incompletely and terminates in a blind pouch because the cervix and upper vagina, like other müllerian derivatives, atrophy under the inhibitory influence of testicular AMH. The testes develop normally but are located intraabdominally, in the inguinal canal, or in the labioscrotal folds. Wolffian ducts develop to a variable extent, but their derivatives are usually rudimentary.

At puberty, secondary sexual characteristics remain female. Breasts develop but there is no menarche. Pubic and axillary hair growth does not appear. Infertility is irreversible.

Complete absence of androgen receptor develops because of deletion of a large segment of the 3′ terminus of the androgen receptor gene; single nucleotide replacement that inactivates the splicing and leads to the synthesis of an altered receptor mRNA and the synthesis of defective protein; and introduction of premature termination codons into the sequence of the receptor protein (reviewed by McPhaul

et al., 1991b). Single amino acid substitutions within the receptor protein may cause changes in the hormone-binding domain, inactive protein, or proteins that are unstable in the binding process.

Qualitative abnormalities that occur in the presence of normal amounts of receptor protein include receptor thermal instability, accelerated ligand dissociation, and defective receptor up-regulation for either testosterone or dihydrotestosterone or both. Qualitative abnormalities are common but heterogeneous.

Clinical features of androgen resistance occur occasionally in receptor-positive individuals. *Receptor-positive* androgen resistance includes deletions of exons and single nucleotide substitutions, resulting in the normal binding of hormone but inactive complex formation as determined in assays of receptor function (McPhaul et al., 1991a). Postreceptor binding events also may be affected since in some cases the ligand seems unable to stimulate the transcription of the androgen-responsive reporter gene.

From all these recent data on molecular biology, succinctly summarized in the review article by McPhaul et al. (1991b), it is evident that the defects underlying the syndrome of androgen receptor deficiency may develop from a bewildering spectrum of mutations and genetic mechanisms. A complete correlation between the clinical findings and the data on molecular biology is still imprecise.

Clinical findings. The clinical picture is variable, and the presentations include a broad spectrum of phenotypes, from apparent females with internal testes to normal males suffering from infertility only. In between there are numerous intermediate forms showing incomplete virilization or ambiguous genitalia (Griffin and Wilson, 1980). According to McPhaul et al. (1991b), these conditions can be pathogenetically grouped into four broad categories:

1. The absence of specific dihydrotestosterone binding (receptor negative)
2. Decreased binding (quantitative receptor defect)
3. Qualitatively abnormal binding (qualitative receptor defect)
4. No receptor binding abnormalities (receptor positive)

These categories correspond to traditional nomenclature:

1. Complete testicular feminization
2. Incomplete testicular feminization
3. Reifenstein's syndrome
4. Infertile males (Griffin and Wilson, 1980)
5. Males with gynecomastia and preserved fertility (Grino et al., 1988)

Testicular feminization involves 46, XY males who have complete end-organ resistance to androgens and show no androgen receptor activity (Griffin and Wilson, 1980). These individuals have female external genitalia and a vaginal pouch but no cervix, uterus, or fallopian tubes.

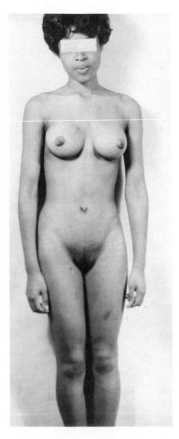

Fig. 3-24. Complete testicular feminization. The patient has well developed breasts and scant pubic hair.

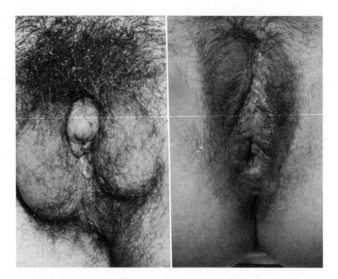

Fig. 3-25. Partial androgen resistance. Ambiguous external genitalia with testes in the labioscrotal folds. Note pubic hair and rudimentary vagina. Following the removal of the testes and vaginoplasty the external genitalia appear phenotypically female. (From Drobnjak, 1974).

The testes are well developed and typically intraabdominal or in the inguinal canal. At puberty, breasts develop, the labia minora grow, but menarche does not occur. Pubic and axillary hair is sparse or nonexistent (Fig. 3-24).

Partial androgen resistance comprises a heterogeneous group. The external genitalia are ambiguous or incompletely virilized (Fig. 3-25). Müllerian derivatives do not develop, whereas wolffian structures give rise to an epididymis and testicular excretory ducts. At puberty, gynecomastia develops and virilization is scant.

The term *Reifenstein's syndrome* is used for patients with ambiguous genitalia, hypospadias, hypogonadism, and gynecomastia (Bowen et al., 1965). This syndrome, however, cannot be separated with confidence from other forms of partial androgen insensitivity, and it is best to consider it as part of the phenotypic spectrum of the syndrome. The same holds true for variants of partial androgen resistance described by Lubs, Gilbert-Dreyfus, Rosenwater, and Walker (Grumbach and Conte, 1992). These familial conditions vary considerably from one kindred to another with considerable individual phenotypic variance among the members of the same affected family.

Males with androgen insensitivity have the normal male habitus. When the androgen receptor defects are mild,

they cause no development abnormalities or grossly visible changes. In these phenotypically normal males, infertility may be the only evidence of the congenital defect (Aiman et al., 1979). In some instances these infertile men are diagnosed during the study of families whose other members show more pronounced forms of androgen insensitivity. Isolated cases have been reported (Aiman and Griffin, 1982).

Hormonal findings. Blood LH and testosterone levels are elevated already in infancy. At puberty, there is an increased pulse frequency and amplitude of spikes of LH accompanied by elevated blood levels of testosterone (Grumbach and Conte, 1992). FSH levels vary and are within normal limits or slightly elevated. Plasma estradiol is elevated because of increased testicular secretion and peripheral conversion of androstenedione and testosterone to estradiol. Castration causes an additional elevation of LH and FSH. Androgen receptor assays show decreased or undetectable binding of testosterone and/or dihydrotestosterone. Other functional defects can be detected. Molecular probes have made it possible to further characterize the subtle defects in these patients (McPhaul et al., 1991a,b).

Pathologic findings. Patients with complete testicular feminization have testicles (Fig. 3-26). In 70% of cases they are intraabdominal, in 20% of cases inguinal, and in a minority of cases asymmetrically located (inguinal on one side and abdominal on the other) or retroperitoneal (Rutgers and Scully, 1991). On gross examination these testes appear normal but are usually multinodular on cross section. The testes are attached to a fibromuscular body on the medial pole and an adnexal cyst on the contralateral side. The fibromuscular body represents a vestigial uterus.

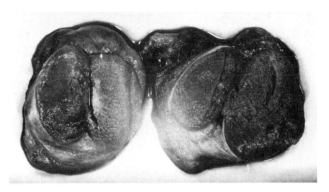

Fig. 3-26. Intraabdominal testes removed from a patient with testicular feminization. (From Drobnjak, 1974).

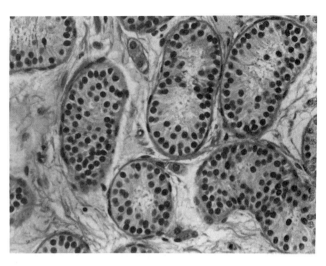

Fig. 3-27. The testis in testicular feminization syndrome is composed of tubules lined by immature Sertoli cells.

A fallopian tube or its remnants are found in a third of all cases. Most patients have a vaginal pouch; upper vaginal development is exceptional (Dodge et al., 1985).

Rutgers and Scully (1991) recognized four histologic patterns in their study of more than 40 cases of testicular feminization: diffuse tubulostromal, lobular tubulostromal, mixed diffuse, and lobular tubulostromal with a predominantly stromal pattern. In 50% of cases the tubules are enveloped by Leydig cells and some spindle cells (tubulostromal pattern); in 20% of cases there are small lobules composed of a few tubules surrounded by Leydig cells or spindle cells in a loose fibrous stroma-lobular tubulostromal pattern. In the remaining cases, one half showed a mixed tubulostromal lobular pattern and the other half contained stroma composed of spindle cells resembling ovaries. The tubules are small and filled with immature Sertoli cells (Fig. 3-27). Larger tubules with a central lumen and scattered spermatogonia may be seen in 30% of cases, usually those that have a tubulostromal pattern. One third of all testes have harmartamatous nodules composed of Sertoli cells, tubules, and Leydig cells. Approximately 10% of the testes contain tumors, which include Sertoli and Leydig cell tumors, fibromas, malignant sex cord cell tumors, and seminomas and embryonal carcinoma (reviewed by Rutgers and Scully, 1991). These tumors may be benign or malignant and may attain considerable size in older patients (Damjanov et al., 1976). Carcinoma in situ has been recorded in a significant number of cases (Skakkebaek, 1979; Nogales et al., 1981; Müller and Skakkebaek, 1990). A definite tendency to give rise to invasive germ cell neoplasia is evidenced. In one case, for example, one testis contained carcinoma in situ and the contralateral testis contained a seminoma (Hurt et al., 1989). The overall risk for developing tumors in complete testicular feminization is in the range of 10%, but it may increase to 30% in older patients (Manuel et al., 1976).

The incomplete forms of androgen insensitivity present with a variety of pathologic changes involving the external and internal genital organs (Amrhein et al., 1977). Histo-

logic changes in the testes have not been systematically studied, but in general they seem to be similar to those reported in complete testicular feminization. Virilized patients show less aberration from the normal male phenotype, and their testes may show considerable preservation of normal male architectural features. Spermatogenesis is impaired except in the mildest cases (McPhaul et al., 1991b).

Deficiency of 5-α-reductase

Definition. Deficiency of 5-α-reductase is an autosomal recessive form of male pseudohermaphroditism characterized by normal development of the testes and wolffian ducts with ambiguous external genitalia.

Pathogenesis. This is a genetically heterogeneous disorder based on an inborn deficiency of 5-α-reductase. This enzyme converts testosterone in androgen-sensitive tissues to dihydrotestosterone, a more potent androgen. In affected individuals the conversion of testosterone to dihydrotestosterone is highly inefficient or almost undetectable (Peterson et al., 1977).

Dihydrotestosterone is essential for the virilization of the fetal external genitalia. In male fetuses deficient in 5-α-reductase, the urogenital sinus remains open, often forming a single perineal orifice. However, the internal female organs do not develop. Testes and wolffian ducts develop, but the prostate and seminal vesicles are missing. At puberty, most patients exhibit selective signs of masculinization, the mechanism of which remains poorly understood (Conte and Grumbach, 1989).

Clinical findings. Genetic male infants are born with ambiguous genitalia and depending on the extent of masculinization may be assigned a male or female gender (Imperato-McGinley et al., 1982 and 1991). In most instances there is a pseudovagina, a perineoscrotal hypospadias, or

> **Congenital syndromes marked by hypogonadotropic hypogonadism**
>
> Isolated gonadotropin deficiency
> Kallmann syndrome (LRH deficiency and anosmia)
> Prader Willi syndrome
> Pituitary dwarfism
> Isolated LH deficiency (fertile eunuch syndrome)
> Isolated FSH deficiency
> Laurence-Moon-Bardet-Biedl syndrome
> Ataxia-hypogonadism syndrome
> Nevoid basal cell carcinoma syndrome
> Crandall syndrome
> Acrocephalosyndactyly syndromes
> Ichthyosis-hypogonadism syndrome

Modified from Castro-Magana M et al. Urology 1990; 35:195, with permission.

perineoscrotal hypospadias with a single perineal orifice and microphallus. Testes are located in the labioscrotal folds or in the inguinal canal. Wolffian ducts develop into an epididymis and vas deferens. At puberty, virilization occurs with enlargement of the phallus and development of scrotal rugae and hyperpigmentation; testicular descent occurs in some individuals (Imperato-McGinley et al., 1982). Deepening of the voice and increased muscle mass have also been noted, but the prostate remains nonpalpable. None of the reported patients developed gynecomastia. Facial hair growth and acne were recorded in some patients but not in others affected within a single family, which indicates a considerable heterogeneity within the same kindred (Imperato-McGinley et al., 1982 and 1991). The reasons for this selective virilization are not understood.

Hormonal findings. The diagnosis of 5-α-reductase deficiency can be made in children by measuring the ratio of 5β to 5α testosterone metabolites in the urine (Conte and Grumbach, 1989). In adult patients the plasma testosterone is within the normal male range, but the dihydrotestosterone levels are decreased and the testosterone to dihydrotestosterone ratio is abnormal. Patients typically show high urinary etiocholanole/androsterone and C_{19} and C_{21} 5β/5α metabolite ratios (Imperato-McGinley et al., 1991). Decreased conversion of exogenous testosterone to dihydrotestosterone and decreased 5-α-reductase in genital skin fibroblasts are used to confirm the diagnosis.

Pathologic findings. In adults, inguinal or labioscrotal testes resemble cryptorchid testes with variable degrees of tubular atrophy, interstitial fibrosis, and Leydig's cell hyperplasia. Spermatogenesis has been described in descended testes (Imperato-McGinley et al., 1982); however, there are no fertile patients on record (Scully, 1991).

Persistent müllerian duct syndrome

This familial condition inherited as an X-linked or autosomal recessive disorder is marked by normally developed external male genital organs, male genital ducts, and a fully developed uterus and fallopian tubes (Sheehan et al., 1985). This condition may be a consequence of deficient AMH synthesis or impaired AMH action during fetal life, which results in incomplete involution of müllerian duct derivatives in an otherwise normal male. The uterus and fallopian tubes are typically located in an inguinal hernia, which accounts for the commonly used synonym *hernia uteri inguinalis* (Nilson, 1939). The testes may be normally located in the scrotum and histologically normal or inguinally located and showing typical histologic features of cryptorchidism (Scully, 1991). As in normal individuals, impaired spermatogenesis is a feature of cryptorchid testes, whereas the patient with scrotal testes may be fertile.

CONGENITAL HYPOGONADOTROPIC HYPOGONADISM

Several congenital syndromes present with hypogonadotropic hypogonadism, some of which are listed in the box at left.

Kallmann's syndrome

Kallmann's syndrome is a genetically determined form of hypogonadotropic hypogonadism with anosmia that affects 1 in 10,000 to 1 in 60,000 persons. Some patients also have cleft lip or cleft palate, and suffer from deafness. The patients show eunochoid body proportions and hypoplastic genitalia (Fig. 3-28). X-linked autosomal recessive inheritance has been demonstrated in some families that exhibit Xp22.3 deletion (Ballabio et al., 1989). A gene named KALIG-1 (Kallmann's syndrome interval gene 1) Localized in this region of X chromosome seems to be deleted in some families (Bick et al., 1992). In other families the syndrome may be autosomally transmitted with sex limitation to males (White et al., 1983). A peculiar discordant appearance of Kallmann's syndrome in identical twins (Hipkin et al., 1990) further illustrates the complexities of the inheritance of this syndrome, which is apparently genetically heterogeneous.

It was proposed that Kallmann's syndrome is a disturbance of migration of fetal neurons from the olfactory placode (Bick et al., 1992). Since the olfactory placode contains precursors of the olfactory nerves and the luteinizing hormone–releasing hormone cells of the hypothalamus, the defect results in anosmia and selective gonadotropin deficiency. Gonadotropins in blood are low and remain at prepubertal levels even in postpubertal patients who do not show the typical pulsatile pattern of gonadotropin secretion (Wu et al., 1991). Gonadotropin deficiency is variable, however, and may be complete or partial; and differentially may affect FSH or LH. Complete gonadotropin deficiency leads to marked hypogonadism. The seminiferous tubules appear immature (Fig. 3-29). However, a partial defect marked by relative preservation of FSH secretion may be associated with spermatogenesis. These patients tend to have gynecomastia; some have been fertile, which accounts for their being called fertile eunuchs (Santen et

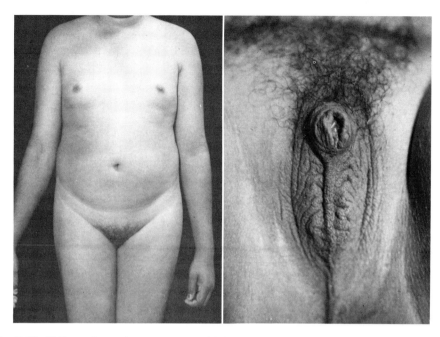

Fig. 3-28. Kallmann's syndrome presents with hypogonadism. This patient has micropenis and cryptorchidism. (Modified from Castro-Magana M et al. Urology 1990; 35:195, with permission).

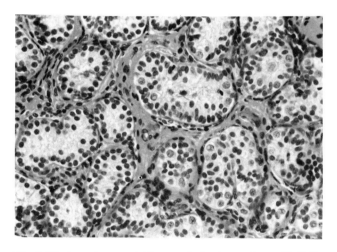

Fig. 3-29. Immature seminiferous tubules in a patient with Kallmann's syndrome.

al., 1971). These patients respond well to treatment of infertility with chorionic gonadotropin (Finkel et al., 1985).

Prader-Willi syndrome

Hypogonadism and hypogenitalism are common features of Prader-Willi syndrome, which is a congenital multisystemic disorder. In 50 to 70% of cases it is associated with an interstitial deletion of the proximal long arm of chromosome 15 (reviewed by Butler, 1990). The condition usually appears sporadically, but it may occur in several members of the same family as well (Lubinsky et al., 1987). Children suffering from this syndrome are born with hypotonia, have small hands and feet, and exhibit morbid obesity during childhood. Mental retardation is a

constant feature. Boys show cryptorchidism, scrotal hypoplasia, and micropenis, whereas girls show hypoplastic labia minora and clitoris. Menarche is late or does not occur; males are infertile. Seminiferous tubules are atrophic and do not show signs of spermatogenesis after puberty. These gonadal findings are considered to be a consequence of inadequate gonadotropin secretion from the hypothalamus.

The linkage between the chromosomal deletion and the clinical syndrome is poorly understood. The issue is complicated even more by the fact that half of all patients do not have chromosomal changes. Some patients with deletions of the long arm of chromosome 15 do not have Prader-Willi syndrome, whereas others have Angelman's syndrome, Williams's syndrome, or hypomelanosis of Ito (Butler, 1990). It is, however, of interest that in Prader-Willi syndrome the deletions involve the chromosome 15, whereas in the Angelman's syndrome it is the maternal chromosome 15 that is affected. Maternal uniparental disomy for chromosone 15, in which both copies of this chromosome are inherited from the mother, is demonstrable in 60% of cases (Mascari et al., 1992). All these findings suggest parental imprinting of this locus (Magenis et al., 1990). Because patients with Angelman's syndrome do not have hypogonadism, the role of the genes on chromosome 15 in regulating directly or indirectly the development of gonads and external genitalia remains poorly understood.

Laurence-Moon-Bardet-Biedl syndrome

This autosomal recessive syndrome is characterized by obesity, retinitis pigmentosa, mental retardation, occasional polydactyly or syndactyly, and renal disease in about 50% of cases (Dekaban et al., 1972). Green et al. (1989) consider Bardet-Biedl syndrome a subset of the

---

X-linked mental retardation associated with testicular changes

Macroorchidism

Fragile X syndrome
X-linked mental retardation with marfanoid habitus
Atkin-Flaitz syndrome

Hypogonadism

Börjeson's syndrome (microgenitalia, gynecomastia, hypogonadism)
Aarskog's syndrome (shawl scrotum, cryptorchidism)
FG syndrome (cryptorchidism, hypospadias)
Simpson-Golabi-Behmel syndrome (cryptorchidism)
Lowe's syndrome (cryptorchidism)
Juberg-Masardi syndrome (rudimentary scrotum, cryptorchidism, micropenis)
RuD's syndrome (hypogonadism)
Renpenning's syndrome (microorchidism)
Chudley MR syndrome (cryptorchidism, microorchidism)
Norrie's disease (cryptorchidism)

Modified from the review article of Glass IA. J Med Genet 1991; 28:361, with permission, which contains the references for all the above listed syndromes.

Laurence-Moon-Biedl syndrome, but because hypogonadism appears in both conditions, the two syndromes are considered together in this context. The symptoms are primarily seen in boys who show delayed sexual maturation. Micropenis, hypospadias, or cryptorchidism are common. Testes show varying degrees of atrophy of seminiferous tubules (Toledo et al., 1977). Although it was generally held that testicular atrophy is a consequence of central hypothalamic hypogonadism (Perez-Palacios et al., 1977), some patients have hypergonadotropic hypogonadism consistent with a primary testicular failure (Toledo et al., 1977). It thus appears that the gonadal pathology in the Laurence-Moon-Bardet-Biedl syndrome shows variability, reflecting a primary testicular or hypothalamic disorder or both.

Other syndromes of hypogonadotropic hypogonadism

Several congenital syndromes with malformations involving multiple organs and hypogonadotropic hypogonadism have been listed by Santen (1991) and Hedinger (1991) and are discussed briefly. These include Rud's syndrome, Möbius's syndrome, hypogonadotropism with ataxia, congenital ichthyosis (Lynch's syndrome), multiple lentigines syndrome (Gorlin's syndrome), Carpenter's syndrome of progressive hearing loss and alopecia, and Kraus-Ruppert syndrome of microcephaly, syndactyly, and hypoplasia of hypothalamic centers. Several X-linked mental deficiency syndromes were reviewed by Glass (1991). (See the box above.)

Congenital syndromes marked by hypergonadotropic hypogonadism

Alström's syndrome
Myotonic dystrophy
Sohval-Soffer syndrome
Van Benthem's syndrome
Börjeson's syndrome
Ichthyosis-hypogonadism syndrome

Modified from Castro-Magana M et al. Urology 1990; 35:195, with permission.

AUTOSOMAL ABNORMALITIES ASSOCIATED WITH GONADAL CHANGES

Gonadal pathology has been noted in conjunction with numerous numerical and structural autosomal chromosomal abnormalities (Skakkebaek et al., 1973). Ovarian pathology is common in trisomy 18 (Russell and Altshuler, 1975) and trisomy 21–related Down's syndrome (Hojager et al., 1978). Russell and Altshuler (1975) described the ovaries in trisomy 18 as dysplastic and noted that the number of oocytes and primordial follicles was decreased; that the surface mesothelium formed plexiform invaginations; that the granulosa cells formed solid cords, some of which were in continuity with epithelial invaginations; and that some follicles were cystic while others were atretic and dysplastic and surrounded with prominent basement membranes.

Ataxia telangiectasia, which is marked by frequent chromosomal breaks, is associated with a paucity of small antral follicles and ovarian atrophy (Miller and Chatten, 1967), which may be related to hormonal or immune disturbances that characterize this syndrome.

Deletion of the short arm of chromosome 11 is associated with complex development malformations affecting the kidney, testes, and external genitalia (Martinez-Mora et al., 1989). This indicates that the short arm of chromosome 11 carries genes that are involved in regulating the morphogenesis of the genital organs, but the nature of these genes has not been elucidated. Affected individuals are at a risk for developing Wilms and germ cell tumors. Primary gonadal failure in these congenital syndromes is accompanied by hypersecretion of gonadotropins. Other congenital syndromes of hypergonadotropic hypogonadism are listed in the box above.

REFERENCES

Abad L, Parrilla JJ, Marcos J, Gimeno F, Bernal AL: Male pseudohermaphroditism with 17 alpha-hydroxylase deficiency: A case report. Br J Obstet Gynecol 1980; 87:1162.

Abbas NE, Toublanc JE, Boucekkine C, Toublanc M, Affara NA, Job JC, Fellous M: A possible common origin of "Y" negative human XX males and XX true hermaphrodites. Hum Genet 1989; 84:356.

Affara NA, Ferguson-Smith MA, Magenis RE, Tolmie JL, Boyd E, Cooke A, Jamieson D, Kwok K, Mitchell M, Snadden L: Mapping testis determinants by an analysis of Y-specific sequences in males with apparent XX and XO karyotypes and females with XY karyotypes. Nucleic Acids Res 1987; 15:7325.

Ahmad KN, Dykes JR, Ferguson-Smith MA, Lenox B, Macks WS: Leydig cell volume in chromatin-positive Klinefelter's syndrome. J Clin Endocrinol Metab 1971; 33:517.

Aiman J, Griffin JE: The frequency of androgen receptor deficiency in infertile men. J Clin Endocrinol Metab 1982; 54:725.

Aiman J, Griffin JE, Gazak JM, Wilson JD, MacDonald PC: Androgen insensitivity as a cause of infertility in otherwise normal men. N Engl J Med 1979; 300:223.

Amrhein JA, Klingensmith GJ, Walsh PC: Partial androgen insensitivity: The Reinfenstein syndrome revisited. N Engl J Med 1977; 297:350.

Anderson CT, Carlson IH: Elevated plasma testosterone and gonadal tumors in two 46XY "sisters." Arch Pathol 1975; 99:360.

Anderson S, Berman DM, Jenkins EP, Russell DW: Deletion of steroid 5α-reductase 2 gene in male pseudohermaphroditism. Nature 1991; 354:159.

Andersson M, Page DC, de la Chapelle A: Chromosome Y-specific DNA is transferred to the short arm of X chromosome in human XX males. Science 1986; 233:86.

Armendares S, Salamanca F, Cantu JM: Familial true hermaphrodism in three siblings: Clinical cytogenetic, histologic and hormonal studies. Hum Genet 1975; 29:93.

Arnholdt IJP, Mendoca BB, Bloise W, Toledo SPA: Male pseudohermaphroditism resulting from Leydig cell hypoplasia. J Pediatr 1985; 106:1057.

Austin CR, Edwards RG: Mechanisms of Sex Differentiation in Animals and Man. London, Academic Press, 1981.

Azziz R, Zacur HA: 21-Hydroxylase deficiency in female hyperandrogenism: Screening and diagnosis. J Clin Endocrinol Metab 1989; 69:577.

Bailey JM, Pillard RC: A genetic study of male sexual orientation. Arch Gen Psychiatry 1991; 48:1089.

Ballabio A, Bardoni B, Carrozzo R, Andrea G, Bick D, Campbell L, et al.: Contiguous gene syndromes due to deletions in the distal short arm of the human X chromosome. Proc Natl Acad Sci USA 1989; 86:10001.

Bandmann H-J, Breit R, Perwein E (Eds): Klinefelter's syndrome. Berlin, Springer-Verlag, 1984.

Bardin CW, Catterall JF: Testosterone: A major determinant of extragenital dimorphism. Science 1981; 211:1285.

Berg FD, Kurzl R, Hinrichsen MJ, Zander J: Familial 46XY pure gonadal dysgenesis and gonadoblastoma/dysgerminoma: Case report. Gynecol Oncol 1989; 32:261.

Berkovitz GD, Fechner PY, Zacur HW, Rock JA, Snyder HM, Migeon CJ, Perlman EJ: Clinical and pathologic spectrum of 46,XY gonadal dysgenesis: Its relevance to the understanding of sex differentiation. Medicine 1991; 70:375.

Berkovitz GD, Rock JA, Urban MD, Migeon CR: True hermaphroditism. Johns Hopkins Med J 1982; 151:290.

Bernstein R, Koo GC, Wachtel SS: Abnormalities of the X chromosome in human 46,XY females siblings with dysgenetic ovaries. Science 1980; 207:768.

Berta P, Hawkins JR, Sinclair AH, Taylor A, Griffiths BL, Goodfellow PN, Fellous M: Genetic evidence equating SRY and the testis determining factor. Nature 1990; 348:448.

Berthezane F, Forest MG, Grimaud JA: Leydig cell agenesis: A cause of male pseudohermaphroditism. N Engl J Med 1976; 295:969.

Bick D, Franco B, Sherins RJ, Heye B, Pike L, Crawford J et al. Brief report: Iatragenic deletion of the KALIG-1 gene in Kallmann's syndrome. N Engl J Med 1992; 326: 1752.

Birnbaum MD, Rose LI: Late onset adrenocortical hydroxylase deficiencies associated with menstrual dysfunction. Obstet Gynecol 1984; 63:445.

Bowen P, Lee CSN, Migeon CJ: Hereditary male pseudohermaphroditism with hypogonadism, hypospadias, and gynecomastia (Reifenstein's syndrome). Ann Intern Med 1965; 62:252.

Boyar RM, Wu RHK, Kapen S, Hellman L, Weitzman ED, Finkelstein JW: Clinical and laboratory heterogenaeity in idiopathic hypogonadotropic hypogonadism. J Clin Endocrinol Metab 1976; 43:1268.

Brody BL, Wentz AC: Late onset congenital adrenal hyperplasia: A gynecologist's perspective. Fertil Steril 1987; 48:175.

Brown DM, Markland D, Dehner LP: Leydig cell hypoplasia: A cause of male pseudohermaphroditism. J Clin Endocrinol Metab 1978; 46:1.

Brown GR: A review of clinical approaches to gender dysphoria. J Clin Psychiatry 1990; 51:57.

Brown CJ, Goss SJ, Lubahn DB, Joseph DR, Wilson EM, French FS, Willard HF: Androgen receptor locus on the human X chromosome: Regional localization to Xg 11-12 and description of a DNA polymorphism. Am J Hum Genet 1989; 44:264.

Bulmer D: The development of the human vagina. J Anat 1957; 91:490.

Burke EF, Gilbert E, Uehling DT: Adrenal rest tumor of the testis. J Urol 1973; 109:649.

Butler MG: Prader-Willi syndrome: Current understanding of cause and diagnosis. Am J Med Genet 1990; 35:319.

Byskov AG: Differentiation of mammalian embryonic gonad. Physiol Rev 1986; 66:71.

Carr DH, Haggar RA, Hart AG: Germ cells in the ovaries of XO female infants. Am J Clin Pathol 1968; 49:521.

Carter JN, Tyson JE, Tolis G, Van Vliet S, Faiman C, Friesen HG: Prolactin-secreting tumors and hypogonadism in 22 men. N Engl J Med 1978; 293:847.

Case Records of the Massachusetts General Hospital (Case 13-1990). N Engl J Med 1990; 322:917.

Castro-Magana M, Bronsther B, Angulo MA: Genetic forms of male hypogonadism. Urology 1990; 35:195.

Cathelineau G, Brerault JL, Fiet J, Julien R, Dreux C, Canivet J: Adrenocortical 11-β-hydroxylation defect in adult women with postmenarchial onset of symptoms. J Clin Endocrinol Metab 1980; 51:287.

Chan-Cua S, Freidenberg G, Jones KL: Occurrence of male phenotype of genotypic females with congenital virilizing adrenal hyperplasia. Am J Med Genet 1983; 34:406.

Chandley AC: The chromosomal basis of human infertility. Br Med Bull 1979; 35:181.

Chandley AC, Edmond P: Meiotic studies on a subfertile patient with a ring Y chromosome. Cytogenetics 1971; 10:295.

Chang HJ, Clark RD, Bachman H: The phenotype of 45, X/46, XY mosaicism: An analysis of 92 prenatally diagnosed cases. Am J Hum Genet 1990; 46:156.

Clark EB: Neck web and congenital heart defects: A pathogenetic association in 45 X-O Turner syndrome? Teratology 1984; 29:355.

Clark RV, Albertson BD, Munabi A, Cassorla F, Aguilera G, Warren DW, Sherins RJ, Loriaux DL: Steroidogenic enzyme activities, morphology, and receptor studies of testicular adrenal rest in a patient with congenital adrenal hyperplasia. J Clin Endocrinol Metab 1990; 70:1408.

Conte FA, Grumbach MM: Pathogenesis, classification, diagnosis and treatment of anomalies of sex. In Endocrinology, 2nd ed, vol 3, edited by DeGroot LJ et al. Philadelphia, WB Saunders, 1989, p 1810.

Court-Brown WM, Mantle DJ, Buckton KE: Fertility in an XY/XXY male married to a translocation heterozygote. J Med Genet 1964; 1:35.

Cunnah D, Perry L, Dacie JA, Grant DB, Lowe DG, Savage MO, Besser GM: Bilateral testicular tumours in congenital adrenal hyperplasia: A continuing diagnostic and therapeutic dilemma. Clin Endocrinol 1989; 30:141.

Cussen LJ, MacMahon RA: Germ cells and ova in dysgenetic gonads of a 46-XY female dizygotic twin. Am J Dis Child 1979; 133:373.

Damjanov I, Klauber G: Microscopic gonadoblastoma in a dysgenetic gonad in an infant. An ultrastructural study. Urology 1980; 15:606.

Damjanov I, Nesbitt KA, Reardon MP, Vidone RA: Giant Sertoli cell adenoma in testicular feminization syndrome. Obstet Gynecol 1976; 48:624.

de la Chapelle A: The etiology of maleness in XX men. Hum Genet 1981; 58:105.

de la Chapelle A: Sex chromosomes and abnormalities. In Principles and Practice of Medical Genetics, edited by Emery AEH, Rimoin DL, 2nd ed, Edinburgh, Churchill Livingstone, 1990, p 193.

Degenhart HJ: Prader's syndrome (congenital lipoid adrenal hyperplasia). Pediatr Adolesc Endocrinol 1984; 13:125.

Dekaban NS, Parks JS, Ross GT: Laurence-Moon syndrome: Evaluation of endocrinological function and phenotypic concordance and report of cases. Med Ann DC 1972; 41:687.

Dewhurst J: Fertility in 47,XXX and 45,X patients. J Medical Genet 1978; 15:132.

Disteche CM, Casanova M, Saal H, Friedman C, Sybert V, Graham J, Thuline H, Page DC, Fellous M: Small deletions of the short arm of the Y chromosome in 46, XY females. Proc Natl Acad Sci USA 1986; 83:7891.

Dodge ST, Finkelston MS, Miyazawa K: Testicular feminization with incomplete Mullerian regression. Fertil Steril 1985; 43:937.

Donahoe PK, Crawford JD, Hendren WH: Mixed gonadal dysgenesis, pathogenesis and management. J Pediatr Surg 1979; 14:287.

Drobnjak P: Interseksualizam. Zagreb, Jugoslavenska Akademija Znanosti i Umjetnosti, 1974.

Duck SC, Katayama KP: Danazol may cause female pseudohermaphroditism. Fertil Steril 1981; 35:230.

Eckstein B, Cohen S, Farkas A, Rosler A: The nature of the defect in familial male pseudohermaphroditism in Arabs of Gaza. J Clin Endocrinol Metab 1989; 68:477.

Eddy AA, Mauer SM: Pseudohermaphroditism, glomerulopathy and Wilms tumor (Drash syndrome): Frequency in end stage renal failure. J Pediatr 1985; 106:584.

Editorial: Klinefelter's syndrome. Lancet 1988; 1:1316.

Editorial: Transsexualism. Lancet 1991; 338:603.

Eicher EM, Washburn LL: Inherited sex reversal in mice: Identification of a new primary sex-determining gene. J Exp Zool 1983; 228:297.

Ellis NA: The human Y chromosome. Semin Dev Biol 1991; 2:231.

Espiner EA, Veale AMO, Sands VE, Fitzgerald PH: Familial syndrome of streak gonads and normal male karyotype in five phenotypic females. N Engl J Med 1970; 283:6

Ferguson-Smith MA: The prepubertal testicular lesion in chromatin-positive Klinefelter's syndrome (primary microorchidism) as seen in mentally handicapped children. Lancet 1959; 1:219.

Ferguson-Smith MA: Karyotype-phenotype correlations in gonadal dysgenesis and their bearing on the pathogenesis of malformations. J Med Genet 1965; 2:142.

Ferguson-Smith MA: Genotype-phenotype correlations in individuals with disorders of sex determination and development including Turner's syndrome. Semin Dev Biol 1991; 2:265.

Ferguson-Smith MA, Cooke A, Affara NA, Boyd E, Tolmie JL: Genotype-phenotype correlations in XX males and their bearing on current theories of sex determination. Hum Genet 1990; 84:198.

Finkel DM, Phillips JL, Synder PJ: Stimulation of spermatogenesis by gonadotropins in men with hypogonadotropic hypogonadism. N Engl J Med 1985; 313:651.

Fisher EMC, Beer-Romero P, Brown LG, Ridley A, McNeil JA, Lawrence JB, et al: Homologous ribosomal protein genes on the human X and Y chromosomes: Escape from X inactivation and possible implications for Turner's syndrome. Cell 1990; 63:1205.

Gartler SM, Liskay RM, Campbell RK, Sparkes R, Gant N: Evidence for two functional X chromosomes in human oocytes. Cell Diff 1972; 1:215.

Gartler SM, Waxman SH, Giblett E: An XX/XY human hermaphrodite resulting from double fertilization. Proc Natl Acad Sci U S A 1962; 48:332.

George FW, Wilson JD: Sex determination and differentiation. In The Physiology of Reproduction, vol I, edited by Knobil E, Neill JD. New York, Raven Press, 1988, p 3.

German J, Simpson JL, Chaganti RSK, Summit RL, Reid LB, Merkatz IR: Genetically determined sex-reversal in 46,XY humans. Science 1978; 202:53.

Giagulli VA, Vermeulen A: Leydig cell function in infertile men with idiopathic oligospermic infertility. J Clin Endocrinol Metab 1988; 66:62.

Glass IA: X linked mental retardation. J Med Genet 1991; 28:361.

Goodfellow P, Lovell-Badge R: Introduction: Sex determination and the mammalian Y chromosome. Semin Dev Biol 1991; 2:229.

Gooren L: The endocrinology of transsexualism: A review and commentary. Psychoneuroendocrinology 1990; 15:3.

Gooren L: Improvement of spermatogenesis after treatment with the antiestrogen tamoxifen in a man with incomplete androgen insensitivity syndrome. J Clin Endocrinol Metab 1989; 68:1207.

Gordon DL, Krmpotic E, Thomas W, Gandy HM, Paulsen CA: Pathologic testicular findings in Klinefelter's syndrome 47,XXY vs 46,XY/47,XXY. Arch Intern Med 1972; 130:726.

Gorski RA: Sexual differentiation of the endocrine brain and its control. In Brain endocrinology, 2nd ed., edited by Motta M, New York, Raven Press, 1991, p 71.

Graham JM, Bashir AS, Stark RE, Silbert A, Walzer S: Oral and written language abilities of XXY boys: Implications for anticipatory guidance. Pediatrics 1988; 81:795.

Graham RA, Seif MW, Aplin JD, Li TC, Cooke ID, Rogers AW, Dockery P: An endometrial factor in unexplained infertility. BMJ 1990; 300:1428.

Grammatico P, Buttoni U, DeSanctis S, Sulli N, Tonanzi T, Onorio AC, et al: A male patient with 48,XXYY syndrome: Importance of distinction from Klinefelter's syndrome. Clin Genet 1990; 38:74.

Green JS, Parfrey PS, Cramer BC, Johnson G, Heath O, McManamon PJ, O'Leary E, Pryse-Phillips W: The cardinal manifestations of Bardet-Biedl syndrome, a form of Laurence-Moon-Biedl syndrome. N Engl J Med 1989; 321:1002.

Griffin JE: Androgen resistance—the clinical and molecular spectrum. N Engl J Med 1992; 326:611.

Griffin JE, Wilson JD: The syndrome of androgen resistance. N Engl J Med 1980; 302:198.

Griffin JE, Wilson JD: Disorders of the testes and the male reproductive tract. In Williams Textbook of Endocrinology, 8th ed., edited by Wilson JD, Foster DW, Philadelphia, WB Saunders, 1991, p 799.

Grino PB, Griffin JE, Cushard WG Jr, Wilson JD: A mutation of the androgen receptor associated with partial androgen resistance, familial gynecomastia, and fertility. J Clin Endocrinol Metab 1988; 66:754.

Grumbach MM, Conte FA: Disorders of sex differentiation. In Williams Textbook of Endocrinology, 8th ed., edited by Wilson JD, Foster DW, Philadelphia, WB Saunders, 1992, p 853.

Hall BD, Spranger JW: Campomelic dysplasia: Further elucidation of a distinct entity. Am J Dis Child 1980; 134:285.

Hall JG, Gilchrist DM: Turner syndrome and its variants. Pediatr Clin North Am 1990; 37:1421.

Hamerton JL, Canning N, Ray M, Smith S: A cytogenetic survey of 14,069 newborn infants: Incidence of chromosomal anomalies. Clin Genet 1975; 8:223.

Hart WR, Burkons DM: Germ cell neoplasms arising in gonadoblastoma. Cancer 1979; 43:669.

Hassold T, Benham F, Leppert M: Cytogenetic and molecular analysis of sex-chromosome monosomy. Am J Hum Genet 1988; 42:534.

Hedinger CE, Dhom G: Pathologie des männlichen Genitale, Berlin, Springer-Verlag, 1991.

Hipkin LJ, Casson IF, Davis JC: Identical twins discordant for Kallmann's syndrome. J Med Genet 1990; 27:198.

Hojager B, Peters H, Byskov AG, Faber M: Follicular development in ovaries of children with Down's syndrome. Acta Paediatr Scand 1978; 67:637.

Hook EB, Warburton D: The distribution of chromosomal genotypes associated with Turner's syndrome: Live birth prevalence rates and evidence for diminished fetal mortality and severity in genotypes associated with structural X abnormalities or mosaicism. Hum Genet 1983; 64:24.

Hsueh WA, Hsu TH, Federman DD: Endocrine features of Klinefelter's syndrome. Medicine 1978; 57:447.

Hurt WG, Bodurtha JN, McCall JB, Ali MM: Seminoma in pubertal patient with androgen insensitivity syndrome. Am J Obstet Gynecol 1989; 161:530.

Imperato-McGinley J, Akgun S, Ertel NH, Sayli B, Shackleton C: The coexistence of male pseudohermaphrodites with 17-ketosteroid reductase deficiency and 5-α-reductase deficiency within a Turkish kindred. Clin Endocrinol 1987; 27:135.

Imperato-McGinley J, Miller M, Wilson JD, Peterson RE, Shackleton C, Gajdusek DC: A cluster of male pseudohermaphrodites with 5α-reductase deficiency in Papua, New Guinea. Clin Endocrinol 1991; 34:293.

Imperato-McGinley J, Peterson RE, Gautier T, Sturla E: Male pseudohermaphroditism secondary to 5α-reductase deficiency: A model for the role of androgens in both the development of the male phenotype and the evolution of a male gender identity. J Steroid Biochem Mol Biol 1979; 11:637.

Imperato-McGinley J, Peterson RE, Stoller R: Male pseudohermaphroditism secondary to 17-hydroxysteroid dehydrogenase deficiency: Gender role change with puberty. J Clin Endocrinol Metab 1979; 49:391.

Imperato-McGinley J, Peterson RE, Gautier T, et al.: Hormonal evaluation of a larger kindred with complete androgens insensitivity: Evidence for secondary 5-α-reductase deficiency. J Clin Endocrinol Metab 1982; 54:931.

Jäger RJ, Anvret M, Hall K, Scherer G: A human XY female with a frame shift mutation in the candidate testis determining gene SRY. Nature 1990; 348:452.

Jäger RJ, Ebensperger C, Fraccaro M, Scherer G: A ZFY-negative 46, XX true hermaphrodite is positive for the Y pseudoautosomal boundary. Hum Genet 1990; 85:666.

Jockenhovel F, Khan SA, Nieschlag E: Diagnostic value of bioactive FSH in male infertility. Acta Endocrinol 1989; 121:902.

Jones HW, Ferguson-Smith MA, Heller RH: Pathologic and cytogenetic findings in true hermaphroditism: Report of 6 cases and review of 23 cases from the literature. Obstet Gynecol 1965; 25:435.

Josso N, Vigier B, Magre S, Picard J-Y: Anti-Mullerian hormone and gonadal development. Semin Dev Biol 1991; 2:285.

Jost A: A new look at the mechanisms controlling sexual differentiation in mammals. Johns Hopkins Med J 1972; 130:38.

Kaneko N, Kawagoe S, Hiroi M: Turner's syndrome—reviews of the literature with reference to a successful pregnancy outcome. Gynecol Obstet Invest 1990; 29:81.

Kim MH, Gumpel JA, Graff P: Pregnancy in a true hermaphrodite. Obstet Gynecol (Suppl) 1973; 53:40S.

Kinsey AC, Pomeroy WB, Martin CE: Sexual Behavior in the Human Male. Philadelphia, WB Saunders, 1948.

Klinefelter HF: Background of the recognition of Klinefelter's syndrome as a distinct pathologic entity. Am J Obstet Gynecol 1973; 116:436.

Klinefelter HF, Reifenstein EC, Albright F: Syndrome characterized by gynecomastia, aspermatogenesis, without A-Leydigism, and increased excretion of follicle stimulating hormone. J Clin Endocrinol 1942; 2:615.

Koopman P, Gubbay J, Vivian N, Goodfellow P, Lovell-Badge R: Male development of chromosomally female mice transgenic for Sry. Nature 1991; 351:117.

Kraus CM, Turksoy N, Atkins L, McLaughlin C, Brown LG, Page DC: Familial premature ovarian failure due to an interstitial deletion of the long arm of the X chromosome. N Engl J Med 1987; 317:125.

Krishnamurthy S, Adcock LL, Okagaki T: Endometrial carcinoma following estrogen-progestogen therapy in Turner's syndrome. A case report and review of the literature. Gynecol Oncol 1977; 5:291.

Larco RV, Jones KL, Benirschke K: Coarctation of the aorta in Turner syndrome. A pathologic study of fetuses with nuchal cystic hygromas, hydrops fetalis, and female genitalia. Pediatrics 1988; 81:445.

Ledbetter DH, Mascarello JT, Riccardi VM, Harper VD, Airhart SD, Strobel RJ: Chromosome 15 abnormalities and the Prader-Willi syndrome: A follow-up report of 40 cases. Am J Hum Genet 1982; 34:278.

Lee PA, Muzur T, Danish R, Amrhein J, Buzzard RM, Money J, Migeon CJ: Micropenis. I. Criteria, etiologies and classification. Johns Hopkins Med J 1980; 146:156.

LeVay S: A difference in hypothalamic structure between heterosexual and homosexual men. Science 1991; 253:1034.

Lieblich JM, Rogol AD, White BJ, Rosen SW: Syndrome of anosmia with hypogonadotropic hypogonadism (Kallmann syndrome). Clinical and laboratory studies in 23 cases. Am J Med 1982; 73:506.

Lippe B: Turner syndrome. Endocrinol Metab Clin North Am 1991; 20:121.

Lippe BM: Physical and anatomical abnormalities in Turner syndrome. In Turner Syndrome, edited by Rosenfield RG, Grumbach RG, New York, Marcel Dekker, 1990, p 183.

Lippe B, Geffner ME, Dietrich RB, Boechat MI, Kangarloo H: Renal malformations in patients with Turner syndrome: Imaging in 141 patients. Pediatrics 1988; 82:852.

Louka MH, Ross RD, Lee JH, Lewis GC: Endometrial carcinoma in Turner's syndrome. Gynecol Oncol 1978; 6:294.

Lubahn DB, Joseph DR, Sullivan PM, Willard HF, French FS, Wilson EM: Cloning of human androgen receptor complementary DNA and localization to the X chromosome. Science 1988; 240:327.

Lubinsky M, Zellweger H, Greenswag L, Larson G, Hansmann I, Ledbetter D: Familial Prader-Willi syndrome with apparently normal chromosomes. Am J Med Genet 1987; 28:37.

Lubs HA Jr: Testicular size in Klinefelter's syndrome in men over fifty. N Engl J Med 1962; 267:326.

Lyon AJ, Preece MA, Grant DB: Growth curve for girls with Turner syndrome. Arch Dis Child 1985; 60:932.

Mackay AM, Pattigrew N, Symington T, Neville AM: Tumors of dysgenetic gonads (gonadogenic aspects). Cancer 1974; 34:1108.

Magenis RE, Toth-Fejel S, Allen LJ, Black M, Brown MG, Budden S, et al.: Comparison of the 15 q deletions in Prader-Willi and Angelman syndromes: Specific regions, extent of deletions, parental origin, and clinical consequences. Am J Med Genet 1990; 35:333.

Manuel M, Katayama KP, Jones HW Jr: The age of occurrence of gonadal tumors in intersex patients with a Y chromosome. Am J Obstet Gynecol 1976; 124:293.

Martinez-Mora J, Audi L, Toran N, Isnard R, Castellvi A, Perez Iribarne M, Egozcue J: Ambiguous genitalia, gonadoblastoma, aniridia and mental retardation with deletion of chromosome 11. J Urol 1989; 142:1298.

Mascari MJ, Gottlieb W, Rogan PK, Butbr MG, Waller DA, Armour JAL, et al: The frequency of uniparental disomy in Prader-Willi syndrome. N Engl J Med 1992; 326:1599.

Massa G, Vanderschueren-Lode-Weyckx M, Malvaux P: Linear growth in patients with Turner syndrome. I. Influence of spontaneous puberty and parental height. Eur J Pediatr 1990; 149:246.

Massarano AA, Adams JA, Preece MA: Ovarian ultrasound appearances in Turner syndrome. J Pediatr 1989; 144:568.

Matlai P, Berl V: Trends in congenital malformations of external genitalia. Lancet 1985; 1:108.

Matsumoto T, Taku K, Miiki T, Harada N, Niikawa N: XY translocation in a boy with ichthyosis, hypogonadism, short stature and mental retardation. Clin Genet 1991; 39:156.

McKusick VA: Mendelian Inheritance in Man, 7th ed. Baltimore, Johns Hopkins, 1986.

McLaren A: Sexual differentiation: Of MIS and the mouse. Nature 1990; 345:111a.

McLaren A: Sexual determination: What makes a man a man? Nature 1990; 346:216b.

McLaren A: Development of the mammalian gonad. The fate of the supporting cell lineage. Bioessays 1991; 13:151a.

McLaren A: Sex determination: The making of male mice. Nature, 1991;351:96b.

McLaughlin B, Barrett P, Finch T, Devlin JG: Late onset adrenal hyperplasia in a group of Irish females who presented with hirsutism, irregular menses and/or cystic acne. Clin Endocrinol 1990; 32:57.

McPhaul MJ, Marcelli M, Tiley WD, Griffin JE, Isidro-Gutierrez RF, Wilson JD: Molecular basis of androgen resistance in a family with a qualitative abnormality of the androgen receptor and responsive to high dose androgen therapy. J Clin Invest 1991; 87:1413a.

McPhaul MJ, Marcelli M, Tilley WD, Griffin JE, Wilson JD: Androgen resistance caused by mutations in the androgen receptor gene. FASEB J 1991; 5:2910b.

Merchant H: Rat gonadal and ovarian organogenesis with and without germ cells: An ultrastructural study. Dev Biol 1975; 44:1.

Medina M, Castorena G, Herrera J, Bermudez JA, Zarate A: Modulation of luteinizing hormone secretion by estrogens in patients with Reifenstein's syndrome. Fertil Steril 1989; 52:239.

Metley C: Predicting intellectual functions in 47,XXY boys from characteristics of sibs. Clin Genet 1987; 32:24.

Mishell DR, Davajan V, Lobo RA (Eds): Infertility, Contraception and Reproductive Endocrinology, 3rd ed. Boston, Blackwell Scientific, 1991.

Miller ME, Chatten J: Ovarian changes in ataxia telangiectasia. Acta Paediatr Scand 1967; 56:559.

Miller WL: Gene conversions, deletions and polymorphisms in congenital adrenal hyperplasia. Am J Hum Genet 1988; 42:4.

Miller WL: Congenital adrenal hyperplasia. Endocrinol Metab Clin North Am 1991; 20:721.

Money J: Paraphilias: Phenomenology and classification. Am J Psychother 1984; 38:164.

Moorthy AV, Chesney RW, Lubinsky M: Chronic renal failure and XY gonadal dysgenesis: "Frasier" syndrome: A commentary on reported cases. Am J Med Genet (Suppl) 1987; 3:297.

Morris JM, Mahesh VB: Further observations on the syndrome "testicular feminization." Am J Obstet Gynecol 1963; 87:731.

Mozaffarian GA, Higley M, Paulsen CA: Clinical studies in an adult male patient with "isolated follicle stimulatory hormone (FSH) deficiency." J Androl 1983; 4:393.

Mulaikal RM, Migeon CJ, Rock JA: Fertility rates in female patients with congenital adrenal hyperplasia due to 21-hydroxylase deficiency. N Engl J Med 1987; 316:178.

Müller J, Skakkebaek NE: Gonadal malignancy in individuals with sex chromosome anomalies. Birth Defects 1990; 26:247.

Munsterberg A, Lovell-Badge R: Expression of the mouse anti-Mullerian hormone gene suggests a role in both male and female sexual differentiation. Development 1991; 113:613.

Muzsnai D, Feinberg M: Mixed endodermal sinus tumor of the ovary in the Swyer's syndrome patient. Gynecol Oncol 1980; 10:230.

Navot D, Laufer N, Kopolovic J, Rabinowitz R, Birkenfeld A, Lewin A et al: Artificially induced endometrial cycles and establishment of pregnancies in the absence of ovaries. N Engl J Med 1986; 314:806.

Netley C: Predicting intellectual functioning in 47,XXY boys from characteristics of sibs. Clin Genet 1987; 32:24.

New MI, Speiser PW: Genetics of adrenal steroid 21-hydroxylase deficiency. Endocr Rev 1986; 7:331.

Newell ME, Lippe BM, Ehrlich RM: Testes tumors associated with congenital adrenal hyperplasia: A continuing diagnostic and therapeutic dilemma. J Urol 1977; 117:256.

Nielsen J, Sillesen I, Hansen KB: Fertility in women with Turner's syndrome: A case report and review of the literature. Br J Obstet Gynecol 1979; 86:833.

Nielsen J, Wohlert M: Sex chromosome abnormalities found among 34,910 newborn children: Results from a 13 year incidence study in Arhus, Denmark. Birth Defects 1991; 26:209.

Nilson O: Hernia uteri inguinalis beim Manne. Acta Chir Scand 1939; 83:231.

Nistal M, Panigua R: Testicular and Epididymal Pathology. New York, Thieme-Stratton, 1984.

Nogales FF, Toro M, Ortega I, Fulwood HR: Bilateral incipient germ cell tumours of the testis in the incomplete testicular feminization syndrome. Histopathology 1981; 5:511.

Ogata T, Matsuo S, Saito M, Prader A: A testicular lesion and sexual differentiation in congenital lipoid adrenal hyperplasia. Helv Paediatr Acta 1988; 43:531.

Opitz JM, Pallister PD: Brief historical note: The concept of "gonadal dysgenesis." Am J Med Genet 1979; 4:333.

Pallister PD, Opitz JM: The Perrault syndrome: Autosomal recessive ovarian dysgenesis with facultative non-sex-limited sensorineural deafness. Am J Med Genet 1979; 4:239.

Palmer CG, Reichmann A: Chromosomal and clinical findings in 110 females with Turner's syndrome. Hum Genet 1976; 35:35.

Palmer MS, Sinclair AM, Berta P, Ellis NA, Goodfellow PN, Abbas NA, Fellous M: Genetic evidence that ZFY is not the testis-determining factor. Nature 1989; 342:937.

Pang S, Lerner AJ, Stoner E, Levine LS, Oberfield SE, Engel I, New MI: Late onset adrenal steroid 3β-HSD deficiency. I. A cause of hirsutism in pubertal and postpubertal females. J Clin Endocrinol Metab 1985; 60:428.

Pang SY, Wallace MA, Hofman L, Thuline HC, Dorche C, Lyon IC et al: Worldwide experience in newborn screening for classical congenital adrenal hyploplasia due to 21-hydroxylase deficiency. Pediatrics 1988; 81:866.

Pecile V, Filippi G: Screening for fra(k) mutation and Klinefelter syndrome in mental institutions. Clin Genet 1991; 39:189.

Pereira ET, Cabral de Almeida JC, Gunha ACYRG, Patton M, Taylor R, Jeffery S: Use of probes for ZFY, SRY and the Y pseudoautosomal boundary in XX males, XX true hermaphrodites and an XY female. J Med Genet 1991; 28:591.

Perez-Palacios G, Uribe M, Scaglia H, Lisker R, Pasapera A, Maillard M, Medina M: Pituitary and gonadal function in patients with the Laurence-Moon-Biedl syndrome. Acta Endocrinol 1977; 84:191.

Peterson RE, Imperato-McGinley J, Gautier T, Sturla E: Male pseudohermaphroditism due to steroid 5-α-reductase deficiency. Am J Med 1977; 64:170.

Petit C, de la Chapelle A, Levilliers J, Castillo S, Noel B, Weissenbach J: An abnormal terminal X-Y interchange accounts for most but not all cases of human XX maleness. Cell 1987; 49:595.

Philip J, Lundsteen C, Owen D, Hirshhorn K: The frequency of chromosome aberrations in tall men with special reference to 47,XYY and 47,XXY. Am J Hum Genet 1976; 28:404.

Price WH, Clayton JF, Colyer S, De Mey R, Wilson J: Mortality ratios, life expectancy and causes of death in patients with Turner's syndrome. J Epidemiol Community Health 1986; 40:97.

Rabinovici J, Jaffe RB: Development and regulation of growth and differentiated function in human and subhuman primate fetal gonads. Endocrinol Rev 1990; 11:532.

Rajfer J, Walsh PC: Mixed gonadal dysgenesis-dysgenetic male pseudohermaphroditism. Pediatr Adolesc Endocrinol 1981; 8:105.

Rangnekar GV, Loya BM, Goswami LK, Sengupta LK: Premature centromeric divisions and prominent telomeres in a patient with persistent Mullerian duct syndrome. Clin Genet 1990; 37:69.

Ranke MB, Blum WF, Haug F, Rosendahl W, Attanasio A, Enders H et al: Growth hormone, somatomedin levels and growth regulation in Turner's syndrome. Acta Endocrinol 1987; 116:305.

Ranke MB, Pfluger, Rosendahl W: Turner's syndrome. Spontaneous growth in 150 cases and review of the literature. Eur J Pediatr 1983; 141:81.

Ratcliffe SG: The sexual development of boys with chromosome constitution 47,XXY (Klinefelter's syndrome). Clin Endocrinol Metab 1982; 11:703.

Rimoin DL, Schimke RN (Eds): Genetic Disorders of the Endocrine Glands. St. Louis, CV Mosby, 1971.

Robboy SJ, Miller T, Donahoe PK, Jahre C, Welch WR, Haseltine FP, Miller WA, Atkins L, Crawford JD: Dysgenesis of testicular and streak gonada in the syndrome of mixed gonadal dysgenesis: Perspective derived from a clinicopatholgic analysis of 21 cases. Hum Pathol 1982; 13:700.

Rodriguez-Rigau LJ, Smith KD: Gynecomastia. In Endocrinology, 2nd ed, edited by De Groot LJ et al, Philadelphia, WB Saunders, 1989; p 2207.

Rosen GF, Vermesh M, D'Ablaing G, Wachtel S, Lobo RA: The endocrine evolution of a 45, X true hermaphrodite. Am J Obstet Gynecol 1987; 157:1272.

Rosenfeld RG, Grumbach MM (Eds): Turner's syndrome. New York, Marcell Dekker, 1990.

Rösler A, Kohn G: Male pseudohermaphroditism due to 17β-hydroxysteroid dehydrogenase deficiency: Studies on the natural history of the defect and effect of androgens on gender role. J Steroid Biochem 1983; 39:663.

Rösler A, Lieberman E, Cohen T: High frequency of congenital adrenal hyperplasia (classic 11 beta-hydroxylase deficiency) among Jews from Morocco. Am J Med Genet 1992; 42:827.

Rudd NL, Klimek ML: Familial caudal dysgenesis: Evidence for a major dominant gene. Clin Genet 1990; 38:170.

Russell P, Altshuler G: The ovarian dysgenesis of trisomy 18. Pathology 1975; 7:149.

Rutgers JL, Scully RE: Pathology of the testis in intersex syndromes. Semin Diagn Pathol 1987; 4:257.

Rutgers JL, Scully RE: The androgen insensitivity syndrome (testicular feminization): A clinicopathologic study of 43 cases. Int J Gynecol Pathol 1991; 10:126.

Saito S, Kumamoto Y: The number of spermatogonia in various congenital testicular disorders. J Urol 1989; 141:1166.

Santen RJ: Male hypogonadism. In Reproductive Endocrinology: Physiology, Pathophysiology and Clinical Management, edited by Yen SSC, Jaffe RB, Philadelphia, WB Saunders, 1991, p 733.

Santen RJ, Leonard JM, Sherins RJ, Gandy HM, Paulsen CA: Short- and long-term effects of clomiphene citrate on the pituitary-testicular axis. J Clin Endocrinol Metab 1971; 33:970.

Savage MO, Lowe DG: Gonadal neoplasia and abnormal sexual differentiation. Clin Endocrinol 1990; 32:519.

Schwartz IS, Cohen CJ, Deligdisch L: Dysgerminoma of the ovary associated with true hermaphroditism. Obstet Gynecol 1980; 56:102.

Schwartz ID, Root AW: The Klinefelter syndrome of testicular dysgenesis. Endocrinol Clin North Am 1991; 20:152.

Scully RE: Gonadoblastoma: A review of 74 cases. Cancer 1970; 25:1340.

Scully RE: Gonadal pathology of genetically determined diseases. In Pathology of Reproductive Failure, edited by Kraus FT, Damjanov I, Kaufman N, Baltimore, Williams & Wilkins, 1991, p 257.

Serhal PF, Craft IL: Oocyte donation in 61 patients. Lancet 1989; 1:1185.

Serra GB, Perez-Palacios G, Jaffe RB: De novo testosterone biosynthesis in the human fetal testis. J Clin Endocrinol Metab 1970; 30:128.

Shah KD, Kaffe S, Gilbert F, Dolgin S, Gertner M: Unilateral microscopic gonadoblastoma in a prepubertal Turner mosaic with Y chromosome material identified by restriction fragment analysis. Am J Clin Pathol 1988; 90:622.

Sheehan SJ, Tobbia IN, Ismail MA, Kelly DG, Duff FA: Persistent Mullerian duct syndrome. Review and report of 3 cases. Br J Urol 1985; 57:548.

Siebenmann RE: Pathology of gonads and adrenal cortex in the intersex. Prog Pediatr Surg 1983; 16:149.

Sigg C, Hedinger CE: Ultrastructure of the testis in Klinefelter's syndrome. In Klinefelter's syndrome, edited by Bandmann HJ, Breit R, Perwein E, Berlin, Springer-Verlag, 1984, p 137.

Simpson JL: Disorders of sexual differentiation. New York, Academic Press, 1976.

Simpson JL: Gonadal dysgenesis and abnormalities of the human sex chromosomes: Current status of phenotypic karyotypic correlations. Birth Defects 1975; 11:23.

Simpson JL: Male pseudohermaphroditism: Genetics and clinical delineation. Hum Genet 1978; 44:1.

Simpson JL, Blagowidow N, Martin AO: XY gonadal dysgenesis. Genetic heterogeneity based upon observations, H-Y antigen status and segregation analysis. Hum Genet 1981; 58:91.

Simpson JL, Christakos AC, Horwith M, Silverman FS: Gonadal dysgenesis in individuals with apparently normal chromosomol complements. Tabulation of cases and compilation of genetic data. Birth Defects 1971; 7:215.

Singh DN, Hara S, Foster HW, Grimes EM: Reproductive performance in women with sex chromosome mosaicism. Obstet Gynecol 1980; 55:608.

Singh RP, Carr DH: The anatomy and history of XO human embryos and fetuses. Anat Rec 1966; 155:369.

Sinisi AA, Perrone L, Quarto C, Barone M, Bellastella A, Faggiano M: Dysgerminoma in 45,X Turner syndrome. Report of a case. Clin Endocrinol 1988; 28:187.

Skakkebaek NE: Carcinoma-in-situ of testis in testicular feminization syndrome. Acta Pathol Microbiol Immunol Scand (A) 1979; 87:87.

Skakkebaek NE, Hulten M, Philip J: Quantification of human seminiferous epithelium IV. Histological studies in 17 men with numerical and structural autosomal aberrations. Acta Pathol Microbiol Scand (A) 1973; 81:112.

Skordis NA, Stetka DG, MacGillivray MH, Greenfield SP: Familial 46,XX males coexisting with familial 46,XX true hermaphrodites in same pedigree. J Pediatr 1987; 110:244.

Soderstrom KO: Ultrastructure of the testis in Klinefelter's syndrome. Arch Androl 1984; 13:113.

Sohval AR: The syndrome of pure gonadal dysgenesis. Am J Med 1965; 38:615.

Solish SB, Goldsmith MA, Voutilainen R, Miller WL: Molecular characterization of a Leydig cell tumor presenting as congenital adrenal hyperplasia. J Clin Endocrinol Metab 1989; 69:1148.

Speiser PW, Dupont B, Rubinstein P, Piazza A, Kastelan A, New MI: High frequency of nonclassical steroid 21-hydroxylase deficiency. Am J Hum Genet 1985; 37:650.

Speiser PW, New MI: Genotype hormonal phenotype in nonclassical 21-OH hydroxylase deficiency. J Clin Endocrinol Metab 1987; 64:86.

Speroff L, Glass RH, Kase NG: Clinical Gynecologic Endocrinology and Infertility, 4th ed, Baltimore, Williams & Wilkins, 1989.

Spitz IM, Diamant Y, Rosen E, Bell J, David MB, Polishuk W, Rabinowitz D: Isolated gonadotropin deficiency. A heterogeneous syndrome. N Engl J Med 1974; 290:10.

Strachan T: Molecular pathology of congenital adrenal hyperplasia. Clin Endocrinol 1990; 32:373.

Swaab DF, Hoffman HA: Sexual differentiation of the human hypothalmus: Ontogeny of the sexually dimorphic nucleus of the preoptic area. Brain Res Dev Brain Res 1988; 44:314.

Szamborski J, Obrebski T, Starzynska J: Germ cell tumors in monozygous virus with gonadal dysgenesis and 46 XY karyotype. Obstet Gynecol 1981; 58:120.

Talerman A: Gonadoblastoma and dysgerminoma in two siblings with dysgenetic gonads. Obstet Gynecol 1971; 38:416.

Talerman A, Verp MS, Senekjian E, Gilewski T, Vogelzang N: True hermaphrodite with bilateral ovotestes, gonadoblastoma and dysgerminomas, 46,XX/46,YY karyotype and successful pregnancy. Cancer 1990; 66:2668.

Tannenbaum M: Ultrastructural pathology of adrenal cortex. Pathol Ann 1973; 8:109.

Tarter TH, Kogan SJ: Contralateral testicular disease after unilateral testicular injury. Current concepts. Semin Urol 1988; 6:120.

Thilen A, Larsson A: Congenital adrenal hyperplasia in Sweden 1969–1986. Prevalence symptoms and age at diagnosis. Acta Paediatr Scand 1990;79:168.

Toledo SP, Medeiros-Netoga, Knobel M, Mattar E: Evaluation of the hypothalamic-pituitary gonadal function in the Bardet-Biedl syndrome. Metabolism 1977; 26:1277.

Toscano V, Balducci R, Bianchi P, Mangiantini A, Sciarra F: Ovarian 17-ketosteroid reductase deficiency as a possible cause of polycystic ovarian disease. J Clin Endocrinol Metab 1990; 71:288.

Valenta LJ, Elias AN: Male hypogonadism due to hyperestrogenism. N Engl J Med 1986; 314:186.

van Nickerk WA, Retief AE: The gonads of human true hermaphrodites. Hum Genet 1981; 58:117.

van Niekerk WA: True hermaphroditism. An analytic review with report of 3 new cases. Am J Obstet Gynecol 1976; 126:890.

Vigier B, Forest MG, Eychenne B, Bezard J, Garrigou O, Robel P, Josso N: Anti-Mullerian hormone produces endocrine sex reversal of fetal ovaries. Proc Natl Acad Sci U S A 1989; 86:3684.

Wallace TM, Levine HS: Mixed gonadal dysgenesis. A review of 15 patients reporting single cases of malignant intratubular germ cell neoplasia of the testis, endometrial adenocarcinoma, and a complex vascular anomaly. Arch Pathol Lab Med 1990; 114:679.

Walzer S, Bashir AS, Silbert AR: Cognitive and behavioral factors in the learning disabilities of 47,XXY and 47,XYY boys. Birth Defects 1991; 26:45.

Wang C, Baker HWG, Burger HG, deKretser DM, Hudson B: Hormonal studies in Klinefelter's syndrome. Clin Endocrinol 1975; 4:399.

Weissenbach J, Goodfellow PN, Smith KD: Report of the committee of the genetic constitution of the Y chromosome. Cytogenet Cell Genet 1989; 51:438.

White BJ, Rogal AD, Brown KS, Lieblich JM, Rosen SW: The syndrome of anosmia with hypogonadotropic hypogonadism: A genetic study of 18 new families and a review. Am J Med Genet 1983; 15:417.

White PC, New MI, DuPont B: Congenital adrenal hyperplasia. N Engl J Med 1987; 316:1519.

Wilson JD, Foster DW (Eds): Williams Textbook of Endocrinology, 8th ed. Philadelphia, WB Saunders, 1992.

Wilson JD, George FW, Griffin JE: The hormonal control of sexual development. Science 1981; 211:1278.

Wilson JD, Griffin JE, George FW, Leshin M: The role of gonadal steroids in sexual differentiation. Recent Prog Horm Res 1981; 37:1.

Wischusen J, Baker HWG, Hudson B: Reversible male infertility due to congenital adrenal hyperplasia. Clin Endocrinol 1981; 14:571.

Wu FCW, Butler GE, Kelnar CJH, Stirling HF, Huhtaniemi I: Patterns of pulsatile luteinizing hormone and follicle-stimulating hormone secretion in prepubertal (midchildhood) boys and girls and patients with idiopathic hypogonadotropic hypogonadism (Kallmann's syndrome): A study using an ultrasensitive time-resolved immunofluorometric assay. J Clin Endocrinol Metab 1991; 72:1229.

Yanase T, Simpson ER, Waterman MR: 17-α-Hydroxylase/17,20-lyase deficiency: From clinical investigation to molecular definition. Endocrinol Rev 1991; 12:91.

Yeh J, Rebar RW, Liu JH, Yen SSC: Pituitary function in isolated gonadotropin deficiency. Clin Endocrinol 1989; 31:375.

Zachmann M, Tassinari D, Prader A: Clinical and biochemical variability of congenital adrenal hyperplasia due to 11-β-hydroxylase deficiency. A study of 25 patients. J Clin Endocrinol Metab 1983; 56:222.

Zah W, Kalderon AE, Tucci JR: Mixed gonadal dysgenesis: A case report and a review of the world literature. Acta Endocrinol 1975; 197(Suppl):3.

Zerah M, Schram P, New MI: The diagnosis and treatment of nonclassical 3-β-HSD deficiency. Endocrinologist 1991; 1:75.

Chapter 4

DEVELOPMENTAL ANOMALIES OF THE REPRODUCTIVE ORGANS

Developmental anomalies of the reproductive organs can be divided into two major groups: (1) those linked to single gene defects or chromosomal or developmental syndromes and (2) those that occur sporadically without any obvious link to well-defined syndromes.

The genetic and chromosomal causes of these anomalies have been discussed in Chapter 3. This chapter deals with sporadic developmental anomalies involving the testes, epididymis and excretory ducts, accessory genital glands, scrotum, and penis, i.e., organs that develop from five fetal primordia: genital ridge, mesonephros (wolffian duct and tubules), müllerian duct, urogenital sinus, and genital tubercle (Table 4-1).

ANOMALIES OF THE TESTIS
Cryptorchidism

The term *cryptorchidism* was derived from the Greek words *cryptos* (hidden) and *orchis* (testis) to denote a spectrum of developmental anomalies affecting the scrotal descent of the fetal testes and resulting in their inappropriate positioning. Cryptorchidism generally is used as a synonym for undescended testes, which may be further classified into the following categories:

1. True cryptorchidism
    Abdominal testes
    Inguinal testes
    Suprascrotal testes
    Obstructed testes
2. Ectopic testes
    Under this heading some authors include *retractile* testes, a normal physiologic variant that does not necessitate treatment and represents a variant of normal development found in 10% of boys. An additional group known as *gliding* testes (Hadziselimovic, 1983) or *ascending* testes (Robertson et al., 1988) is occasionally included as an intermediate group between cryptorchid and retractile testes.

Incidence. Testicular descent into the scrotum occurs during the last 3 months of intrauterine life, and in most boys it has been completed by the time of birth. However, in 4% to 6% of boys, testicular descent has not been completed (Scorer, 1964; Chilvers et al., 1984), and either there are no palpable testes in the scrotum or the testes retract into the inguinal canal on palpation. Approximately 20% to 30% of premature babies weighing less than 2500 g have undescended tests (Scorer, 1964; JRHCSG, 1986[a]). However, most of these undescended testes descend during the first 3 months of postnatal life and essentially all do by the end of the first year (Scorer and Farrington, 1971). Thus, if the diagnosis of cryptorchidism is

Table 4-1. Developmental origin of reproductive organs

Fetal structure	Male	Both male and female	Female
Genital ridge	Testis Rete testis (Gubernaculum testis)		Ovary Rete ovarii† Round ligament of uterus
Mesonephros			
Mesonephric tubules	Efferent ductules Aberrant ductules† Paradidymis†		Epoöphoron† Aberrant ductules† Paraoöphoron†
Mesonephric duct	Epididymis Appendix epididymis† Vas deferens Ejaculatory duct Seminal vesicle	Ureter Renal pelvis and collecting tubules Trigone of bladder	Duct of the epoöphoron† Gartner's duct†
Müllerian duct	Appendix testis† Prostatic utricle† Colliculus seminalis		Oviducts Uterus Cervix and upper vagina
Urogenital sinus	Prostate Bulbourethral glands of Cowper Scrotum	Bladder Urethra	Lower vagina Vulva Bartholin's glands Paraurethral glands of Skene
Genital tubercle	Penis		Clitoris

Modified from Gray and Skandalakis. Embryology for Surgeons. Philadelphia, WB Saunders, 1972.
*Embryonic remnants
†Structures that involute during development.

made at a 3-month examination or at 1 year of age, the overall incidence is between 1% and 2% (Scorer and Farrington, 1971). The frequency of cryptorchidism is somewhat higher among preterm than term babies (Scorer and Farrington, 1971).

Chilvers et al. (1984) reported a doubling of frequency of undescended testes in England and Wales from 1962 to 1981. The reasons for this increase are not clear, and a comprehensive study of epidemiology and pathogenetically and clinically important aspects of cryptorchidism is being conducted by the John Radcliffe Hospital Cryptorchidism Study Group (JRHCSG, 1986 [a–c]).

Etiology and pathogenesis. Since 1786, when John Hunter wrote the first major monograph addressing testicular descent into the scrotum, there have been numerous attempts to provide scientific explanation for cryptorchidism. Hunter's dilemma was to determine whether the testis is abnormal and thus does not descend normally or whether the abnormalities noticed in the testis were secondary to its incomplete descent. This dilemma remains incompletely resolved. Three theories prevail:

1. *Gonadal dysgenesis*—This theory suggests that the descent does not occur because the testis is abnormal.
2. *Mechanical*—This hypothesis links cryptorchidism purely to mechanical factors that interfere with testicular descent.

3. *Endocrine*—This theory purports that the maldescent reflects hormonal defects in the developing fetus.

In extreme cases, such as those with an obviously obliterated inguinal canal or with hypothalamic-pituitary disorders or gonadal dysgenesis, the developmental, mechanical, or endocrine etiologies of testicular maldescent are intuitively obvious. However, in most sporadic cases of cryptorchidism such explanations are not so readily apparent.

It is generally accepted that cryptorchidism reflects a disturbance of fetal testicular descent during intrauterine life (reviewed by Hutson and Donahoe, 1986). Testicular descent encompasses three phases:

1. Caudal displacement of the intraabdominal testis because of cranial migration and subsequent regression of the metanephros
2. Transabdominal movement of the testis from the posterior abdominal wall to the inguinal region
3. Descent of the testis through the inguinal canal into the scrotum.

The first phase is completed by 7 weeks, the second by 12 weeks, and the third between 7 months and birth. Disturbance during the last phase accounts for most cases of cryptorchidism.

Several hypotheses have been proposed to explain

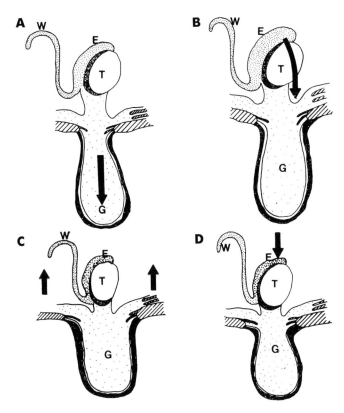

Fig. 4-1. Theories on the transinguinal passage of testes during fetal development. **A,** Traction hypothesis. **B,** Epididymal push hypothesis. **C,** Differential growth hypothesis. **D,** Abdominal pressure hypothesis. (Modified from Hutson JM, Donahoe PK. Endo Rev 1976; 7(3), with permission).

transinguinal passage of the testes (Hutson and Donahoe, 1986; Rajfer, 1987; Editorial, Lancet, 1989):

1. Traction hypothesis
2. Epididymal push hypothesis
3. Differential growth hypothesis
4. Abdominal pressure hypothesis
5. Endocrine hypothesis

The presumptive explanation of testicular maldescent based on these hypotheses schematically is presented in Figure 4-1. However early abnormal developmental events, i.e., those that interfere with normal gonadogenesis or intraabdominal movement of gonads, can also result in testicular maldescent.

The traction theory is based on the assumption that the gubernaculum testis and the cremaster muscle mediate testicular descent by pulling the testis into the scrotum. This hypothesis is based on comparative anatomic studies, and although it may explain the descent of testes in some animals, extrapolation of these data to humans is unwarranted (Rajfer, 1987). There is no evidence that the human fetal gubernaculum, which is composed of loose connective tissue, exerts any traction on the testis. In fact, it appears to act more like a guide than a pulley (Hadziselimovic and Herzog, 1987). The role of the cremaster muscle in testic-

ular descent is even more tenuous since the only function of this muscle appears to be related to retraction of the testes rather than its pulling the testis into the scrotum.

The *epididymal push hypothesis* postulates a propulsive action of the epididymis on the developing testis. Although cryptorchidism often accompanies developmental anomalies of the epididymis in experimental animals, any interference with wolffian duct development may cause cryptorchidism. It is unlikely that this mechanism accounts for more than a small number of human cases of cryptorchidism.

The *differential growth hypothesis* suggests that the difference in the growth of testes and the gubernaculum on the one hand and the body wall on the other leads to an upward growth of the inguinal canal, which finally encloses the relatively immobile testis. However, since there is no evidence that the gubernaculum grows more slowly than the body as a whole, this theory remains highly speculative.

The *abdominal pressure hypothesis* relates testicular descent to increased intraabdominal pressure generated by the growing viscera. Intraabdominal pressure has been shown to play an important role in testicular descent in experimental animals, but its function during human development remains incompletely appreciated (Hutson and Donahoe, 1986).

There are several *endocrine hypotheses,* all of which are based on overwhelming evidence that endocrine factors play a crucial role in regulating normal testicular descent (reviewed by Hutson et al. 1990). An intact hypothalamic-pituitary-testicular axis seems to be essential for normal testicular development and descent; cryptorchidism is a constant feature of hypogonadotropic hypogonadism (Rajfer, 1987). Besides gonadotropins, sex hormones and the anti-müllerian hormone (AMH) have been implicated. Hutson and Donahoe (1986) have proposed a biphasic model of testicular descent suggesting that the AMH regulates the transabdominal migration of the testes to the internal inguinal ring, whereas dihydrotestosterone plays a crucial role during the transinguinal passage of the testis. Clinical data from patients with persistent müllerian duct syndrome and testicular feminization support this model. Experimental data on mice treated prenatally with estrogens further support this hypothesis, since it is known that estrogens prevent müllerian ducts from involuting, likely by inhibiting the action of AMH on its target organs. Since exposure of male fetuses to estrogen or diethylstilbestrol in utero is related to an increased frequency of testicular maldescent, it seems plausible that sex hormones and AMH influence testicular descent during fetal life.

Clinical studies of the association of cryptorchidism to other disorders provide evidence for the role of central neuroendocrine and local anatomic factors. Cryptorchidism is common in patients suffering from mental retardation, cerebral palsy (Cortada and Kousseff, 1984), and de-

Partial list of congenital malformations and developmental syndromes associated with cryptorchidism

Chromosomal syndromes
  XXXXY
  Trisomy 13
  Trisomy 18
  Trisomy 21
  Deletion of long arm of chromosome 21
  Deletion of short arm of chromosome 4
Acrocephalosyndactyly
Basal cell nevus syndrome
Carpenter's syndrome
Cockayne's syndrome
Cornelia de Lange's syndrome
Fanconi's syndrome
Fraser's syndrome
Hallermann-Streiff syndrome
Lenz's microphthalmia
Leopard syndrome
Meckel's syndrome
Noonan's syndrome
Occulocerebrorenal syndrome of Lowe
Opitz's syndrome
Osteochondritis dissecans
Prader-Willi syndrome
Prune-belly syndrome
Rubinstein-Taybi syndrome
Russell-Silver syndrome
Smith-Lemli-Opitz Syndrome
van Beuthrem syndrome
Zellweger syndrome

Based on data compiled by Nistal and Paniagua, 1984.

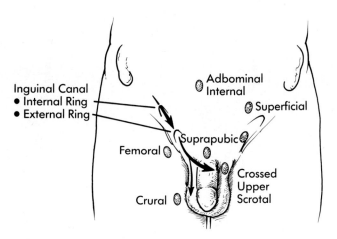

Fig. 4-2. Most common locations of ectopic testes. (Modified from Fonkalsrud and Mengel, 1981, with permission).

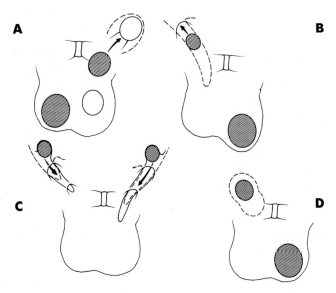

Fig. 4-3. Four types of cryptorchid testes. **A,** High scrotal testes. **B,** Intracanalicular testes. **C,** Intraabdominal testes. **D,** Obstructed testes. (Modified from Scorer CG, Farrington GH. Congenital Deformities of the Testis and Epididymis. New York, Appleton-Century Crofts, 1971, with permission).

velopmental anomalies of the central nervous system (Kropp and Voeller, 1981).

Familial cases of cryptorchidism have been reported (Jones and Young, 1982). An increased incidence of cryptorchidism has been reported among close relatives; 1.5% to 4% of fathers and 6.2% brothers of an affected propositus likewise have cryptorchidism (Czeizel et al., 1981a and b). However, the discordance of cryptorchidism in identical twins indicates that in most instances there are no genetic causes of cryptorchidism. An increased incidence of undescended testes is a feature of at least 40 congenital disorders (Griffin and Wilson, 1992). Some of the syndromes commonly associated with cryptorchidism have been reviewed by Nistal and Paniagua (1984) and are listed in the box above.

The association of cryptorchidism with developmental anomalies of the urogenital system such as ureteral duplication (Fram et al., 1982), posterior ureteric valves (Krueger et al., 1980), and hypospadias (Shima et al., 1979) indicates that local morphogenetic disturbances affecting the embryonic field. Malformations of the epididymis are es-

pecially common, reflecting the close relationship of the testis and its appendages during development (Koff and Scaletscky, 1990).

An increased incidence of cryptorchidism (5.5%) was found after exposure to diethystilbestrol in utero (Gill et al., 1979). Although Depue (1984) suggested that endogenous hyperestrinism in obese women might be related to cryptorchidism in offspring, Davies et al. (1986) doubt that endogenous hyperestrinism plays a significant role. These authors likewise found no adverse effects from oral contraceptives taken within 1 year before conception. They did, however, report a possible link with placental insufficiency, as evidenced by the positive correlation between the incidence of threatened abortions and cryptorchidism in offspring. They speculated that this correla-

Table 4-2. Fertility of men with cryptorchidism

Author	Year	Age (yr) at treatment*	Definition of Fertile	Number of Fertile Men with Bilateral Cryptorchidism/total	(%)	Unilateral Number of Fertile Men with Unilateral Cryptorchidism/Total	(%)
Hand	1956	(2–73)	Pregnancy	15/24	(63%)	47/61	(77%)
Albescu et al.	1971	11 (6–15)	60 million sperm/ml	11/22	(50%)	20/21	(95%)
Werder et al.	1976	11 (5–17)	40 million sperm/ml	4/14	(29%)	20/23	(87%)
Richter et al.	1976	NR	20 million sperm/ml	19/50	(38%)	15/28	(54%)
Dickerman et al.	1979	NR	12 million sperm/ml	2/21	(10%)	18/47	(38%)
Gilhooly et al.	1984	8 (1–13)	Pregnancy	16/45	(36%)	80/100	(80%)
Chilvers et al.	1986	NR	20 million sperm/ml	82/331	(25%)	343/600	(57%)
Total				149/507	(29%)	543/800	(62%)

From data compiled by Rajfer, 1990.
*Mean age is given if available; range is in parentheses; NR = not reported.

Table 4-3. Sperm counts in patients with a history of cryptorchidism

	Treatment	Number of azoospermic men/total (%)	Number of oligospermic men/total (%)	Number of azoospermic + oligospermic men/total (%)
Unilateral	None	1/14 (7%)	9/14 (64%)	27/61 (44%)
	Orchiopexy with or without hCG	72/519 (14%)	124/406 (31%)	257/600 (43%)
Bilateral	None	16/20 (80%)	4/20 (20%)	20/20 (100%)
	Orchiopexy with or without hCG	105/248 (42%)	76/248 (31%)	249/331 (75%)

Modified from Chilvers C et al. J Pediatr Surg 1986; 21:691, with permission.

tion may reflect decreased levels of maternal human chorionic gonadotropin (hCG) and reduced fetal testosterone.

In summary, the data from the literature do not provide a definitive explanation for cryptorchidism. One safely can say that there is no single cause and that in most instances the defect is the end result of an interaction between hormonal and local morphogenetic events.

Clinical findings. The diagnosis of cryptorchidism is made by palpating the scrotum. If no testes can be palpated, one must decide whether the condition represents cryptorchidism, testicular ectopia, or retractile testes. By definition, a cryptorchid testis is located within the normal path of testicular descent and cannot be repositioned manually into the scrotum (Jarow, 1990). Ectopic testes are found outside the normal path of descent (Fonkalsrud and Mengel, 1981). They may form an abnormal mass adjacent to a normally descended testis with an impalpable testis contralaterally (Dickinson and Hewett, 1991). Most often, ectopic testes present as an inguinal or femoral hernia, a midline mass, or a mass in the upper scrotum or crural region (Fig. 4-2).

Cryptorchid testes must be distinguished from retractile testes. The latter can be brought easily into the scrotum but retract upon release into the inguinal canal because of an overactive cremasteric reflex. Retractile testes account

for most cases of cryptorchidism referred to pediatric surgeons (Abney and Keel, 1990).

Cryptorchidism can be bilateral or, more commonly, unilateral. Scorer and Farrington (1971) recognize four types of cryptorchid testes (Fig. 4-3):

1. Intraabdominal testes, not accessible to palpation, which account for 10% of cases.
2. Intracanalicular testes, located in the inguinal canal, account for 20% of cases.
3. High scrotal testes which account for 40% of cases.
4. Obstructed testes, those retained by connective tissue cords between the inguinal pouch and the scrotal inlet, which account for 30% of cases.

Since the abnormality can be recognized early in life, surgery typically is performed between the child's first and second birthdays for cosmetic reasons and prevention of the most important postpubertal complication—infertility (Jarow, 1990). The reported beneficial effects of orchiopexy vary from one study to another (Table 4-2 and Table 4-3). The results of treatment are better for unilateral cryptorchid testes than bilateral ones (Table 4-4). Infertility is more common in men with bilateral cryptorchidism. Interestingly, however, men with unilateral cryptorchidism frequently show abnormal spermatogenesis in the contralat-

Table 4-4. Effect of age at treatment on sperm count*

Reference	Age at treatment for bilateral cryptorchidism		Age at treatment for unilateral cryptorchidism	
	<8 years (%)	>9 years (%)	<8 years (%)	>9 years (%)
Hortling et al., 1967	5/9 (56)	9/13 (69)	2/5 (40)	3/14 (21)
Knorr, 1979	8/11 (73)	27/38 (71)	11/13 (85)	28/59 (47)
Wojciechowski et al., 1977	29/36 (81)	12/12 (100)	31/71 (44)	20/35 (57)
Total	42/56 (75)	48/63 (76)	44/89 (49)	51/108 (47)

Modified from Chilvers C et al. J Pediatr Surg 1986; 21:691, with permission.
*Number in the table are (azoospermic cases + oligospermic cases)/(total cases).

eral descended testis. The role of adjuvant hormonal therapy, usually with gonadotropin-releasing hormone (GnRH) antagonists, remains to be evaluated fully (Palmer, 1991).

Cryptorchidism is associated with an increased incidence of testicular cancer. According to Strader et al. (1988), the relative risk is 5.9. In unilateral cryptorchidism the undescended testis is at a higher risk for neoplasia, but the incidence of tumors in the contralateral testis is also increased.

Orchiopexy in early life does not eliminate the risk of cancer. Carcinoma in situ is found in 2% to 3% of men with a history of cryptorchidism (Giwercman et al., 1989). Overall, the risk is higher with bilateral cryptorchidism and is highest in men with abdominal testes and those who did not have orchiopexy in infancy (Palmer, 1991). Approximately 10% of all men with testicular cancer have had cryptorchidism (Whitaker, 1988).

Pathology. Cryptorchid testes generally are smaller than normal even after orchiopexy. Their size varies and depends primarily on their original site of retention. Puri and Sparnon (1990) reported the following values: Normal adult testes have a volume of 20.8 ± 4.3 ml; repositioned abdominal testes measure 4.9 ± 3.5 ml; intracanalicular 9.8 ± 4.4 ml; and those from the superior inguinal pouch 17.0 ± 4.9 ml. The contralateral testis of patients with unilateral cryptorchidism has the same volume as a normal testis.

The histologic appearance of cryptorchid testes varies depending on the age of the patient and the extent of injury. In normal boys a surge of luteinizing hormone and follicle-stimulating hormone occurs at 60 to 90 days postpartum (Fig. 4-4). This surge stimulates the infant's Leydig cells to proliferate (Hadziselimovic et al., 1986). Stimulated Leydig cells secrete testosterone. Androgens induce the first transformation of gonocytes into dark spermatogonia, which represent precursors of spermatocytic cells. In cryptorchidism the surge of gonadotropins is blunted, and the usual sequelae do not occur. Understimulated Leydig cells do not release enough testosterone to effect transformation of the infant's gonocytes. Thus, cryptorchid testes have fewer Leydig cells and more fetal gonocytes than age-matched normal testes. The total number of germ cells in the cryptorchid testis is comparable to the number of germ cells in control testes, but the ratio of differentiated gonocytes to spermatogonia is at the fetal level (Huff et al., 1991). The second wave of differentiation, i.e., transformation of dark spermatogonia into primary spermatocytes at the age of 3 years, also is defective, and this contributes further to the reduced number of germ cells in the adult testis (Huff et al., 1989). The obvious differences between the cryptorchid testes and the age-matched control testes become apparent during the third year of life (Hedinger, 1982). Whereas the number of germ cells increases in normal prepubertal testes, the number of germ cells in cryptorchid testes remains low (Fig. 4-5). Bilateral cryptorchid testes are identical to unilateral cryptorchid testes in this respect, although in the latter cases, the scrotal testes show normal germ cell counts (Hedinger, 1982). Abdominal testes show an even more pronounced reduction of germ cells (Salle et al., 1968). Retractile testes, considered by some to be the mildest form of testicular maldescent, have germ cell counts only mildly reduced (Saito and Kumamoto, 1989). Thus, it follows that the degree of testicular maldescent correlates with the extent of germ cell injury and ultimately with reproductive potential.

Histopathologic changes in cryptorchid testes have been studied systematically (Nistal et al., 1980; Hedinger, 1982; Schindler et al., 1987; Huff et al., 1989; Cortes and Thorup, 1991). The changes vary from one case to another and depend on the age of the patient, location of the testis, and the mode of treatment (Figs. 4-6 to 4-8).

A semiquantitative system for the evaluation of testicular lesions in the testes at the time of orchiopexy has been devised by Nistal et al. (1980). This classification takes into account the tubular fertility index (TFI = tubules with germ cells expressed as the percentage of all tubules) (Mack et al., 1961; Lipshultz et al., 1976); the number of Sertoli cells per tubular cross section; and the mean tubular diameter (MTD).

Nistal et al. (1980) consider germinal cell hypoplasia as slight, moderate, or marked if the tubular fertility index is greater than 50%, 30% to 50%, or less than 30%, respec-

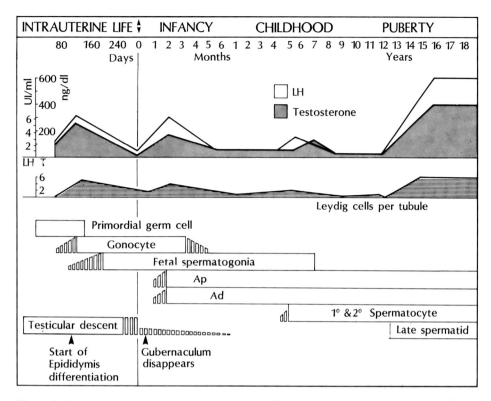

Fig. 4-4. Testicular development in relationship to LH and testosterone secretion in early life. (From Hadziselimovic, 1991).

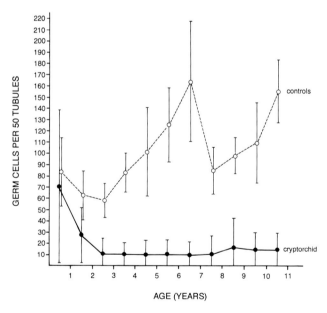

Fig. 4-5. Cryptorchid testes. Contain fewer germ cells than normal testes. (Modified from Hedinger CE. Eur J Pediatr 1982; 139:266, with permission).

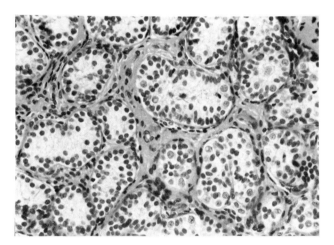

Fig. 4-6. Cryptorchid testis from a 2-year-old boy contains a reduced number of germ cells.

tively. The Sertoli cell index (SCI) allows one to classify testes as normal for age or as showing Sertoli's cell hypoplasia (less than one third below normal for the patient's age) or Sertoli cell hyperplasia (one third above normal for the patient's age). It should be noted that SCI decreases

from 40 ± 3 at birth to 10 ± 1 in adulthood (Hadziselimovic and Seguchi, 1974). Tubular hypoplasia is considered mild if the reduction of the MTD is less than 30% and severe if the reduction is 30% or more. Focal tubular lesions such as hypoplastic tubules and megatubules, ring tubules, and calcospherites are also taken into account.

On the basis of these criteria, Nistal et al. (1980) have

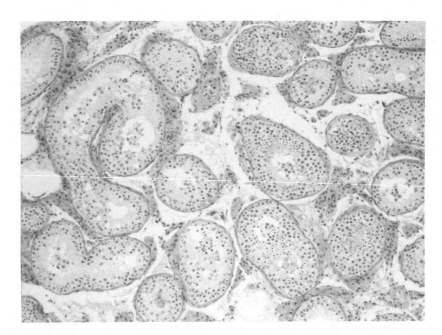

Fig. 4-7. Postpubertal cryptorchid testis shows a lack of spermatogenesis, interstitial edema and fibrosis.

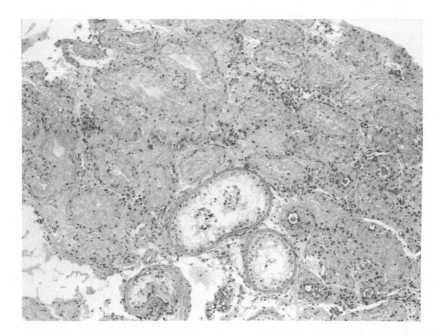

Fig. 4-8. Cryptorchid testis from an adult man shows extensive fibrosis and tubular hyalinization.

classified prepubertal cryptorchid testes into four categories as follows:

I. Minimal changes, characterized by normal TFI, normal SCI, normal MTD, or mild tubular hypoplasia with some focal lesions, such as megatubules or calcospherites.

II. Marked germinal hypoplasia, evidenced by a markedly reduced TFI; SCI is normal; MTD shows signs of slight or marked tubular hypoplasia; focal lesions such as ring tubules or calcospherites are present.

III. Diffuse tubular hypoplasia, evidenced in reduced TFI and MTD; SCI indicates Sertoli cell hypoplasia; megatubules and calcospherites are commonly found.

IV. Diffuse Sertoli cell hyperplasia, evidenced by an increased SCI; TFI is variable, ranging from marked to severe hypoplasia. The MTD varies

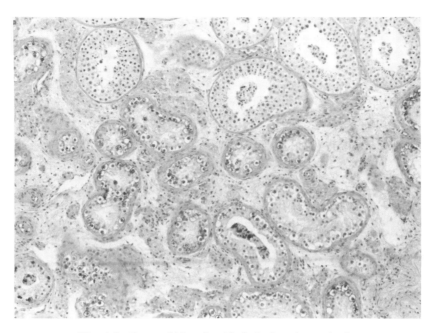

Fig. 4-9. Cryptorchid testis with foci of carcinoma in situ.

from normal to slight to marked hypoplasia. Sertoli cells often are pseudostratified and prominently expand the tubules. The TFI is variable, reflecting marked to severe hypoplasia. The MTD varies in a range from normal to severe hypoplasia. Ring tubules, megatubules, and calcospherites are seen focally. Vacuolated Leydig cells are seen in testes that have undergone biopsy during the first year of life.

Using these criteria, Nistal et al. (1980) classified testes from 203 patients and found that 26% showed type I lesions, 24% type II lesions, 33% type III lesions, and 17% type IV lesions. Type III and IV lesions are more often accompanied by focal dysgenesis of seminiferous tubules and abnormal forms of tubules. Type I lesions predominate in obstructed testes, type II and III lesions in high scrotal or intracanalicular testes, and type IV lesions in intraabdominal testes. The long-term follow-up, which is incomplete in the study of Nistal et al. (1980), indicates that spermatogenesis evolves normally only in testes with type I lesions.

Approximately 25% of descended testes show the same lesions as the unilateral cryptorchid testis. In bilateral cryptorchid testes, 80% show identical lesion types. Contralateral scrotal testes show the same abnormalities as the cryptorchid testes. Even the descended prepubertal testes have a reduced total number of germ cells and delayed maturation as evidenced by a lack of transformation of dark spermatogonia into spermatocytes (Huff et al., 1989).

Additional findings. In a considerable number of patients, testicular maldescent is accompanied by epididymal abnormalities (Koff and Scaletsky, 1990). These primarily present as abnormalities of size, shape, or positioning of the head, body, and tail of the epididymis. In a minority of cases there is separation of the testis from the epididymis and constriction or atresia of the excretory ducts. In approximately 15% of cases there is an inguinal hernia (Nistal and Paniagua, 1984); a small number of patients may have concomitant hydrocele. An incarcerated inguinal hernia may cause testicular ischemia, but these changes are distinct from those seen in cryptorchid testes (Hadziselimovic et al., 1991).

Testicular torsion is an important complication. It may occur even prenatally and may account for a certain number of congenital cases of unilateral agenesis of the testis (Huff et al., 1991).

Cryptorchid testes in adults show a marked reduction in spermatogenic cells (Blumer and Hedinger, 1989; Giwercman et al., 1989). Untreated and surgically repositioned testes show essentially identical changes. Blumer and Hedinger (1989) could not find any germ cells in orchidectomy specimens from 52% of the cryptorchid men they examined and in 46% of cryptorchid men with orchiopexy. Giwercman et al. (1989) found advanced spermatogenesis in only 37% of cryptorchid testes. Orchiopexy apparently has almost no beneficial effect on spermatogenesis. The one normal scrotal testis, however, usually is enough to preserve fertility (Gilhooly et al., 1984; Fallon and Kennedy, 1985).

Approximately 2% to 3% of adult cryptorchid testes contain atypical germ cells arranged in nests of carcinoma in situ (Fig. 4-9). It has been argued that orchiopexy should be performed as soon as possible to prevent subsequent malignancy, but it seems that even early surgical repositioning of cryptorchid testes does not decrease the risk of cancer (Giwercman et al., 1989). It is not possible to

Table 4-5. Syndromes of fetal testicular insufficiency in 46, XY individuals

Timing of injury (stage of fetal life in weeks)	Syndrome	Gonadal pathology	External genitalia	Internal genitalia
<8	46, XY Pure gonadal dysgenesis	Streak gonad	Female	Female
8–10	46, XY Gonadal dysgenesis	Streak gonad or testicular remnants	Female or ambiguous	Female or ambiguous
12–14	Anorchia	No testes or fibrous remnants	Male	Male
>14	Rudimentary testes	Rudimentary testes	Male (micropenis)	Male

predict from biopsies at the time of orchiopexy which testes will retain spermatogenic cells, which will undergo complete involution and atropy, and which will give rise to tumors. Most likely, the final outcome depends on several factors: the degree of immaturity and the developmental arrest, the location of the testis, and the timing of the orchiopexy. The possibility that some cryptorchid testes are dysgenetic, as proposed by Sohval (1957), and therefore carry an inherent predisposition to neoplasia irrespective of their location cannot be excluded.

Anorchia

Anorchia is defined as congenital absence of one or both testes in genetically male individuals who have otherwise normal male genitalia. Unilateral anorchia is also called monorchia or unilateral testicular regression syndrome (Smith et al., 1991).

Incidence and pathogenesis. Bilateral anorchia occurs in 1 of 20,000 males, and monorchia in 1 of 5000 (Bobrow and Gough, 1970). Unilateral anorchia is a consequence of abnormal morphogenesis of the testis or testicular injury during intrauterine life. Current evidence favors the latter hypothesis, suggesting that in most instances the testis disappears because of an infarction (Smith et al., 1991). Unilateral developmental anomalies involving the kidney and seminal vesicles are occasionally associated with ipsilateral monorchia (Das and Amar, 1980).

Bilateral anorchia also may be a consequence of testicular regression after an intrauterine insult or developmental event affecting the developing testes. In the study of Smith et al. (1991), 2.5% of cases of testicular regression syndrome were bilateral. The occurrence of anorchia in several members of the same family has also been reported (Hall et al., 1975).

Bilateral anorchia is closely related to several other developmental syndromes such as the vanishing testes syndrome, embryonic testicular regression syndrome, XY gonadal dysgenesis, XY gonadal agenesis, and rudimentary testis syndrome (Grumbach and Conte, 1992). These terms describe a spectrum of partially overlapping developmental anomalies in which the testis has either disappeared or regressed to a nonfunctioning rudiment during fetal development. If the testis does not develop in a 46, XY individual

or involutes before the eighth week of fetal life, i.e., before the masculinization of external genitalia has been initiated, the genitalia will be phenotypically female and the syndrome will correspond to 46, XY gonadal dysgenesis. Damage to fetal testes between the eighth and tenth weeks of gestation results in gonadal agenesis or dysgenesis with female (Coulam, 1978) or ambiguous external genitalia (Sarto and Opitz, 1973). Testicular involution between weeks 12 and 14 of intrauterine life, i.e., after masculinization of external genitalia is completed, is associated with anorchia and male external genital organs (Goldberg et al., 1974). Incomplete regression of fetal testes after the early critical periods results in rudimentary testes, micropenis, and male ejaculatory ducts (Bergada et al., 1962; Najjar et al., 1974). An overview of embryolnic events leading to anorchia and related developmental syndromes caused by presumptive fetal testicular damage or insufficiency is outlined in Table 4-5 (Coulam, 1978; Grumbach and Conte, 1992).

Pathology. Histologic findings of tissue removed during exploration usually are nonspecific. Kogan et al. (1986) have studied 65 cases of monorchia and have found that only 14% of their cases were devoid of testicular tissue or müllerian remnants that would suggest true agenesis of the testis. In 69%, a blind-ended spermatic cord was found usually with a fibrovascular nubbin. These nubbins contained wolffian structures (83%) and calcifications or hemosiderin (20%). Smith et al. (1991) have performed a comprehensive study of testicular remnants in 75 patients with unilateral anorchia and 2 patients with bilateral anorchia. In 79% of the cases they identified an intrascrotal vas deferens; in 36% an epididymis; and in 4% residual seminiferous tubules. The typical gonadal residues consisted of fibrovascular tissue in which the investigator could identify adipose tissue in 44%, nerve tissue in 56%, and atrophic striated muscle in 57% of cases. In two cases a well-demarcated fibrous nodule was found. Calcifications and iron pigment deposits were seen in 42% of cases, occasionally accompanied by a giant cell reaction. These findings suggest that unilateral anorchia represents, indeed, testicular regression and likely is caused by a prenatal vascular incident, probably a hemorrhagic infarction. The theory of an intrauterine vascular occlusion is indirectly supported by the fact that a testicular remnant resides on the left in 60% to 80% of cases (Honoré, 1978; Smith et al., 1991), which correlates well with a greater susceptibility of left-sided testes to torsion and infarction (Burge, 1987). These explanations of anorchia are conjectural, however, and the true cause of testicular regression is not evident in most cases.

The contralateral testis in monorchia is anatomically normal and usually shows compensatory enlargement (Koff, 1991). The extent of hypertrophy depends on the magnitude of testicular volume reduction, the age of injury, and the status of the descended testis. This finding is clinically important and provides the surgeon exploring the scrotum with the possibility of making a diagnosis of unilateral anorchia or cryptorchidism—a dilemma that can be solved definitively only by laparoscopy (Guiney et al., 1989). The scrotal testis is enlarged in the former condition and normal sized in the latter.

Histologically, the descended testis shows an increased number of Leydig cells, more germ cells, and a higher rate of transformation of adult dark spermatogonia into primary spermatocytes than in the contralateral descended testis of patients with unilateral cryptorchidism (Huff et al., 1991). These data are consistent with a mechanical explanation for monorchia and support the notion that the pathogenesis of unilateral anorchia differs from that of unilateral cryptorchidism. The descended testes in monorchia function normally and most adults are fertile.

Polyorchidism

Polyorchidism is a developmental anomaly resulting in supernumerary testes. This is a rare urologic curiosity with less than 60 documented cases recorded in the literature (Rudy, 1989). Most cases show triorchidism, and only one histologically verified case of tetraorchidism is on record (Snow et al., 1985).

Leung (1988) reviewed the pathogenesis of this condition and concluded that all cases could be explained by invoking transverse division or doubling of the genital ridge during gonadogenesis, probably by a peritoneal fibrous band. The third testis may be located in the scrotum above or below the normal testes, in the inguinal canal, in the abdominal cavity, or in the groin (Leung, 1988; Rudy, 1989). The supernumerary testis usually has its own epididymis. The epididymis may have no connection to an excretory duct, or it may extend into a vas deferens that is in most cases confluent with the normal testis on the same side. Reduplication of the vas deferens also has been reported (Fig. 4-10).

Polyorchidism does not cause infertility per se. However, it may be associated with other scrotal anomalies such as hydrocele, torsion, and varicocele. It predisposes to infection and torsion of the testis to which it is attached (Rudy, 1989). It is most important not to mistake this anomaly for a tumor. Surgical removal should be carefully

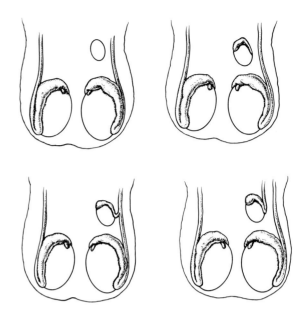

Fig. 4-10. Different forms of polyorchidism. (From Leung AKC. Am Fam Phys 1988; 38:153, © Bert Oppenheim. Redrawn with permission).

planned to avoid overtreatment and inadvertent damage to the normal testes, excretory ducts, and intrascrotal vasculature.

Various testicular and paratesticular anomalies

Hamartomas, inclusions, embryonic rests, and related developmental anomalies have little impact on fertility. Nevertheless, such lesions can be misdiagnosed on gross examination or histologic examination of tissues removed during surgical evaluation of infertile patients. Detailed descriptions of these lesions can be found in the monographs on urogenital pathology of Nistal and Paniagua (1984), Hill (1989), and Murphy (1989) or in clinical textbooks of urology (Gillenwater et al., 1991).

Embryonic remnants

Appendix testis (hydatid of Morgagni) is a cystic structure varying in diameter from a few millimeters to several centimeters and attached to the anterior side of the upper pole of the testis. It represents a blind residue of the proximal portion of the müllerian duct, and it is found in more than 90% of men. Histologically, it is composed of fibromuscular tissue strands lined by cuboidal cells forming glandlike structures that resemble oviductal epithelium. This epithelial lining is in continuity with the mesothelium of the tunica vaginalis.

Appendix epididymis is a cystic structure attached to the head of the epididymis. This remnant of the wolffian duct is found in 25% of men. It is composed of fibromuscular tissue encircling glandlike spaces, which are lined with columnar vacuolated cells.

Aberrant ducts (Haller's organ) are derived from incompletely involuted mesonephric ducts. They are located

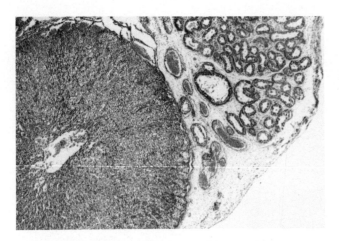

Fig. 4-11. Adrenal choristoma in adronogenital syndrome.

Causes of hydrocele

1. Congenital
   Incomplete closure of processus vaginalis
   Persistent inclusion of processus vaginalis in the cord
2. Infectious
   Sexually transmitted
   Filariasis
3. Tumors
4. Trauma
5. Iatrogenic
   Scrotal surgery
   Renal transplantation
6. Idiopathic

along the body of the epididymis and are lined by cuboidal or columnar epithelium.

Paradidymis comprises a group of small ducts derived from the remnants of the caudal portion of the mesonephric ducts; hence, they are histologically indistinguishable from the aberrant ducts. The paradidymis is found in the spermatic cord.

Testicular and epididymal appendages are usually asymptomatic, although occasionally they necessitate scrotal exploration because of enlargement, cystic dilatation, or even torsion (Virdi et al., 1991).

Choristomas

Adrenal choristomas, according to Dahl and Dahn (1962), are small yellow nodules composed of adrenal cells that can be found along the spermatic cord or epididymis, on the tunica albuginea, or in the testis of 15% of newborn males. They vary in size up to several millimeters. In adrenogenital syndrome, adrenal rests may assume tumorlike proportions (Fig. 4-11) and cannot be readily distinguished from Leydig cell tumors (Rutgers et al. 1988, Knudsen et al. 1991). An ectopic pheochromocytoma of the spermatic cord was described by Eusebi and Masserilli in 1971.

In *splenic choristomas,* splenic tissue may be attached to the testis or paratesticular structures, almost always on the left side. Splenic gonadal fusion may be continuous when the splenic fragment is linked to the normal spleen by a fibrous strand or may be discontinuous (Ceccacci and Tosi, 1981; Gouw et al., 1985). This anomaly is often associated with cryptorchidism, hernias, and multiple congenital malformations.

Cysts

Hydrocele is defined as fluid between the layers of the space of the scrotum lined by the tunica vaginalis. Hydrocele is common in children and is usually related to incomplete closure of the processus vaginalis or its incomplete obliteration. It is often associated with an inguinal hernia. In adults, hydrocele may accompany other intrascrotal and several extrascrotal diseases and/or events (box above).

The lumen of the hydrocele contains serous fluid; the cavity is lined with mesothelium (Nistal and Paniagua, 1984). Infected hydroceles contain turbid fluid, and their wall is thickened because of chronic inflammation. Acute hydrocele is usually a symptom of an underlying disease but in itself it has no effect on fertility (Politoff et al.; 1990). Bilateral long-standing hydrocele, especially if infected, may cause testicular atrophy and inflammation or compression of the epididymis.

Epidermoid cysts are keratin-filled inclusion cysts lined with squamous epithelium. These may be found in the testis or epididymis, accounting for approximately 1% of all surgically resected testicular masses (Malek et al., 1986). On average, epidermoid cysts measure 1 cm in diameter, although occasionally they may expand up to 10 cm in diameter.

Simple cysts are dilated epithelium-lined spaces measuring 5 to 15 mm in diameter found in the testis or the epididymis. These cysts may be detected by ultrasonography (Kratzik et al., 1989). Most of these cysts are either inclusion or retention cysts derived from various scrotal structures and are lined with nondescript flattened, squamous, columnar, or transitional epithelium (Tammela et al., 1991).

Spermatoceles are protrusions of the epididymis that are filled with milky fluid and lined by cuboidal epithelium. They stem from the efferent ducts. Spermatozoa in various stages of degeneration typically are found in the lumen.

Congenital cystic dysplasia, or multicystic dysplasia of the hilar portion of the testis and epididymis, is a rare congenital anomaly described by Leissring and Oppenheimer (1973). It seldom occurs but always is associated with renal agenesis (Nistal et al., 1984; Wegmann et al., 1984).

Acquired cystic dilatation of the rete testis has been described in patients undergoing chronic dialysis (Nistal et al., 1989).

CONGENITAL ANOMALIES OF THE EPIDIDYMIS AND VAS DEFERENS

Anomalies of the epididymis and vas deferens can be classified as follows:

1. Configurational anomalies of size, shape, and positioning
2. Congenital aplasia, obliteration, or interruption
3. Obstruction
4. Duplication

Anomalies of the epididymis and ductus deferens may present as isolated defects or in conjunction with other anomalies of wolffian duct derivatives. Some cases are associated with congenital defects of the seminal vesicles (Hirsch and Lipshultz, 1985; Goldstein and Schlossberg, 1988). A significant number of cryptorchid testes are associated with epididymal anomalies (Marshall and Shermeta, 1979; Heath et al., 1984; Koff and Scaletscky, 1990).

Configurational anomalies of the epididymis

The normal epididymis is closely apposed to the lateral side of the testis. The head of the epididymis is tightly attached to the upper pole of the testis, whereas the body can be drawn apart from the testis by inserting a finger into what is appropriately called the digital fossa (Scorer and Farrington, 1971). The tail is held firmly caudally by the connective tissue remnants of the gubernaculum.

Scorer and Farrington (1971) classify epididymal aberrations into five categories:

1. Extended epididymis
2. Detached epididymis
3. Angled epididymis
4. Disruption of the continuity of vas or epididymis
5. Epididymis with mesorchium

All these anomalies are encountered more frequently in men with cryptorchidism than in men with normally located testes. Scorer and Farrington (1971) analyzed 54 epididymal abnormalities and described 69% as extended, 13% as having a detached epididymal tail, 17% showing total detachment, and 9% having an acutely angled epididymal body. Some cases had more than one anomaly.

Epididymal positioning that is anterior rather than lateral to the testis occurs in 10% to 15% of males (Beccia et al., 1976). It is not clear whether this has any impact on fertility.

Congenital aplasia, obstruction, or interruption of the epididymis

Congenital defects of the epididymis may present in several forms (Scorer and Farrington, 1971; Kroovand and Perlmutter, 1981) (Fig. 4-12). They include:

1. Agenesis of all mesonephric duct derivatives.
2. Interruption of vasa efferentia or nonunion of the globus major of the epididymis and the testis. Vasa

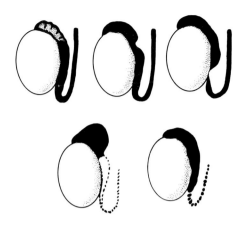

Fig. 4-12. Congenital defects of the epididymis. (Modified from Nistal and Paniagua, 1984; and Scorer and Farrington, 1971).

efferentia may end in blind loops, and the fibrous strands connecting the testis with the epididymis do not contain patent ducts.
3. Cystic dilatation of the head of the epididymis with obliteration of the rete-epididymal junction.
4. Constriction of the midportion of the body of the epididymis with agenesis or atresia of the ducts. This may cause complete separation of the head from the body of the epididymis.
5. Agenesis or atresia of the tail of the epididymis and the vas deferens.
6. Distal ectopia of epididymal tissue (Ayano et al., 1982).

The most common cause of obstructive azoospermia is the absence of the vas deferens followed by obstruction of the distal epididymis and obstruction between the head of the epididymis and rete testis.

Congenital anomalies of the vas deferens

Scorer and Farrington (1971) classify congenital defects of the vas deferens into the following categories:

1. Obliteration of a short segment of the vas that is transformed into a fibrous streak
2. Complete agenesis of a short segment of the vas
3. Failure of the vas to canalize, although it appears continuous and normal on external examination
4. Complete agenesis of the vas beyond a short stump that is attached to the tail of the epididymis

Congenital defects of the epididymis or the vas deferens may be unilateral or bilateral (Girgis et al., 1969). Sporadic as well as familial cases have been described (Schellen and Van Straaten, 1980; Padron and Mas, 1991).

Ipsilateral renal agenesis is found in 79% of cases of unilateral agenesis of the vas deferens (Donahue and Fauver, 1989). These findings reflect a disturbance in the development of the mesonephric (wolffian) duct derivatives; i.e., the ureteric bud and the primordium of the vas deferens. The ureteric bud does not grow cranially to reach the metanephrogenic blastema, and does not induce kidney formation, and the primordium of the vas deferens and epididymis does not interconnect with the testis.

Bilateral agenesis of the vas deferens is encountered with bilateral renal agenesis (Potter's syndrome), but that condition usually is lethal. Sporadic bilateral agenesis of the vas deferens accounts for about 10% of primary obstructive azoospermia (Girgis et al., 1969). Remarkable results have been reported by using epididymal sperm from men with these obstructions for in vitro fertilization (Silber et al., 1990), indicating that bilateral agenesis of vas deferens is not an untreatable cause of infertility any longer.

Complex obstructions of excretory ducts

Approximately 80% of patients with cystic fibrosis are sterile and show atresia of mesonephric duct derivatives (Holsclaw et al., 1971). Numerous abnormalities have been described, including obliteration and atresia of the efferent ductules, epididymal ducts, and vas deferens. Seminiferous tubules show atrophy, and spermatogenesis is abnormal. The pathogenesis of these changes is not fully understood. Ductal obstruction with inspissated secretions during fetal life or early childhood is one possible explanation. Periorchitis due to meconium may also develop early in life (Dehner et al., 1986). Cystic fibrosis gene may affect formation of the vas deferens and epididymis, and it appears that the congenital bilateral absence of the vas deferens could be a manifestation of cystic fibrosis (Anguiano et al., 1992).

Young's syndrome, or obstructive azoospermia and chronic sinobronchial infection, is another poorly understood cause of infertility related to a defect of sperm transport (Young, 1970). Handelsman et al. (1984) have suggested that the obstruction of the epididymis in these patients is caused by abnormal viscous seminal fluid. Typically, the head of the epididymis is expanded by sperm, whereas the body is obstructed with inspissated secretions. The reasons for the accumulation of secretions are not known. Theoretically, the secretions could be a consequence of abnormal absorption or propulsion secondary to ciliary dyskinesis. In contrast to patients with Kartagener's syndrome who show marked ultrastructural changes underlying ciliary immotility, the spermatozoa of patients with Young's syndrome show relatively minor quantitative changes (Wilton et al., 1991). However, it is possible that even these minor changes are sufficient to produce dysfunction of ciliary cells in the bronchi and epididymis and thus cause abnormal intraluminal fluid flow.

Male offspring of women who took diethylstilbestrol during pregnancy may have fertility problems. These are in part due to the obstruction of cystically dilated epididymal ducts and in part due to other gonadal and genital tract anomalies observed in these individuals (Bibbo and Gill, 1981; Whitehead and Leither, 1981).

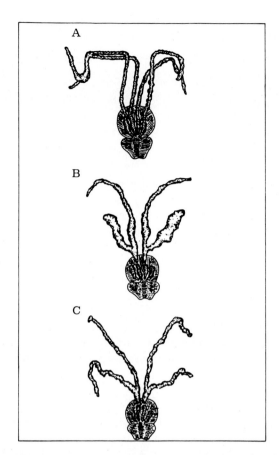

Fig. 4-13. Variations in the size and shape of seminal vesicles. (Modified from Papp G. Acta Chirurgia Hungaria 1988; 29:263, with permission).

Duplication

Duplication of the vas deferens has been described with polyorchidism (Leung, 1988). Duplicated vas deferens may be associated with anomalies of seminal vesicles (Redman et al., 1983).

ANOMALIES OF THE SEMINAL VESICLES, THE EJACULATORY DUCTS, AND THE PROSTATE

Seminal vesicles and ejaculatory duct evolve jointly from the mesonephric (wolffian) duct. The primordia appear during the thirteenth week of fetal life as buds of the mesonephric duct. These epithelial strands proliferate and undergo complex branching and recanalization until the ampullae of seminal vesicles and the ejaculatory duct are formed in the last trimester of pregnancy (Gray and Skandalakis, 1972). Seminal vesicles have a complex morphogenesis and assume several forms, which are considered to represent variations of the normal (Papp, 1988) (Fig. 4-13).

Anomalies of seminal vesicles are not common. These have been reviewed in monographs by Hill (1989) and Hedinger and Dhom (1991) and include:
1. Agenesis and atresia
2. Ectopia
3. Abnormal connections with adjacent structures

Agenesis of seminal vesicles may be unilateral or bilateral and is frequently associated with developmental anomalies of the vas deferens (Hirsch and Lipshultz, 1985). In a study of 26 men with absence of the vas deferens, Goldstein and Schlossberg (1988) found normal seminal vesicles in 46%, unilateral absence or hypoplasia in 31%, and bilateral hypoplasia or absence in 23% of cases. Donahue and Fauver (1989) state that unilateral agenesis of the vas deferens often is associated with renal agenesis, which is understandable since both the ureter and the vas deferens originate from the wolffian duct. However, these authors have not examined the status of seminal vesicles in their patients. On the basis of common embryologic origin, one could predict that some, if not most of these patients, also have ipsilateral developmental defects of the seminal vesicles. Several cases of unilateral renal agenesis associated with ipsilateral seminal vesicle agenesis or cystic malformations are on record (Beeby, 1974; Donohue and Greenslade, 1973).

Developmental defects may lead to *atresia* of the vesicles or ejaculatory ducts and cystic dilatation of the ampulla. Unilateral and especially bilateral agenesis of the seminal vesicles is therefore often associated with obstructive azoospermia. Ejaculate typically lacks fructose, which is secreted by seminal vesicles. The defect is diagnosed best by ultrasonography (Hirsch and Lipshultz, 1985) or computer-assisted tomography (Goldstein and Schlossberg, 1988). On the basis of these data, patients may be further evaluated for retroperitoneal exploration or reconstructive surgery.

Ectopic seminal vesicles and *abnormal communications* of seminal vesicles with the ejaculatory duct, urinary bladder, or ureters are rare and usually reflect complex developmental disturbances affecting the wolffian duct derivatives (Das and Amar, 1980; Redman et al., 1983). Older literature and European contributions to the study of these anomalies have been reviewed by Dhom in the monograph by Hedinger and Dhom (1991).

The *genesis* of the prostate is extremely rare and of minimal practical significance (Gray and Skandalakis, 1972). It may occur sporadically or as a part of complex syndromes affecting the urogenital tract. Moermann et al. (1984) have described congenital hypoplasia of the prostate causing urethral obstruction in children with the prune-belly syndrome.

ANOMALIES OF THE PENIS AND SCROTUM

Anomalies of the penis occur as part of complex developmental syndromes or are isolated and sporadic lesions.

The critical period for the differentiation of external genitalia is from the tenth to the twentieth week of intrauterine life. The genital tubercle and the urogenital sinus begin to develop in the same way in males and females and initially do not show any sexual dimorphism. The genital tubercle gives rise to the penis or clitoris. The urogenital sinus closes to form the scrotum and penile urethra or,

in females, differentiates into the vestibule of the vulva.

Penile anomalies of size, shape, and location and penile urethral anomalies can be classified as follows:

Anomalies of the penis

1. Agenesis
2. Micropenis
3. Penile duplication
4. Penile torsion and curvatures

Anomalies of the penile urethra

1. Epispadias
2. Hypospadias
3. Duplication of the penile urethra
4. Atresia and stenosis of the urethra and urethral valves

Anomalies of the scrotum

1. Scrotal hypoplasia
2. Scrotal ectopia
3. Bifid scrotum
4. Penoscrotal transposition

These conditions are rarely seen by pathologists, and a detailed discussion of genital morphology, clinical presentations, and treatment modalities can be found in specialized textbooks of urology (Walsh et al., 1986; Ashcraft, 1990; Gillenwater et al., 1991).

Agenesis of the penis

Agenesis of the penis is an extremely rare anomaly that occurs at a rate of 1 in 10 to 30 million (Kessler and McLaughlin, 1973). In most reported cases a fully formed scrotum is present and contains testes, whose function appears preserved (Gautier et al., 1981). Penile agenesis may be combined with an absent scrotum and several complex urogenital anomalies or multisystemic syndromes (Hensle, 1991); the urethra opens into the perineum just anterior to the rectum or into the rectum itself (Richart and Benirschke, 1960; Gray and Skandalakis, 1972). In a few patients the urethral meatus or urethra is surrounded by a small amount of cavernous erectile tissue.

Micropenis and *microphallus* are the terms used to describe a normally formed penis that is 2.5 standard deviations below the norm for age (Hensle, 1991). Some authors use the term microphallus for the ambiguous organ with hypospadias typical of pseudohermaphroditism and distinguish it from micropenis, which does not show hypospadias (Lee et al., 1980). Micropenis occurs in several forms (Fig. 4-14) and should be distinguished from *webbed* or *buried* penis in which the penis may be of normal size but is covered by the skin of the scrotum (Crawford, 1977). In newborn boys the stretched penis measures at least 2 cm. The measurements for other age groups are given in Table 4-6.

As stated by Lee et al. (1980), micropenis is not a diag-

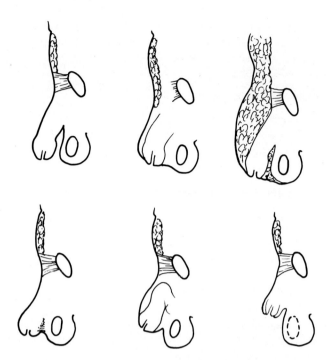

Fig. 4-14. Micropenis. (Modified from Maizels M et al. Surgical correction of the buried penis. J Urol 1986; 136:268, with permission. © Williams & Wilkins, 1986).

Table 4-6. Length of the penis, measured from the pubis to the tip in normal males

Age	Mean + SD (cm)	Mean − 2.5 SD (cm)
Newborn, 30 weeks	2.5 ± 0.4	1.5
Newborn, 34 weeks	3.0 ± 0.4	2.0
Newborn, term	3.5 ± 0.4	2.4
0–5 months	3.9 ± 0.8	1.9
1–2 years	4.7 ± 0.8	2.6
2–3 years	5.1 ± 0.9	2.9
3–4 years	5.5 ± 0.9	3.3
4–5 years	5.7 ± 0.9	3.5
5–6 years	6.0 ± 0.9	3.8
6–7 years	6.1 ± 0.9	3.9
7–8 years	6.2 ± 1.0	3.7
8–10 years	6.3 ± 1.0	3.8
Adult	13.3 ± 1.6	9.3

Adapted from Hensle, 1991. The table is based on the original data of Feldman and Smith, 1975 and Schonfeld and Beebe, 1942.

nosis but a sign. In their series of 45 patients, micropenis was a symptom of hypogonadotropic hypogonadism (31%), primary testicular failure (24%), and androgen insensitivity (7%) and was considered to be idiopathic in 36% of cases. The syndromes commonly associated with micropenis are listed in the box above right. Hormonal treatment usually gives good results, and most patients develop an erectile adult penis with normal length (Danish et al., 1980; Reiley and Woodhouse, 1989).

Penile duplication

Penile duplication is not a single entity and it presents in several forms (Gray and Skandalakis, 1972; Hensle,

---

Syndromes associated with micropenis

1. Hypogonadotropic hypogonadism
   Kallmann's syndrome
   Prader-Willi syndrome
   Laurence-Moon-Biedl syndrome
2. Primary hypogonadism
   Klinefelter's syndrome
3. Androgen insensitivity
4. Others
   Carpenter's syndrome
   Cornelia de Lange's syndrome
   Down's syndrome
   Fanconi's pancytopenia
   Fetal hydantoin syndrome
   Hallermann-Streiff syndrome
   Long-arm 18 deletion
   Noonan's syndrome
   Smith-Lemli-Opitz syndrome
   Williams's syndrome

Modified from Lee PA et al. John Hopkins Med J 1980; 146:156.

1991). The spectrum of anomalies ranges from bifurcation of the shaft and duplication of the glands to complete diphallia with two separate scrotums (Hensle, 1991). Frequently, other genitourinary anomalies occur simultaneously. Surgical reconstruction may require complex interventions and often is not entirely satisfactory.

Penile torsion and curvatures

Penile torsion and curvatures are usually asymptomatic but if marked may interfere with erection and require surgical correction (Hensle et al., 1991).

Anomalies of the penile urethra

The penile urethra is formed with the closure of the urethral plate by the outer and inner genital folds and the preputial fold. The raphe forms at the base of the penis, and the orifice of the urethra at the tip of the penis (Fig. 4-15). Incomplete or defective closure of the primordium of the penile urethra leads to hypospadias, the most important malformation of the penile urethra. Other anomalies, such as epispadias, duplication of the penile urethra, atresia, and stenosis of the urethra, are less common (Gray and Skandalakis, 1972).

Hypospadias denotes defects of the penile urethra in which the urethral orifice is located on the ventral side of the penis proximal to the normal site. *Epispadias* refers to the urethral orifice on the dorsum of the penis. *Atresia* refers to congenital obstruction of any part of the urethra but most often of the entire penile and glandular urethra. It may be associated with *urethral valves,* which although more common in the posterior urethral may occur in other parts as well. *Duplication of the urethra, accessory urethras,* and *blind urethral canals* attached to the normal urethra are rare anomalies (Gray and Skandalakis, 1972)

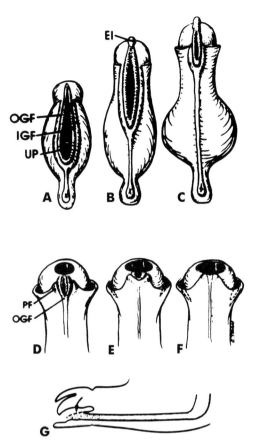

Fig. 4-15. Embryology of penile and glanular urethra. The inner and outer genital folds cover the urethral plate (UP) and form the raphe (**A-C**). The glanular urethra is a compound of ectodermal pit at tip of glans and open end of the ureteral groove. **D** through **F** show further closure of the groove by outer genital and preputial folds and orifice of the central pit in the glans. **G** shows the breakdown *(arrow)* of the intervening septum to create one orifice, the fossa navicularis, and the lacuna magna (OGF indicates outer genital folds; IGF, inner genital folds; PF, preputial folds; UP, urethral plate; and EI, ectodermal tag marking site of ectodermal ingrowth). *Arrow* in G also indicates site of "anastomosis" between the ectodermal pit and the urethral groove. (From Sommer JT, Stephens FD. J Urol 1980; 124:94, by permission).

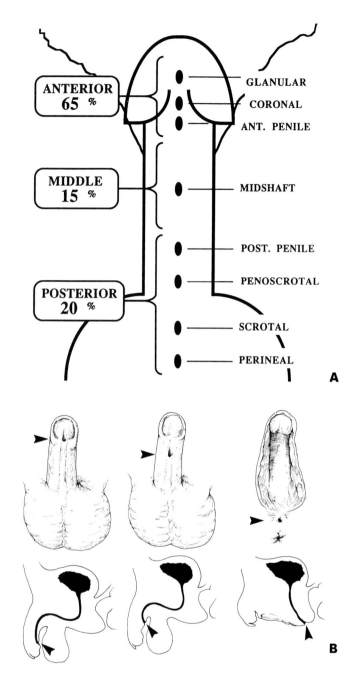

Fig. 4-16. A, Classification of hypospadias. (From Keating MA and Duckett JW. In Nyhus LM (Ed). Surgery Annual 1990. Appleton-Century Crafts, 1990, by permission). **B,** Artist's drawing of these forms of hypospadia. (From Welch, 1962, with permission).

reflecting abnormal formation of the penile urethra. Connective tissue *chordae*, i.e., condensed connective tissue distal to a hypospadias, may also present as an isolated defect. All these anomalies tend to be associated with other urogenital developmental defects.

The incidence of hypospadias is between 3 and 4.7 per 1000 newborn males (Czeizel and Toth, 1990). Polygenic inheritance has been suggested by observing that the incidence is increased among siblings and in offspring of affected individuals (Bauer et al., 1981). It is also more common in monozygotic twins than in singletons (Roberts and Lloyd, 1973) and in children born to women exposed to progestins during pregnancy (Czeizel and Toth, 1990), which suggests that placental insufficiency or hormonal influences may be pathogenetically important.

Several classifications of hypospadias have been pro-

posed (reviewed by Duckett, 1991). For practical purposes, Duckett favors a simple classification into three categories (Duckett, 1989; Keating and Duckett, 1990; Duckett, 1990).

1. Anterior hypospadias (65%), which include glanular, coronal, and anterior penile locations
2. Penoscrotal hypospadias
3. Scrotal and perineal hypospadias (Fig. 4–16).

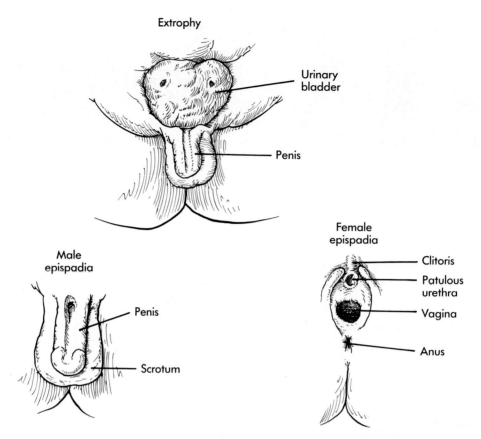

Fig. 4-17. Epispadias and related anomalies in males and females. (Modified from Jeffs RD Lepor H. In Walsh PC (Ed). Campbell's Urology; 5th ed. Philadelphia, WB Saunders 1986, with permission).

All hypospadias are more often associated with other urogenital anomalies, but the posterior hypospadias seem to be more often related to other defects than anterior or middle hypospadias. Among the associated anomalies most prominent are undescended testes and hernias, which occur in about 9% of patients with hypospadias in general and 17% to 32% of patients with posterior hypospadias (Duckett, 1991). Utricullus masculinus is found most often in patients with posterior hypospadias (Devine et al., 1980). Other urogenital anomalies occur in 1.5% to 3% of cases, (Duckett, 1991). The most significant accompanying urinary tract anomalies are renal agenesis, obstruction of the ureteropelvic junction, and urinary reflux (Khuri et al., 1981).

Clinical symptoms of hypospadias fall into four categories (Smith, 1990):

1. Misdirection of urinary stream
2. Inadequate ejaculation
3. Deformity due to chordae
4. Psychological discomfort due to penile abnormality

Great advances have been made in the surgical repair of hypospadias (Smith, 1990; Duckett, 1991). The operation is preferably performed before the age of 1 year, between 3 and 9 months. Normal sexual function can be expected in most patients, despite some complications such as fistula formation, stenosis, stricture, and persistence of chordae that occur in 2% to 7% of treated patients (Smith, 1990; Duckett, 1991).

Epispadias are considerably less common than hypospadias. Isolated epispadias occurs at a rate of 1 in 117,000 newborn males and 1 in 480,000 females (Dees, 1949). Epispadias associated with urinary bladder extrophy may be part of the so-called urinary bladder extrophy-epispadias syndrome, a spectrum of anomalies that develop because of a defective morphogenesis of the cloacal membrane (Jeffs and Lepor, 1986). This occurs in 1 in 10,000 to 50,000 live-born infants. All these anomalies require major reconstructive surgery, and the results depend on the nature of the extent of the developmental defect (Fig. 4-17).

Anomalies of the scrotum

The scrotum develops from labioscrotal folds that begin fusing in the midline over the urethral folds and remain loosely textured laterally to form scrotal swellings (Gray and Skandalakis, 1972). Anomalies of the scrotum relate to the midline fusion and its relationship to the penis (Hensle, 1991). If the scrotum does not develop completely on one or both sides, the anomaly is called *scrotal hypopla-*

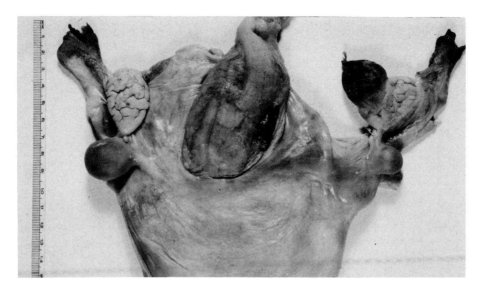

Fig. 4-18. Agenesis of the uterus and fallopian tubes. Both ovaries present. The central structure is the rectum.

sia. Bifid scrotum refers to incomplete midline fusion of the labioscrotal folds and usually is associated with severe hypospadias. *Scrotal ectopia* refers to displacement of the scrotum usually to the site of the inner inguinal canal or anywhere along the buttocks and the inner thigh (Hensle, 1991). *Penoscrotal transposition* is an anomaly characterized by a scrotum that overrides the penis which in itself may be normal or abnormal with regard to its size and shape.

ANOMALIES OF THE FEMALE GENITAL ORGANS

The female genital organs develop from three fetal primordia:

1. The genital ridge that gives rise to the ovary
2. The müllerian ducts, which give rise to the fallopian tubes, uterus, cervix, and upper vagina
3. The urogenital sinus, which gives rise to the lower portion of the vagina, vulva, and external genitalia

Complex anomalies involving the female genitalia associated with gonadal dysgenesis or congenital adrenal dysfunction have been reviewed by Grumbach and Conte (1992) and in Chapter 3. These anomalies often are associated with hormonal imbalance and reproductive failure. Other urinary tract anomalies such as cloacal extrophy also are associated with genital tract defects (Visnesky et al., 1990). Isolated congenital anomalies of the female genital organs are uncommon, or at least they seldom present as the primary cause of infertility. Most important among these are defects in the formation of the vagina and uterus, which include various forms of partial or complete agenesis, atresia, deformities, and incomplete fusion of various parts (box at right).

Developmental anomalies of the female reproductive tract

1. Agenesis
   Vagina
   Uterus
   Fallopian tubes
   Ovary
2. Incomplete fusion of müllerian ducts
   Uterus didelphys
   Bicornuate uterus
   Unicornuate uterus
   Arcuate uterus
   Subseptate uterus
3. Urogenital sinus defects
   Fusion of the labia
4. Sundry conditions
   Transposition
   Fusion
   Ectopia
   Dysplasia

Agenesis

Agenesis of any part of the female genital tract may present as an isolated defect, but, most often, several anomalies present as the so-called Mayer-Rokitansky-Küster-Hauser syndrome (Griffin et al., 1976; Buttram and Gibbons, 1979). This syndrome includes an aplasia of all derivatives of the müllerian ducts (Buttram and Gibbons, 1979). Patients lack one or both fallopian tubes, the uterus, and the upper vagina (Fig. 4-18). The lower vagina typically ends in a dimple, or a short blind-ended pouch 1 to 6 cm in diameter. The ovaries, clitoris, labia minora,

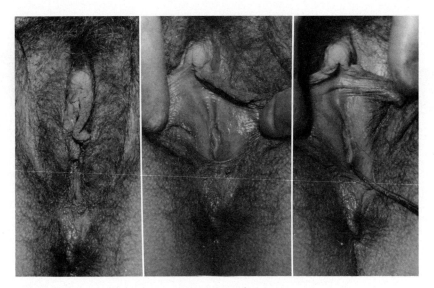

Fig. 4-19. Agenesis of the vagina. Instead of the vagina there is only a blind-ended pouch. The labia and clitoris are normal. (Courtesy P. Drobnjak).

and labia majora are normal (Fig. 4-19). These patients have a normal female phenotype and karyotype. They enter puberty, and although there is normal ovulation, menstrual bleeding does not occur. Renal, skeletal, and other congenital anomalies occur at an increased frequency (Griffin et al., 1976).

Mayer-Rokitansky-Küster-Hauser syndrome is diagnosed by external gynecologic examination, laparoscopy and ultrasonography, or radiologic imaging (Togashi et al., 1987; Fedele et al., 1990). On the basis of these studies, it was found that agenesis is almost never complete and that some rudiments of the müllerian ducts can be found. They variously form fibrous cords, endometrial islands, and cystic structures. In some cases, a unicornuate or cavitary hypoplastic uterine rudiment, which is attached to a fibrotic strand, is found (Fedele et al., 1990).

Women born without a uterus are infertile. For now, surgical reconstruction of the anomalies cannot correct infertility. However, harvesting of oocytes with in vitro fertilization and intrauterine transfer to a surrogate mother remains a viable alternative.

Agenesis of the ovaries may be unilateral or bilateral. The pathogenesis of this rare condition is not fully understood. In some cases, it has been suspected that an autoamputation secondary to torsion of the ovary and the fallopian tube has occurred in utero (Beyth and Bar-on, 1984). The evolution of this adnexal lesion utero has been demonstrated on ultrasonography (Sherer et al., 1990). Calcified residues of such ovaries can be seen radiologically (Kennedy et al., 1981).

Incomplete fusion of müllerian ducts

Müllerian ducts, which normally are paired, symmetric fetal structures, fuse in the midline to form the uterus, cervix, and upper part of the vagina. Various uterine anoma-

lies are the most important abnormalities resulting from incomplete fusion of the müllerian ducts. Septation of the upper vagina, vaginal reduplication, and cervical anomalies also are pathogenetically related to the same developmental defects.

Buttram and Gibbons (1979) have divided müllerian anomalies into several classes. This classification, slightly modified, is used by the American Fertility Society (Fig. 4-20) and includes:

I. Segmental müllerian agenesis or hypoplasia affecting the vagina, cervix, fundus, fallopian tubes, or any combination of these.

II. Unicornuate uterus with or without a rudimentary horn and with or without an endometrial cavity. Furthermore, those with an endometrial cavity may or may not have communications with the opposite horn.

III. Uterus didelphys.

IV. Bicornuate uterus in which the division is partial or complete to the internal os.

V. Septate uterus with a complete septum to the internal or external os.

VI. Arcuate uterus.

VII. Uterus with internal luminal changes, such as a T-shaped uterus, constricting bands, or a widening of the lower two thirds of the uterus, as seen in offspring of women taking diethylstilbestrol during pregnancy. Buttram and Gibbons (1975) have not taken into account vaginal sagittal septa, which most often coexist with class III, IV, and V anomalies.

In the study of 144 patients with müllerian anomalies, Buttram and Gibbons (1979) found approximately one third of cases to be related to diethylstilbestrol. The most

American Fertility Society classification of uterine anomalies

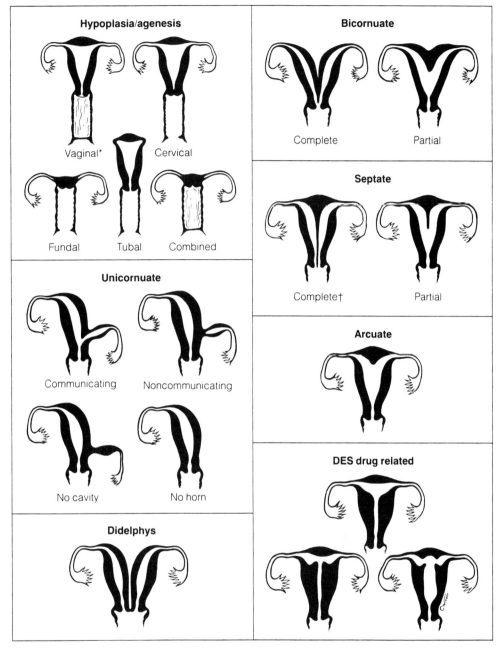

*Uterus may be normal or take a variety of abnormal forms.
†May have two distinct cervices.

Fig. 4-20. Uterine developmental anomalies. (Modified by Chris Wikoff from the American Fertility Society classifications of adnexal adhesions, distal tubal occlusion, tubal occlusion secondary to tubal ligation, tubal pregnancies, Müllerian anomalies, and intrauterine adhesions. Fertil Steril 1988; 49:944. Reproduced with permission of the publisher, The American Fertility Society).

common idiopathic anomaly was a septate uterus. All these anomalies, and especially septate uteri, seem to be associated with pregnancy wastage (Buttram and Gibbons, 1979; Ben-Raphael et al., 1991), although there is no general agreement as to what extent the reproductive performance of these women is impaired (Maneschi et al.,

1991b). Metroplasty and other forms of reconstructive surgery (Damewood and Rock, 1987) or laparoscopic resection of intrauterine septa (Valle et al., 1991) are used to treat infertility problems in such cases.

Müllerian anomalies may be associated with other urogenital developmental defects, most notably unilateral agenesis of the kidney (Wiersma et al., 1976). Females with unilateral renal agenesis frequently have genital anomalies, most often in the form of a didelphic uterus with an obstructed vagina. A double uterus with an obstructed vagina (Maneschi et al., 1991a) and a unicornuate uterus have also been described (Crowther, 1991).

Urogenital sinus defects

Rare defects of the urogenital sinus include fusion, deformities or absence of labia (Gray and Skandalakis, 1972). Imperforate hymen and variants of a normal hymen (Berkowitz et al., 1991) represent minor anomalies of limited significance for the work-up of infertile women.

Sundry conditions

Ectopic ovaries and splenic gonadal fusion are rare anomalies (Meneses and Ostrowski, 1989). Embryonic rests such as Gartner's duct, paroöphoron, epoöphoron, aberrant ductules, vesicular appendages, and hydatid of Morgagni are remnants of the wolffian duct. They are medical curiosities of almost no relevance for the reproductive function of female internal genital organs.

REFERENCES

Abney TO, Keel BA (Eds): The Cryptorchid Testis. Boca Raton, FL, CRC Press, 1990.

Anguiano A, Oates RD, Amos JA, Dean M, Gerrard B, Stewart C et al.: Congenital bilateral absence of the vas deferens: a primarily genital form of cystic fibrosis. JAMA 1992; 267:1794.

Ashcraft KW (Ed): Pediatric Urology. Philadelphia, WB Saunders, 1990.

Atwell JD: Ascent of the testis: fact or fiction? Br J Urol 1985; 57:474.

Ayano Y, Omori K, Ogata J, Ikegami K: Retroperitoneal epididymal structures in adult male. Eur Urol 1982; 8:52.

Bauer SB, Retik AB, Colodny AH: Genetic aspects of hypospadias. Urol Clin North Am 1981; 8:559.

Beccia DJ, Krane RJ, Olson CA: Clinical management of non-testicular intrascrotal tumors. J Urol 1976; 116:476.

Beeby DI: Seminal vesicle cyst associated with ipsilateral renal agenesis: Case report and review of literature. J Urol 1974; 112:120.

Beltran-Brown F, Villeguas-Alvarez F: Clinical classification for undescended testes; experience in 1010 orchidopexies. J Pediatr Surg 1988; 23:444.

Ben-Raphael Z, Seidman DS, Recabi K, Bider D, Mashiach S: Uterine anomalies. A retrospective matched-control study. J Reprod Med 1991; 36:723.

Bergada C, Cleveland WW, Jones HW Jr: Variants of embryonic testicular dysgenesis: Bilateral anorchia and the syndrome of rudimentary testis. Acta Endocrinol 1962; 40:521.

Berkowitz CD, Elvik SL, McCann J, Reinhart MA, Strickland S, Chikuma J: Septate hymen: Variations and pitfalls in diagnosis. Adolesc Pediatr Gynecol 1991; 4:197.

Beyth Y, Bar-on E: Tuboovarian autoamputation and infertility. Fertil Steril 1984; 42:932.

Bibbo M, Gill WB: Screening of adolescents exposed to diethylstilbestrol in utero. Pediatr Clin North Am 1981; 28:379.

Blumer CF, Hedinger CE: Vorkommen von Keimzellen in adulten kryptorchen Hoden. Pathologe 1989; 10:3.

Bobrow M, Gough MH: Bilateral absence of testes. Lancet 1970; 1:366.

Burge DM,: Neonatal testicular torsion and infarction: Aetiology and management. Br J Urol 1987; 59:70.

Buttram VC Jr, Gibbons WE: Müllerian anomalies: A proposed classification (an analysis of 144 cases). Fertil Steril 1979; 32:40.

Ceccacci L, Tosi S: Splenic gonadal fusion; case report and review of the literature. J Urol 1981; 126:558.

Chilvers C, Dudley NE, Gough MH, Jackson MB, Pike MC: Undescended testis: The effect of treatment on subsequent risk of subfertility and malignancy. J Pediatr Surg 1986; 21:691.

Chilvers C, Pike MC, Forman D, Fogelman K, Wadsworth MEJ: Apparent doubling of frequency of undescended testis in England and Wales in 1962–81. Lancet 1984; 2:330.

Connor MH, Styne DM: Familial functional anorchidism: A review of etiology and management. J Urol 1985; 133:1049.

Cooper BJ, Little TM: Orchiopexy: Theory and practice. Br Med J 1985; 291:706.

Cortada X, Kousseff BG: Cryptorchidism in mental retardation. J Urol 1984; 131:674.

Cortes D, Thorup J: Histology of testicular biopsies taken at operation for bilateral maldescended testes in relation to fertility in adulthood. Br J Urol 1991; 68:285.

Coulam CB: Testicular regression syndrome. Obstet Gynecol 1979; 53:44.

Crawford BS: Buried penis. Br J Plast Surg 1977; 30:95.

Crowther ME: Unicornuate uterus. Int J Gynecol Obstet 1991; 34:281.

Czeizel A, Erödi E, Toth J: An epidemiological study on undescended testis. J Urol 1981; 126:524a.

Czeizel A, Erödi E, Toth J: Genetics of undescended testis. J Urol 1981; 126:528b.

Czeizel A, Toth J: Correlation between the birth prevalence of hypospadias and parental subfertility. Teratology 1990; 41:167.

Dahl EV, Bahn RC: Aberrant adrenal cortical tissue near the testis in human infants. Am J Pathol 1962; 40:587.

Damewood MD, Rock JA: Reproductive uterine surgery. Obstet Gynecol Clin North Am 1987; 14:1049.

Danish RK, Lee PA, Mazur T, Amrhein JA, Migeon CJ: Micropenis. II. Hypogonadotropic hypogonadism. Johns Hopkins Med J 1980; 146:177.

Das S, Amar AD: Ureteral ectopia into cystic seminal vesicle with ipsilateral renal dysgenesis and monorchia. J Urol 1980; 124:574.

Davies TW, Williams DRR, Whitaker RH: Risk factors for undescended testis. Int J Epidemiol 1986; 15:197.

Dees JE: Congenital epispadias with incontinence. J Urol 1949; 62:513.

Dehner LP, Scott D, Stocker JT: Meconium periorchitis: A clinicopathologic study of four cases with a review of the literature. Hum Pathol 1986; 17:807.

Depue RH: Maternal and gestational factors affecting the risk of cryptorchidism and inguinal hernia. Int J Epidemiol 1984; 13:311.

Devine CJ, Gonzales-Serva L, Stecker JF Jr: Utricular configuration in hypospadia and intersex. J Urol 1980; 123:407.

Dickinson AJ, Hewett P: Transverse testicular ectopia presenting as strangulated inguinal hernia. Br J Urol 1991; 69:271.

Donohue RE, Fauver HE: Unilateral absence of the vas deferens. A useful clinical sign. JAMA 1989; 261:1180.

Donohue RE, Greenslade NF: Seminal vesicle cyst and ipsilateral renal agenesis. Urology 1973; 2:66.

Duckett JW: Advances in hypospadias repair. Postgrad Med J 1990; 66(Suppl 1):S62.

Duckett JW: Hypospadias. In Adult and Pediatric Urology, 2nd ed., edited by Gillenwater JY, Grayhack JT, Howards SS, Duckett JW. Mosby–Year Book, St. Louis, 1991, p 2103.

Ebbehoj J, Metz P: Congenital penile angulation. Br J Urol 1987; 60:264.

Editorial: Testicular descent revisited. Lancet 1989; 339:360.

Elder JS, Jeffs RD: Suprainguinal ectopic scrotum and associated anomalies. J Urol 1982; 127:336.

Eusebi V, Masserilli G: Pheochromocytoma of the spermatic cord: Report of a case. J Pathol 1971; 105:283.

Fallon B, Kennedy TJ: Long-term follow-up of fertility in cryptorchid patients. Urology 1985; 25:502.

Fedele L, Dorta M, Brioschi D, Giudici MN, Candiani GB: Magnetic resonance imaging in Mayer-Rokitansky-Kuster-Hauser syndrome. Obstet Gynecol 1990; 76:593.

Feldman KW, Smith DW: Fetal phallic growth and penile standards for newborn male infants. J Pediatr 1975; 86:395.

Fonkalsrud EW, Mengel W: The Undescented Testis. Chicago, Year Book, 1981.

Fram RJ, Garnick MB, Retik A: The spectrum of genitourinary abnormalities in patients with cryptorchidism, with emphasis on testicular carcinomas. Cancer 1982; 50:2243.

Gautier T, Salient J, Pena S: Testicular function in 2 cases of penile agenesis. J Urol 1981; 126:556.

Gearhart JP, Donohoue PA, Brown TR, Walsh PC, Berkovitz GD: Endocrine evaluation of adults with mild hypospadias. J Urol 1990; 144:274.

Gilbert J, Clark RD, Koyle MA: Penile agenesis: A fatal variation of an uncommon lesion. J Urol 1990; 143:338.

Gilhooly PE, Meyers F, Lattimer JK: Fertility prospects for children with cryptorchidism. Am J Dis Child 1984; 138:940.

Gill WB, Schumacher GFB, Bibbo M, Strauss FH, Schoenberg HW: Association of diethylstilbestrol exposure in utero with cryptorchidism, testicular hypoplasia and semen abnormalities. J Urol 1979; 122:36.

Gillenwater JY, Grayhack JT, Howards SS, Duckett JW (Eds): Adult and Pediatric Urology, 2nd ed., St. Louis, Mosby–Year Book, 1991.

Girgis SM, Etriby AA, Ibrahim AA, Kahil SA: Testicular biopsy in azoospermia: A review of the last ten years' experience of over 800 cases. Fertil Steril 1969; 20:467.

Giwercman A, Bruun E, Frimodt-Moller C, Skakkebaek NE: Prevalence of carcinomas in situ and other histopathological abnormalities in testes of males with a history of cryptorchidism. J Urol 1989; 142:998.

Golan A, Caspi E: Congenital anomalies of the müllerian tract. Contemp Obstet Gynecol 1992; 37:39.

Goldberg LM, Skaist LB, Morrow JM: Congenital absence of testes: Anorchism and monorchism. J Urol 1974; 111:840.

Goldstein M, Schlossberg S: Men with congenital absence of the vas deferens often have seminal vesicles. J Urol 1988; 140:85.

Gouw ASH, Elema JD, Bink-Boelkens MTE, de Jongh HJ, Tenkate LP: The spectrum of splenogonadal fusion. Case report and review of 84 reported cases. Eur J Pediatr 1985; 144:316.

Gray SW, Skandalakis JE: Embryology for Surgeons. Philadelphia, WB Saunders, 1972.

Griffin JE, Edwards C, Madden JD, Harrod MJ, Wilson JD: Congenital absence of the vagina. Ann Intern Med 1976; 85:224.

Griffin JE, Wilson JD: Disorders of the testes and male reproductive tract. In Williams Textbook of Endocrinology, 8th ed., edited by Wilson JD, Foster DW. Philadelphia, WB Saunders, 1992, p 799.

Grumbach MM, Conte FA: Disorders of sex differentiation. In Williams Textbook of Endocrinology, 8th ed., edited by Wilson JD, Foster DW, Philadelphia, WB Saunders, 1992, p 853.

Guiney EJ, Corbally M, Malone PS: The place of laparoscopy in the management of impalpable testis. Br J Urol 1989; 63:313.

Guiney EJ, McGlinchey J: Torsion of the testis and the spermatic cord in the newborn. Surg Gynecol Obstet 1981; 152:273.

Hadziselimovic F: Cryptorchidism. In Adult and Pediatric Urology, 2nd ed., edited by Gillenwater JY, Graychak JT, Howards SS, Duckett JW, St. Louis, Mosby–Year Book, 1991.

Hadziselimovic F: Cryptorchidism. Management and Implications. Berlin, Springer-Verlag, 1983.

Hadziselimovic F, Hecker E, Herzog B: The value of testicular biopsy in cryptorchidism. Urol Res 1984; 12:171.

Hadziselimovic F, Herzog B: Cryptorchidism. Pediatr Surg Int 1987; 2:132.

Hadziselimovic F, Herzog B, Huff DS, Menardi G: The morphometric histopathology of undescended testes and testes associated with incarcerated inguinal hernia: A comparative study. J Urol 1991; 146:627.

Hadziselimovic F, Seguchi H: Ultramikroskopische Untersuchungen an Tubulus Seminiferus bei Kindern von der Geburt bis zur Pubertät. II. Entwicklung und Morphologie der Sertolizellen. Verh Anat Ges 1974; 68:149.

Hadziselimovic F, Thommen L, Girrard J, Herzog B: The significance of postnatal gonadotropin surge for testicular development in normal and cryptorchid testes. J Urol 1986; 136:274.

Hall JG, Morgan A, Blizzard RM: Familial congenital anorchia. Birth Defects 1975; 11:115.

Handelsman DJ, Conway AJ, Boylan LM, Turtle JR: Young's syndrome: Obstructive azoospermia and chronic sinopulmonary infections. N Engl J Med 1984; 310:3.

Heath AL, Man DWK, Eckstein HB: Epididymal abnormalities associated with maldescent of the testis. J Pediatr Surg 1984; 19:47.

Hedinger CE: Histopathology of undescended testes. Eur J Pediatr 1982; 139:266.

Hedinger C, Dhom G: Pathologie des männlichen Genitale. Berlin, Springer-Verlag, 1991.

Hendren WH, Caesar RE: Chordae without hypospadias: Experience with 33 cases. J Urol 1992; 147:107.

Hensle TW: Genital Anomalies. In Adult and Pediatric Urology, 2nd ed, edited by Gillenwater JY, Graychak JT, Howards SS, Duckett JW, St. Louis, Mosby–Year Book, 1991, p. 2083.

Hill GS (Ed): Uropathology. New York, Churchill Livingstone, 1989.

Hirsch IH, Lipshultz LI: Transrectal ultrasonography elucidates the causes of male infertility. Masters Urol 1985; 1:105.

Holsclaw DS, Perlmutter AD, Jockin H: Genital abnormalities in male patients with cystic fibrosis. J Urol 1971; 106:568.

Honoré LH: Unilateral anorchism. Report of 11 cases with discussion of etiology and pathogenesis. Urology 1978; 11:251.

Huff DS, Hadziselimovic F, Duckett JW, Elder JS, Snyder HM: Germ cell counts in semithin sections of biopsies of 115 unilaterally cryptorchid testes. The experience from the Children's Hospital of Philadelphia. Eur J Pediatr 1987; 146:S25.

Huff DS, Hadziselimovic F, Snyder HM III, Blyth B, Duckett JW: Early postnatal testicular maldevelopment in cryptorchidism. J Urol 1991; 146:624.

Huff DS, Hadziselimovic F, Snyder HM III, Duckett JW, Keating MA: Postnatal testicular maldevelopment in unilateral cryptorchidism. J Urol 1989; 142:546.

Huff DS, Wu H-Y, Snyder HM III, Hadziselimovic F, Blythe B, Duckett JW: Evidence in favor of the mechanical (intrauterine torsion) theory over endocrinopathy (cryptorchidism) theory in the pathogenesis of testicular agenesis. J Urol 1991; 146:630.

Hunter JA: Observations on Certain Parts of the Animal Oeconomy. London, 1786.

Hutson JM, Donahoe PK: The hormonal control of testicular descent. Endocr Rev 1986; 7:270.

Hutson JM, Williams MP, Fallat ME, Attah A: Testicular descent: New insights into its hormonal control. Oxford Rev Reprod 1990; 12:1.

Jackson MB, Gough MH, Dudley NE: Anatomical findings at orchidopexy. Br J Urol 1987; 59:568.

Jarow JP: Cryptorchidism. In Current Problems in Infertility and Impotence, edited by Rajfer J. Chicago, Year Book Medical Publishers, 1990.

Jeffs RD, Lepor H: Management of the exstrophy-epispadias complex and urachal anomalies. In Campbell's Urology, edited by Walsh PC. Philadelphia, WB Saunders, 1986, p 1883.

John Radcliffe Hospital Cryptorchidism Study Group (JRHCSG): Boys with late descending testes: The source of patients with retractile testes undergoing orchidopexy? Br Med J 1986; 293:789a.

John Radcliffe Hospital Cryptorchidism Study Group (JRHCSG): Cryptorchidism: An apparent substantial increase since 1960. Br Med J 1986; 293:1401c.

Jones IRG, Young ID: Familial incidence of cryptorchidism. J Urol 1982; 127:508.

Josso N, Briard M-L: Embryonic testicular regression syndrome: Variable phenotypic expression in siblings. J Pediatr 1980; 97:200.

Kaplan E, Schwachman H, Perlmutter AD: Reproductive failure in males with cystic fibrosis. N Engl J Med 1968; 279:65.

Kaufman A, Guia R, Davila H: Diphallus with third urethra. Urology 1990; 35:257.

Keating MA, Duckett JW: Recent advances in the repair of hypospadias. Surg Annu 1990; 22:405.

Kelami A: Congenital penile deviation and its treatment with the Nesbit-Kelami technique. Br J Urol 1987; 60:261.

Kennedy LA, Pinckney LE, Currarino G, Votteler TP: Amputated calcified ovaries in children. Pediatr Radiol 1981; 141:83.

Kessler WO, McLaughlin AP: Agenesis of penis: Embryology and management. Urology 1973; 1:226.

Khuri FJ, Hardy BE, Churchill BM: Urologic anomalies associated with hypospadias. Urol Clin North Am 1981; 8:565.

Knudsen JL, Savage A, Mobb GE: The testicular "tumour" of androgenital syndrome—a persistent diagnostic pitfall. Histopathology 1991; 19:468.

Koff SA: Does compensatory testicular enlargement predict monorchism? J Urol 1991; 146:632.

Koff WJ, Scaletscky R: Malformations of the epididymis in undescended testis. J Urol 1990; 143:340.

Kogan SJ, Gill B, Bennett B: Human monorchidism: A clinicopathological study of unilateral absent testes in 65 boys. J Urol 1986; 135:758.

Kratzik C, Hainz A, Kuber W, Donner G, Lunglmayr G, Frick J, Schmoller HJ, Amann G: Surveillance strategy for intratesticular cysts: Preliminary report. J Urol 1990; 143:313.

Kroogvand RL, Perlmutter AD: Congenital anomalies of the vas deferens and epididymis. In Pediatric Andrology, edited by Kogan SJ, Hafez ESE, Boston, Martinus Nijhoff, 1981, p 173.

Kropp KA, Voeller KKS: Cryptorchidism in meningomyelocele. J Pediatr 1981; 99:110.

Krueger RD, Hardy BE, Churchill BM: Cryptorchidism in boys with posterior urethral valves. J Urol 1980; 124:101.

Lee PA, Mazur T, Danish R, Amrheim J, Blizzard RM, Money J, Migeon CJ. Micropenia I. Criteria, etiologies and classification. Johns Hopkins Med J 1980; 146:156.

Leissring JC, Oppenheimer RO: Cystic dysplasia of the testis: A unique congenital anomaly studied by microdissection. J Urol 1973; 110:362.

Leung AKC: Polyorchidism. Am Fam Physician 1988; 38:153.

Lipshultz LI: Cryptorchidism in the subfertile male. Fertil Steril 1976; 27:610.

Lipshultz LI, Carminos-Torres R, Greenspan CS, Snyder PJ: Testicular function after unilateral orchidopexy. N Engl J Med 1976; 295:15.

Mack WS, Scott LS, Ferguson-Smith MA, Lennox B: Ectopic testis and true undescended testis: A histological comparison. J Pathol Bacteriol 1961; 82:439.

Maioels M: J Urol 1986; 136:268.

Malek RS, Rosen JS, Farrow GM: Epidermoid cyst of the testis: A critical analysis. Br J Urol 1986; 58:55.

Maneschi M, Maneschi F, Incandela S: The double uterus associated with an obstructed hemivagina: Clinical management. Adolesc Pediatr Gynecol 1991; 4:206a.

Maneschi F, Parlato M, Incandela S, Maneschi M: Reproductive performance in women with complete septate uteri. J Reprod Med 1991; 36:723b.

Marshall FF, Shermeta DW: Epididymal abnormalities associated with undescended testis. J Urol 1979; 121:341.

Menese MF, Ostrowski ML: Female splenic-gonadal fusion of the discontinuous type. Hum Pathol 1989; 20:486.

Moerman P, Fryns JP, Goddeeris P, Lauweryns JM: Pathogenesis of the prune-belly syndrome: A functional urethral obstruction caused by prostatic hypoplasia. Pediatrics 1984; 73:470.

Murphy WM, ed: Urological Pathology. Philadelphia, WB Saunders, 1989.

Najjar SS, Takla RJ, Nassar VH: The syndrome of rudimentary testes: Occurrence in five siblings. J Pediatr 1974; 84:119.

Nistal M, Iniguez L, Paniagua R: Cysts of the testicular parenchyma and tunica albuginea. Arch Pathol Lab Med 1989; 113:902.

Nistal M, Paniagua R: Testicular and Epididymal Pathology. New York, Thieme-Stratton, 1984.

Nistal M, Paniagua R, Diez-Pardo JA: Histologic classification of undescended testes. Hum Pathol 1980; 11:666.

Nistal M, Regadera J, Paniagua R: Cystic dysplasia of the testis. Light and electron microscopic study of three cases. Arch Pathol Lab Med 1984; 108:579.

Nistal M, Santamaria L, Paniagua R: Acquired cystic transformation of the rete testis secondary to renal failure. Hum Pathol 1989; 20:1065.

Orlowski JP, Levin HS, Dyment PG: Intrascrotal Wilms' tumor developing in a heterotopic renal anlage of probable mesonephric origin. J Pediatr Surg 1980; 15:679.

Ostermayer H, Frei A: Nebenhoden und Samenblase als Mündungsort ektoper Harnleiter. Urologe 1981; 20:389.

Padron RS, Mas Y: Familial bilateral vas deferens agenesis. Int J Fertil 1991; 36:23.

Palmer JM: The undescended testicle. Endocrinol Metab Clin North Am 1991; 20:231.

Papp G: Uroandrology II. Andrological significance of the diseases of the seminal vesicle. Acta Chir Hung 1988; 29:263.

Politoff L, Hadziselimovic F, Herzog B, Jenni P: Does hydrocele affect later fertility? Fertil Steril 1990; 53:700.

Popek EJ: Embryonal remnants in inguinal hernia sac. Hum Pathol 1990; 21:339.

Puri P, Nixon HH: Bilateral retractile testes: Subsequent effects on fertility. J Pediatr Surg 1977; 12:563.

Puri P, Sparnon A: Relationship of primary site of testis to final testicular size in cryptorchid patients. Br J Urol 1990; 66:208.

Rajfer J: Hormonal regulation of testicular descent. Eur J Pediatr 1987; 146(Suppl 2):S6.

Rajfer J: Surgical and hormonal therapy for cryptorchidism: An overview. Horm Res 1988; 30:139.

Redman JF, Jacks DC, Golladay ES: Vasal vesical communications. Urology 1983; 22:59.

Reiley JM, Woodhouse CRJ: Small penis and the male sexual role. J Urol 1989; 142:569.

Richart R, Benirschke K: Penile agenesis. Arch Pathol 1960; 70:252.

Roberts CJ, Lloyd S: Observation on the epidemiology of simple hypospadias. Br Med J 1973; 1:768.

Robertson JFR, Azmy AF, Cochran W: Assent to ascent of the testis. Br J Urol 1988; 61:146.

Rudy F: Anomalies of the testis. In Uropathology, vol II., edited by Hill GS, New York, Churchill Livingstone, 1989, p 955.

Rutgers JL, Young RH, Scully RE: The testicular "tumor" of the adrenogenital syndrome. A report of six cases and review of the literature on testicular masses in patients with adrenocortical disorders. Am J Surg Pathol 1988; 12:503.

Saito S, Kumamoto Y: The number of spermatogonia in various congenital testicular disorders. J Urol 1989; 141:1166.

Salle B, Hedinger CE, Nicole R: Significance of testicular biopsies in cryptorchidism in children. Acta Endocrinol 1968; 58:67.

Sarto GE, Opitz JM: The XY gonadal agenesis syndrome. J Med Genet 1973; 10:288.

Schellen TMCM, Van Straaten A: Autosomal recessive hereditary congenital aplasia of the vasa deferentia in four siblings. Fertil Steril 1980; 34:401.

Schindler AM, Diaz P, Cuendet A, Sizonenko, PC: Cryptorchidism: A morphologic study of 670 biopsies. Helv Paed Acta 1987; 42:145.

Schonfeld WA, Beebe GW: Normal growth and variation in the male genitalia from birth to maturity. J Urol 1942; 48:759.

Scorer CG: The descent of the testis. Arch Dis Child 1964; 39:605.

Scorer CG, Farrington GH: Congenital Deformities of the Testis and Epididymis. New York, Appleton-Century-Crofts, 1971.

Sheldon CA, Duckett JW: Hypospadias. Pediatr Clin North Am 1987; 34:1259.

Sherer DM: Prenatal sonographic diagnosis and subsequent management of fetal adnexal torsion. J Ultrasound Med 1990; 9:161.

Shima H, Ikoma F, Terakawa T: Developmental anomalies with hypospadias. J Urol 1979; 122:619.

Silber SJ, Ord T, Balmaceda J, Patrizio P, Asch RH: Congenital absence of the vas deferens: The fertilizing capacity of human epididymal sperm. N Engl J Med 1990; 323:1788.

Sizonenko PC: Cryptorchidism: Introductory remarks. Horm Res 1988; 30:137.

Skoglund RW, McRoberts JW, Ragde H: Torsion of testicular appendages: Presentation of 43 new cases and a collective review. J Urol 1970; 104:598.

Smith ED: Hypospadias. In Pediatric Urology, edited by Ashcraft KW. Philadelphia, WB Saunders, 1990.

Snow BW, Tarry WF, Duckett JW: Polyorchidism: An unusual case. J Urol 1985; 133:483.

Soejima H, Ogawa O, Nomura Y, Ogata J: Pheochromocytoma of the spermatic cord: A case report. J Urol 1977; 118:495.

Sohval AR: Testicular dysgenesis in relation to neoplasm of the testicle. J Urol 1956; 75:285.

Strader CH, Weiss NS, Daling JR: Cryptorchidism, orchiopexy and the risk of testicular cancer. Am J Epidemiol 1988; 127:1013.

Swerdlow AJ, Wood KH, Smith PG: A case-control study of the aetiology of cryptorchidism. J Epidemiol Community Health 1983; 37:238.

Tammela TLJ, Karttunen TJ, Mattila SI, Makarainen HP, Hellstrom PA, Kontturi MJ: Cysts of the tunica albuginea—more common testicular masses than previously thought? Br J Urol 1991; 68:280.

Togashi K, Nishimura K, Itoh K, Fujisawa I, Nakano Y, Torizuka K, Ozasa H, Ohshima M: Vaginal agenesis: Classification by MR imaging. Radiology 1987; 162:675.

Valle JA, Lifchez AS, Moise J: A simpler technique for reduction of uterine septum. Fertil Steril 1991; 56:1001.

Virdi JS, Conway W, Kelly DG: Torsion of the vas aberrans. Br J Urol 1991; 68:435.

Visnesky PM, Texter JH, Galle P, Walker GG, McRae MA: Genital outflow tract obstruction in an adolescent with cloacal exstrophy. Obstet Gynecol 1990; 76:548.

Walker AW, Mills SE: Glandular inclusions in inguinal hernia sacs and spermatic cords: Müllerian-like remnants confused with functional reproductive structures. Am J Clin Pathol 1984; 82:85.

Wallin M, Marshall FF, Fink MP: Aberrant epididymal tissue: A significant clinical entity. J Urol 1987; 138:1247.

Walsh PC ed: Campbell's Urology, 5th ed. Philadelphia, WB Saunders, 1986.

Wegmann W, Illi O, Kummer-Vago M: Zystische Hodendysplasie mit ipsilateraler Nierenagenesie. Schweiz Med Wochenschr 1984; 114:144.

Welch KJ: Hypospadias. In Pediatric Surgery, edited by Benson CD, Mustard WT, Ravitch MM, Snyder WH Jr, Welch KY, Chicago, Year Book, 1962.

Wensing CJG: The embryology of testicular descent. Horm Res 1988; 30:144.

Whitaker RH: Neoplasia in cryptorchid men. Semin Urol 1988; 6:107.

Whitehead ED, Leither E: Genital abnormalities and abnormal semen analysis in male patients exposed to diethylstilbestrol in utero. J Urol 1981; 125:47.

Wiersma AF, Peterson LF, Justerma EJ: Uterine anomalies associated with unilateral renal agenesis. Obstet Gynecol 1976; 47:654.

Wilton LJ, Teichtahl H, Temple-Smith PD, Johnson JL, Southwick GJ, Burger HG, deKretser DM: Young's syndrome (obstructive azoospermia and chronic sinobronchial infection): A quantitative study of axonemal ultrastructure and function. Fertil Steril 1991; 55:144.

Wollin M, Duffy PG, Malone PS, Ransley PG: Buried penis. A novel approach. Br J Urol 1990; 65:97.

Young D: Surgical treatment of male infertility. J Reprod Fertil 1970; 23:541.

Chapter 5

INFECTIOUS CAUSES
OF INFERTILITY

Infections of the male genital tract
  Epididymo-orchitis
  Inflammation of the seminal vesicles, urethra, and prostate
Infections of the female genital tract
  Cervicitis
  Endometritis
  Salpingitis and pelvic inflammatory disease

INFECTIONS OF THE MALE GENITAL TRACT

Infection of the genital organs is an important cause of infertility, especially in women, in whom it may account for up to one third of all identifiable causes of reproductive failure (Rowland, 1980). Obstruction of male excretory ducts as a result of chronic infections is the underlying cause of infertility in less than 10% of azoospermic men (Wong et al., 1973; Greenberg et al., 1978). Nevertheless, since the arguments about the infectious causes of infertility in men have not been settled (Nahoum, 1982; Berger and Holmes, 1986), and since many subfertile men have chronic infections and are treated accordingly, it is reasonable to assume that urogenital infections may affect fertility in men as well as in women.

Epididymo-orchitis

As a result of the anatomic proximity of the testis to the epididymis almost all infections involving one of these organs will spread to the other. Although isolated inflammation of the testis *(orchitis)* or epididymis *(epididymitis)* may occur, and although each of these lesions represents usually the first morphologic signs of infection, in most clinical cases the inflammation is rarely, if ever, limited to one organ. Inflammatory lesions involving the testis and epididymis are, therefore, considered together under the term *epididymo-orchitis* (see box on p. 106).

Epididymo-orchitis can be classified according to several criteria as follows:

1. *Duration*—The inflammation may be acute, chronic, or recurrent.
2. *Etiology*—The inflammation may be caused by bacterial, spirochetal, protozoal, viral, fungal, or parasitic infections.
3. *Route of infection*—The infection may reach the scrotum through an ascending (canalicular), hematogenous, or lymphatic spread or by direct entry of pathogens through wounds.
4. *Morphology*—Histologically, the infection may present as suppuration, abscess, chronic fibrosis, interstitial mononuclear cell infiltrates, or granulomatous inflammation or gumma.

Pathogenesis. Infectious agents may reach the testis and epididymis through several routes. In many cases of epididymitis or orchitis, the route of spread seems obvious as in the case of ascending infection from the common sexually transmitted organisms. In a clinical setting, however, it is often not possible to demonstrate the route of infection, the provenance of the agent or to provide proof of the underlying mechanism. The elucidation of pathogenesis may only be of academic interest in most cases but is important for explaining and treating recurrent infections.

As stated, ascending or canalicular spread of infection is most commonly the route of entry of pathogens transmitted sexually and of those associated with lower urinary tract infections. Foremost among the pathogens of ascending infections are *Neisseria gonorrhoeae, Chlamydia trachomatis, Escherichia coli,* and other gram-negative bacteria. An ascending infection is most often caused by a reflux of infected urine from the urethra into the ejaculatory ducts and ductus deferens (Mikuz and Damjanov, 1982). Such reflux has been documented in children (Kiviat et al., 1972), and it may be the cause of recurrent epididymitis in boys (Megalli et al., 1972). However, epididymitis is less common in this young age group than in adults (Williams

105

Causes of epididymo-orchitis

1. Bacteria
   Neisseria gonorrhoeae
   Escherichia coli
   Mixed flora
   Mycobacterium tuberculosis
   M. leprae
   Haemophilus influenzae
   Salmonella, Brucella
2. Spirochetes
   Treponema pallidum
3. Fungi
   Histoplasma capsulatum
   Blastomyces dermatitidis
   Coccidioides immitis
4. Parasites
   Wuchereria bancrofti
   Schistosoma haematobium
   Echynococcus granulosus
5. Viral
   Mumps virus
   Adenovirus
   Coxsackie virus B
   Cytomegalovirus
6. Idiopathic
   Sarcoidosis
   Malacoplakia
   Granulomatous orchitis
   Xanthogranulomatous orchitis

et al., 1979), and the contribution of urethro-ejaculatory duct reflux in adults has been disputed.

Although it is questionable whether reflux of urine can occur in otherwise healthy persons, there is ample evidence that bacteria can reach the epididymides and testes from the lower urinary tract in patients with chronic urinary tract infection and in those suffering from obstruction of the urinary bladder neck and from neurogenic bladder. Children with congenital malformations of the urethra or posterior urethral valves or anovesical malformations are at a greater risk than others to develop ascending infections of the scrotum (Siegel et al., 1987). Accordingly, it is possible that some men have abnormal mechanisms of micturition, which predispose them to epididymitis (Thind et al., 1990).

It has been shown that there are differences in intravesical pressure between normal men and those with epididymitis. In the bladder's resting state, urine cannot enter the posterior urethra or the vas deferens because the intraurethral pressure exceeds bladder pressure. However, during micturition the pressure equalizes between the urethra and the bladder, and if voiding is strenuous, the increased pressure in the bladder may force urine into the ejaculatory duct (Thind et al., 1990). This explanation seems plausible, but whether it represents the underlying mechanism in most or only some cases of ascending epididymo-orchitis remains to be proven.

Blood-borne infections occur during sepsis or when there is dissemination of microorganisms from foci of inflammation in other organs. Viral orchitis caused by mumps virus (Werner, 1950), *coxsackie virus B* (Freij et al., 1970), or epididymitis caused by cytomegalovirus (McCarthy et al., 1991) develop after hematogenous spread of the infectious agents. Tuberculosis of the epididymis and testis almost always results from the spread of infection from another distant site of primary infection (Ferrie and Rundle, 1983). Epididymo-orchitis caused by *Haemophilus influenzae* (Thomas et al., 1981), *Nocardia* (Wheeler et al., 1986), *Salmonella* (Scott and Cosgrove, 1977), *Toxoplasma* (Nistal et al., 1986), and other microbes or parasites can be traced, in most cases, to hematogenous dissemination.

The *lymphatic* spread of infection from pelvic organs is not always distinct from ascending infection due to canalicular spread through the ejaculatory ducts and vas deferens. This fact is best illustrated by the appearance of epididymo-orchitis in patients suffering from tuberculosis of the kidneys or lower urinary tract (Windblad, 1975). Theoretically, the spread of infection from the kidney could occur through infected urine, but in view of the anatomic connections between the kidney and the genital organs, a lymphatic as well as a hematogenous spread cannot be excluded (Ross et al., 1961; Ferrie and Rundle, 1983). Epididymo-orchitis caused by attenuated tuberculosis bacilli, which has been described after intravesical injection of bacille Calmette-Guérin (BCG) favors the etiology of ascending canalicular infection from the lower urinary tract (George et al., 1991). Parasites that spread through the lymphatics, such as *Wuchereria,* may cause scrotal infection (Das et al., 1983). Schistosomiasis of the testis, epididymis, and vas deferens may reflect lymphatic, venous, canalicular or even hematogenous spread (Houston, 1964; Elbadawi et al., 1979).

Open wounds from traumatic laceration of the testis or scrotum often are entry sites of infection. Likewise, infections after surgery of the scrotum or the inguinal canal may cause epididymo-orchitis.

Inflammation of the testis and epididymis may be a manifestation of several diseases that have an incompletely understood pathogenesis (Klein et al., 1985). Multisystemic diseases, such as the acquired immunodeficiency syndrome (AIDS), can be accompanied by marked pathologic changes in the testis (dePaepe et al., 1989; dePaepe and Waxman, 1989; Yoshikawa et al., 1989; Nistal et al., 1986). These changes reflect, in part, the systemic effects of the viral infection and in part are secondary to infections that have spread to the testis and epididymis through one or more pathways.

Etiology. The primary causative agents of epididymo-orchitis have been changing over the years and generally reflect the prevalance of various infectious diseases in populations (Mittemeyer et al., 1966; Berger et al., 1979; Berger and Holmes, 1986; Melekos and Asbach, 1987). The etiology also is dependent on the age, social habits, sexual orientation, and general health of each patient.

Bacterial epididymo-orchitis is relatively uncommon in children (Hermansen et al., 1980). In this age group, *E. coli* and *Pseudomonas* predominate. In adults less than 35 years of age, sexually transmitted organisms such as *N. gonorrhoeae, Chlamydia,* and *Mycocoplasma* account for most cases (Berger et al., 1979). Untreated gonococcal epididymo-orchitis is a major cause of male infertility in Africa (Berger and Holmes, 1986). In older men, in whom urinary tract infections usually are secondary to obstruction of the bladder neck from prostatic hypertrophy, coliform bacteria are the leading cause of epididymo-orchitis (Berger et al., 1979; Melekos and Asbach, 1987). Other less common causes of bacterial epididymo-orchitis have been reviewed by Nistal and Paniagua (1984), Berger and Holmes (1986), and Hedinger and Dhone (1991) and include *Brucella* spp., *Salmonella* spp., *Streptococcus* spp., *Staphylococcus* spp., *Neisseria meningitidis, Streptococcus pneumoniae, Klebsiella, Actinomyces,* and *Nocardia.*

Certain microorganisms that usually are not linked to urogenital infections appear more often than would be expected in bacterial cultures from patients with epididymo-orchitis. These include principally *H. influenzae* (Thomas et al., 1981; Greenfield, 1986) and *Salmonella* species (Scott and Cosgrove, 1977; Weinstein et al., 1983).

Reports of syphilitic infection of the testis and epididymis were relatively common in the preantibiotic era but are rarely found in current literature (Persaud and Rao, 1977; Dao and Adkins, 1980). Likewise, in accordance with the decreasing incidence of tuberculosis, contemporary literature contains few reports of epididymo-orchitis caused by *M. tuberculosis* (Steinhauser and Wurster, 1975). Isolated case reports of tuberculous epididymo-orchitis published recently deal with unusual presentations such as isolated scrotal tuberculosis without any evidence of disease elsewhere (Stein and Miller, 1983); tuberculosis presenting as hydrocele (Reeve et al., 1974); tuberculosis limited to the spermatic cord (Duckek and Winblad, 1974); and tuberculosis presenting in an atypical clinical setting (Simon and Worthington, 1982).

M. leprae has a predilection to involve testes; testicular leprosy is common in the lepromatous and borderline forms of the disease (Nistal and Paniagua, 1984). Lepra bacilli proliferate in lower temperatures typical of the scrotum, and it is therefore not surprising that orchitis may be the first sign of infection with this acid-fast bacillus (Aktar et al., 1980). However, since leprosy is rare outside tropical, underdeveloped countries and since most patients with leprosy have multisystemic disease (Watson et al., 1974), statistics on the prevalence of lepromatous epididymo-orchitis are inexact and the impact of this infection on fertility remains inadequately documented.

Most *viral* infections of the testis and epididymis usually occur during systemic viremia and are often clinically unrecognized. The paradigm of viral orchitis is the inflammation that occurs during mumps infection (Gall, 1947; Werner, 1950). However, it has been shown that epididymo-orchitis may occur in other viral diseases caused by the adenovirus (Naveh and Friedman, 1975), Epstein-Barr virus (Hanid, 1977), echovirus (Welliver and Cherry, 1978), and cytomegalovirus (McCarthy et al., 1991). Viral infection can affect the testes and epididymides of male fetuses during gestation, as indirectly attested to by the finding of abnormalities in the vas deferens and epididymis of boys known to have had congenital rubella (Priebe et al., 1979). In most viral infections, the testis is more involved than the epididymis (Riggs and Sanford, 1962). Viral inclusions may be found in the epididymis (McCarthy et al., 1991) even without obvious clinical evidence of epididymitis. Bilateral infections are common, although in most cases the infection on one side produces more complaints, giving the impression of unilateral disease.

Fungi rarely cause epididymo-orchitis outside of tropical regions. An only exception is infection with *Histoplasma capsulatum,* which may involve the epididymis and testis during systemic dissemination and rarely as a localized scrotal disease (Monroe, 1974; Kauffman et al., 1981). Most other fungal infections of the testis and epididymis are noted in immunosuppressed persons such as those treated for cancer or those suffering from AIDS (Yoshikawa et al., 1989). Sporadic cases of fungal epididymo-orchitis are nevertheless on record and include infections caused by *Coccidioides immitis* (Gottesman, 1974) and *Blastomyces dermatitidis* (Eickenberg et al., 1975). Microorganisms with features of bacteria and fungi, such as *Nocardia* and *Actinomyces,* also have been reported to cause epididymo-orchitis (Wheeler et al., 1986).

Parasites causing scrotal lesions are important in the tropics but rarely are identified as pathogenetic organisms in temperate climates. Single case reports of epididymal or scrotal schistosomiasis (Honoré and Coleman, 1975), filariasis (Raghavaiah, 1981), and echynococcal infection (Halim and Vaezzadeh, 1980) illustrate the typical pathologic changes associated with parasitic infections of scrotal organs.

Clinical findings. Clinical findings in epididymo-orchitis depend on the predominant involvement of the testis or the epididymis. *Acute epididymitis* has been reviewed comprehensively by Berger (1991). Symptoms depend on the causative agent, the sequence of events that led to scrotal infection, the extent of the inflammatory reaction, and the duration of the disease. Principal symptoms include scrotal pain, tenderness on palpation, edema, and erythema. Usually the presentation is insidious, but one third of all patients have a sudden onset of symptoms. Local pain may be associated with dysuria or radiate into the inguinal region, especially in patients infected with *C. trachomatis* (Berger et al., 1979). A urethral discharge may be found in patients infected with *N. gonorrhoeae* but, surprisingly, only in 50% of cases (Watson, 1979). Berger (1991) recommends the taking of urethral swabs, a first-void midstream urine specimen, and, in refractory cases, epididymal aspirates for culture. This approach is used for patients who have indwelling urethral catheters, for those who do not respond to conventional antibiotic therapy, and for those with recurrent epididymitis and epididymitis of unknown etiology.

Orchitis is dominated by symptoms related to testicular edema and pain caused by the expanding tunica albuginea. Usually, symptoms are not focal but include the entire testicle. Urinary symptoms usually are not prominent; there is no urethral discharge and the urine does not contain pathogenic bacteria. Ultrasonography recently has been used to evaluate testicular enlargement and to help in distinguishing epididymo-orchitis from other lesions, such as torsion, hydrocele, and tumors.

Infertility is an important complication of epididymo-orchitis. Berger and Holmes (1986) reviewed the literature, analyzed their own data, and found that 10% to 40% of all patients with a history of testicular and/or epididymal inflammation, both unilateral and bilateral, were sterile. Testicular atrophy and persistent inflammation could be found to be the underlying cause of subfertility in patients who were studied with biopsy (Nilsson et al., 1968; Wolin, 1971). Even in those patients with predominant epididymitis there are inflammatory changes in the adjacent testicular parenchyma, and it is quite plausible that the contralateral testis may be involved even though there are no clinical signs of bilateral disease.

Reduced fertility and low sperm counts in patients with unilateral epididymo-orchitis are not fully understood. Several hypotheses were proposed but none was generally accepted. The most likely causes, discussed by Berger and Holmes (1986), are as follows:

1. *Unilateral obstruction*—This explanation is difficult to accept, since men with one testis usually have normal sperm counts.
2. *Subclinical bilateral inflammation*—Since infections easily spread from one scrotal compartment to another, bilateral lesions are common and occur more often than clinically recognized.
3. *Sympathetic damage to the contralateral testis*—Circulating autoantibodies to sperm and reduced spermatogenesis in the contralateral testis have been reported by several investigators. Thus, damage may be mediated by immune mechanisms.

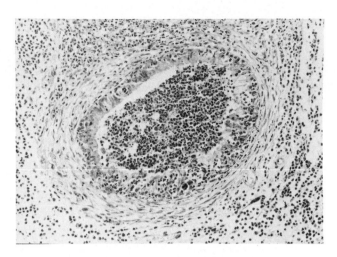

Fig. 5-1. Suppurative epididymo-orchitis.

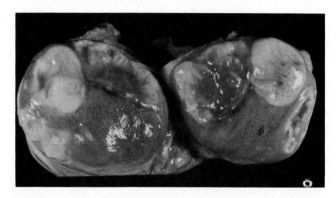

Fig. 5-2. Abscess of the epididymis and testis. (From Mikuz G, Damjanov I. Pathol Annual 1982(I); 17:101, with permission.)

Pathology. Pathologic findings vary from one case to another, but they depend primarily on the nature of the causative agent and the duration of the disease.

Suppurative epididymo-orchitis. This form of inflammation usually is caused by bacteria that spread through the seminal ducts and invade the epididymis (Fig. 5-1). The lumen of the duct contains pus; the wall of the epididymis usually is infiltrated with polymorphonuclear leukocytes. Abscesses may form, thus destroying large portions of the epididymis with extensions into the testis and adjacent scrotal structures (Fig. 5-2). Hydrocele often accompanies this form of inflammation, and its fluid may become infected with the spread of inflammation. The fluid becomes turbid or purulent. In extreme cases the entire scrotum may be filled with pus.

Interstitial epididymo-orchitis. Interstitial infiltrates of mononuclear cells in the testis or epididymis represent the typical reaction to viral infections as seen in mumps orchitis (Gall, 1947; Manson, 1990). In early stages of the orchitis, scattered lymphocytes and plasma cells are noted, though spermatogenesis continues (Fig. 5-3). In older le-

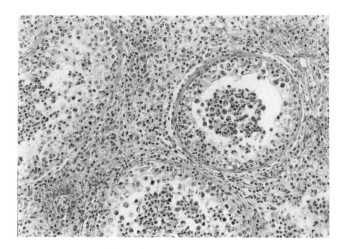

Fig. 5-3. Acute mumps orchitis.

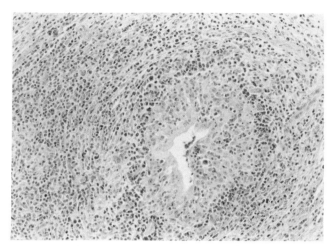

Fig. 5-5. Mumps infection involving the rete testis and epididymis.

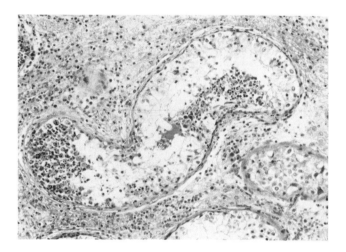

Fig. 5-4. Chronic mumps orchitis.

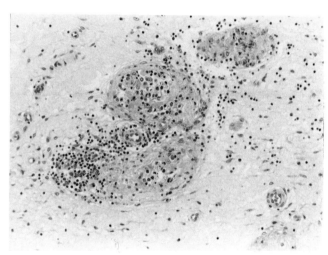

Fig. 5-6. Nonspecific orchitis of unknown origin incidentally discovered in an orchiectomy specimen of a patient with prostate carcinoma.

sions, there is extensive tissue damage evidenced by arrested spermatogenesis and atrophy of the spermatogenic epithelium with tubular hyalinization (Fig. 5-4).

Viral orchitis extends usually to the rete testis and epididymis, which are infiltrated with lymphocytes and plasma cells (Fig. 5-5).

Infiltrates of lymphocytes and plasma cells may be found in the interstitial tissue of the testis and epididymis of older men without clinical evidence of epididymo-orchitis (Fig. 5-6). Such nonspecific inflammation detected in orchiectomy specimens of patients with prostate cancer or at autopsy could represent residues of previous infections or an immune response to testicular and epididymal injury. In most cases, however, it is not possible to provide an unequivocal explanation for such histologic findings.

Granulomatous inflammation. Caseating granulomas composed of epithelioid cells and lymphocytes surrounding foci of necrosis may be caused by *M. tuberculosis, Histoplasma,* or other infectious agents known to cause

such inflammation in other anatomic sites (Fig. 5-7). Extensive destruction of the testis and epididymis occurs in long-lasting infection. Epididymal nodularity or scattered foci of induration in the testis may be seen on gross inspection. On cut surface, larger granulomas appear caseous, whereas the smaller foci appear whitish and firm. The causative agents may be demonstrated by special stains, immunohistochemistry, or bacteriologic culture. If no caustive agents are demonstrated, the differential diagnosis should include systemic granulomatoses, especially sarcoidosis (Fig. 5-8), which may involve the testis and its appendages (Amenta et al., 1981).

Malacoplakia. Malacoplakia is a histologically typical response to injury that may involve the testis (McClure, 1980) or epididymis (Dubey et al., 1988). The etiology of malacoplakia is not known, but generally it is accepted

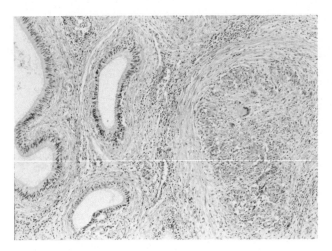

Fig. 5-7. Granulomatous epididymo-orchitis caused by *M. tuberculosis*.

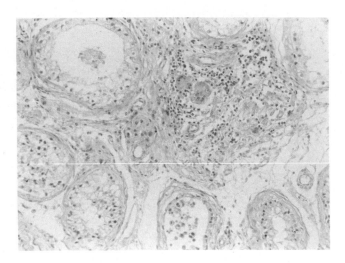

Fig. 5-8. Sarcoidosis of the testis.

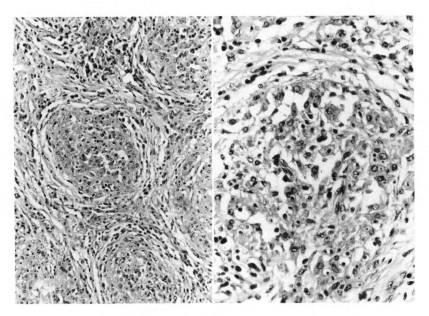

Fig. 5-9. Malacoplakia of the testis.

that it represents a mononuclear cell response to bacterial infection (Damjanov and Katz, 1981). Histologically, the inflammatory lesions are composed of histiocytes, lymphocytes, and plasma cells, which infiltrate the connective tissue, interstitial spaces of the testis, seminiferous tubules, and epididymal ducts (Fig. 5-9). Normal anatomic structures of each organ are obliterated and destroyed by the inflammatory infiltrate. Histiocytes infiltrating the malacoplakic lesions may contain residues of phagocytized bacteria. More often, they typically contain large, round, calcified, cytoplasmic inclusions that are positive on periodic acid–Schiff reaction (PAS) and are rich in iron. These inclusions are known as Michaelis-Gutmann bodies; the histiocytes containing them eponymically are known as von Hansemann cells. On electron microscopy, the Michaelis-

Gutmann bodies appear as concentric layers of mineralized and nonmineralized granular matrix (Fig. 5-10). Biochemically, these bodies are composed of hydroxyapatite crystals. It has been proposed that von Hansemann histiocytes accumulate various materials in their phagolysosomes, and since they cannot digest or evacuate them, this foreign material becomes the nidus for calcification and leads to formation of cytoplasmic microcalcospherites (Damjanov and Katz, 1981).

The diagnosis of malacoplakia is based on finding typical von Hansemann histiocytes with calcified cytoplasmic inclusions (Rinaudo et al., 1977). Testicular infiltrates composed of histiocytes, lymphocytes, and plasma cells that do not contain typical von Hansemann histiocytes are classified as granulomatous orchitis (Aitchison et al.,

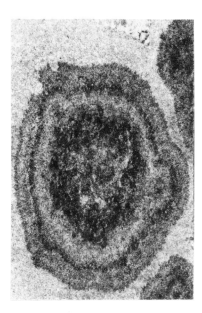

Fig. 5-10. Electron microscopy of the Michaelis-Gutmann body. (From Damjanov I, Katz SM. Pathol Annual 1981(II); 16:103, with permission.)

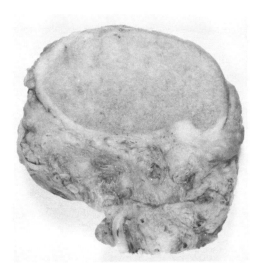

Fig. 5-11. Gumma of testis.

1990). The distinction of malacoplakia from granulomatous orchitis is tenuous, however, and many cases labeled granulomatous orchitis probably represent early malacoplakia devoid of diagnostic Michaelis-Gutmann bodies (Nistal and Paniagua, 1984). Xanthogranulomatous epididymitis described by Wiener et al. (1987) could be yet another variant of the same disease.

Gumma. Gumma is a typical lesion of tertiary syphilis that on rare occasions may occur in the testis or epididymis. It is characterized by central necrosis surrounded by normal tissue components that still preserve their outlines and are surrounded at the periphery with inflammatory infiltrates composed of lymphocytes, plasma cells, histio-

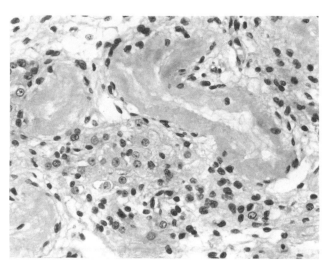

Fig. 5-12. Fibrosis of the testis or tubular hyalinization are late sequelae of chronic epididymo-orchitis.

cytes, and occasional giant cells. The entire testis may be destroyed by chronic inflammation which also involve, the capsule and surrounding structures (Fig. 5-11).

Eosinophilic inflammation. Eosinophilic inflammation is a common reaction to parasites. In addition to numerous eosinophils, typical infiltrates contain lymphocytes and plasma cells. Polymorphonucelar leukocytes forming microabscesses, fibrosis, and foreign body giant cells may be seen as well.

Foreign body giant cell reaction. This reaction often is elicited by dead parasites or the ova that they have deposited in the scrotal tissue.

Fibrosis. Fibrosis is a common sequela of chronic epididymo-orchitis (Fig. 5-12). It may present as focal or diffuse scarring of the testis and epididymis in which the connective tissue replaces the normal tissue components (Fig. 5-13). Interstitial fibrosis of the testis and epididymis surrounding residual atrophic tubules or ductules may be seen. Also, connective tissue capsules encasing the testis or epididymis or chronic abscesses that have developed in any of the scrotal compartments occur (Fig. 5-14). Occasionally, the entire testis and epididymis are destroyed and replaced by multiple abscesses, each of which is encased by a dense fibrous capsule giving the cross-sectioned scrotum a honeycomb appearance.

Inflammation of the seminal vesicles, urethra, and prostate

The impact on fertility of lower urinary tract, seminal vesicle, and prostate infections is debatable. Nevertheless, a clinical work-up of an infertile man would be incomplete without a urologic evaluation, which should document that the organs at the neck of the bladder are normally developed and also that they do not harbor any signs of acute or chronic infection.

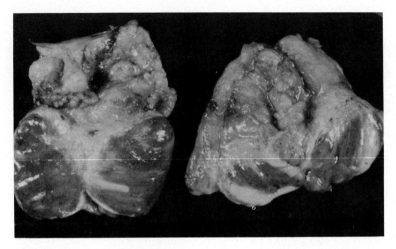

Fig. 5-13. Fibrosis of chronic orchitis.

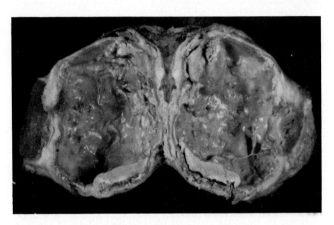

Fig. 5-14. Chronic scrotal abscesses.

Comhaire et al. (1987) consider that a patient has an accessory gland infection if at least two of the following laboratory or clinical findings are present:

1. History of urogenital infection, epididymitis, sexually transmitted disease, and/or abnormalities on rectal examination
2. Abnormal discharge on prostatic massage or abnormal urine
3. More than one million white cells per milliliter found in the ejaculate
4. Pathogenic bacteria in significant numbers isolated and cultured from the urinary tract
5. Abnormal gross appearance, pH, or biochemical profile of seminal fluid

Infections of the seminal vesicles, prostate, urinary bladder, and urethra could affect fertility in several ways:

1. Acute inflammation may influence the viability of spermatozoa and can alter their morphology (Boström, 1971) by virtue of the action of bacteria or the inflammatory cells in the exudate.

2. Inflammation of the seminal vesicles may change the pH of the fluid as well as its composition. This could influence the fertilizing capacity of the spermatozoa.
3. Purulent inflammation could destroy the seminal vesicles; chronic inflammation could obliterate their communication with the urethra. Thus, formation of the normal ejaculate could be prevented since 70% of most of the ejaculate is from the seminal vesicles.
4. Chronic inflammation and scarring in the area of the bladder neck could lead to obstruction of the ejaculatory ducts and obstructive azoospermia.
5. Inflammation of the bladder neck could spread into the ejaculatory ducts and into the epididymis, destroying the epithelium and causing scarring and obstruction of sperm passages.

The prevalence of seminal vesicle inflammation in asymptomatic adults, those with urinary tract infection, or those with infertility is not known. However, there is no reason to believe that seminal vesicles would be spared from infection involving other parts of the lower male urinary tract.

Clinical diagnosis of an abscess involving the seminal vesicles may be made with modern imaging techniques, as shown by Fox et al. (1988), who used computerized, coaxial tomography to corroborate their clinical diagnosis and to monitor the therapy. Whether chronic vesiculitis adversely affects fertility, as proposed by Scarselli et al. (1978), remains to be proved. Furthermore, even if one were to prove that the inflammation of seminal vesicles may cause subfertility, in clinical practice it is a rarely encountered disease.

Prostatitis is a more prevalent disease than vesiculitis, but its impact on fertility remains controversial (Berger and Holmes, 1986). The pathogenesis of prostatitis and various complications of this disease are given in Algorithm 5-1. Boström (1971) found histologic signs of prostatitis in 22% of men younger than 40 years and in 60% of

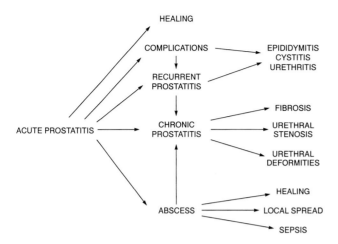

Algorithm 5-1. Consequences of prostatic infection.

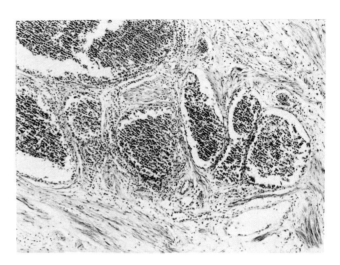

Fig. 5-15. Acute and chronic prostatitis.

those who were older than 40. Such inflammation may be symptomatic or asymptomatic. The causative agents vary and include coliform bacteria, *Chlamydia,* and *Ureaplasma urealyticum* as well as other common sexually transmitted microorganisms (Berger and Holmes, 1986). However, few reliable clinical findings are pathognomic for prostatitis, and the clinical significance of histologic or bacteriologic signs of prostatic inflammation, acute or chronic, cannot be interpreted unequivocally (Gorelick et al., 1988).

Inflammation of the posterior urethra often is associated with prostatitis. It may be caused by coliform bacteria, *Chlamydia,* and other sexually transmitted microorganisms. *N. gonorrhoeae* has a predilection to colonize the periurethral glands, thus accounting for the frequent gonococcal infections of the bulbar urethra and the common occurrence of posterior urethral strictures in untreated cases (Blandy, 1980). Approximately 2% to 5% of all patients with gonorrhea develop that complication. More recent data do not include information on the prevalence of this complication, though it is important clinically to consider it as a cause of obstructive azoospermia in patients with a history of gonococcal infection.

Lees (1990) has summarized the significance of bacteria in human semen and has emphasized that there is a wide disparity in conclusions between various studies, reflecting in part the methodologic differences between different studies and in part the differences in the populations tested. According to Lees (1990), the following important points should be noted:

1. In fertile men there are fewer bacteriologically positive cultures than in age-matched infertile men.
2. Bacterial isolates are more often obtained from men with a history of genital tract infection.
3. Asymptomatic bacteriospermia is greater in men with a history of gonococcal infection than in any other group of patients.
4. Most samples of semen contain bacteria; often two or more different bacteria may be cultured.

5. *Ureaplasma* is more frequently isolated from patients with nonspecific urethritis or gonococcal infection than from those who are asymptomatic and never had sexually transmitted diseases.
6. It is likely that only a few microorganisms cause infertility and that the aerobic gram-positive bacteria probably are not important pathogenetically since they represent normal urethral flora. Similarly, there is no consistent documentation proving the pathogenetic role of *Trichomonas,* a commonly found sexually transmitted organism, in infertility.

Pathologic findings. The pathology of various forms of inflammation involving the seminal vesicles and the prostate has been described in detail in textbooks of urogenital pathology (Murphy, 1989; Petersen, 1992). The histologic findings are nonspecific. In acute inflammation, the gland is infiltrated with polymorphonuclear leukocytes, which also fill the lumen of the glands. Microabscesses are common, and they may become confluent to occupy large portions of the parenchyma, although grossly visible abscesses are uncommon except in diabetic patients. Chronic prostatitis is marked by nonspecific infiltrates of lymphocytes, histiocytes, and plasma cells (Fig. 5-15). Histologically distinct forms of prostatitis, such as granulomatous prostatitis (Epstein and Hutchins, 1984) or eosinophilic prostatitis, do not correspond to any particular clinical picture. Malacoplakia of the prostate is histologically similar to the same disease found elsewhere. It does not have specific clinical findings (Kawamura et al., 1980).

INFECTIONS OF THE FEMALE GENITAL ORGANS

Infections of the female genital organs are among the most important causes of infertility (Sherris and Fox, 1983). Such infections may involve particular parts of the internal reproductive organs or cause inflammation of the entire genital tract, known as pelvic inflammatory disease (PID).

Cervicitis

Cervicitis presents as acute or chronic inflammation of the endocervix, characterized clinically by a mucopurulent exudate in the cervical canal (Paavonen et al., 1985). The diagnosis may be corroborated by colposcopy, microscopic examination of the cervical mucus, and bacteriologic studies. Colposcopy usually reveals erythema and edema of the transformation zone. Cervical smears contain typically more than 10 polymorphonuclear leukocytes per high power field (Brunham et al., 1984). Gram-stained cervical smears may reveal *Chlamydia* (Katz et al., 1989). Bacteriologic data provide the final proof of the infection. The diagnosis may be confirmed by cervical biopsy, but this procedure is usually not performed routinely, espe-

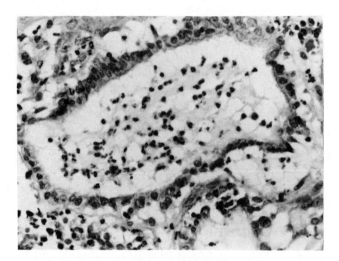

Fig. 5-16. Acute cervicitis.

cially since there is suboptimal correlation between the histologic findings and the clinical data.

Pathologic findings. On the basis of histologic findings, cervicitis may be classified as acute or chronic. However, the correlation between the histologic and clinical data has been poor for several reasons, including:

1. Nonspecific nature of the inflammatory response
2. Frequent coexistence of acute and chronic inflammatory cells
3. Multifactorial etiology of the lesions
4. Inadequate knowledge of the natural history of cervicitis

Acute inflammation is characterized by infiltrates composed of polymorphonuclear leukocytes in the stroma and within the lumen of glands and inside the epithelium (Fig. 5-16). In addition to acute inflammatory cells, almost all cases show signs of chronic inflammation. Occasionally abscesses form, replacing the glands or the stroma. Edema of the stroma and the epithelium is common. Epithelial ulcerations, with or without signs of necrosis, are found occasionally.

Chronic cervicitis is characterized by infiltrates composed of lymphocytes, macrophages, and plasma cells (Fig. 5-17). Occasionally, the infiltrates contain prominent eosinophils, but mast cells are usually inconspicuous. Dense infiltrates may form lymphoid follicles with prominent germinal follicles (Fig. 5-18). Granulomatous cervicitis is found in tuberculosis, sarcoidosis, and histoplasmosis but may be caused by many other pathogens.

Kiviat et al. (1990a) have performed a controlled histopathologic study of endocervicitis in women with bacteriologically proven infectious cervicitis who have clinical ev-

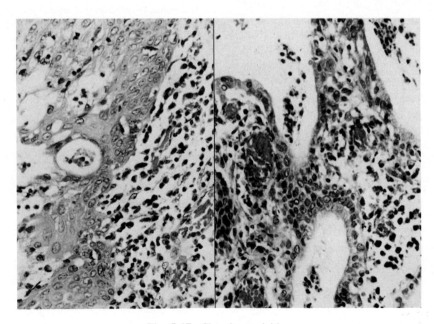

Fig. 5-17. Chronic cervicitis.

idence of mucopurulent cervicitis and those in whom an infectious etiology could not be documented. These authors analyzed epithelial and stromal changes and found that some of these histologic features are very good predictors of infection, which correlated well with the clinical and bacteriologic data (Table 5-1). It is important to note that acute and chronic inflammatory cells occur in both groups, but in general, such infiltrates were more common in women with mucopurulent cervicitis and bacteriologically proven cervical infection than in controls. Chronic inflammatory cells could represent residues of previous infections, but the noninfectious causes of inflammation could not be ruled out. Kiviat et al. (1990a) caution not to

make clinical predictions on the basis of histologic findings alone.

The etiologic diagnosis of cervicitis cannot be made histologically. Certain morphologic features are more frequently associated with certain pathogens. Thus, *C. trachomatis* is associated with follicles that have germinal centers, focal surface ulceration, intraepithelial inflammation of grandular and squamous epithelium, and occasional reactive epithelial atypia and dense stromal inflammation with plasma cells. Necrotic ulcers and inflammatory infiltrates dominated by lymphocytes and histiocytes rather than plasma cells are common in herpes virus infection. Viral nuclear inclusions are not readily visible in tissue

Table 5-1. Prevalence of endocervical histologic features in women with clinically diagnosed mucopurulent cervicitis

Histologic findings	Clinically confirmed mucopurulent cervicitis (%)	Control group (%)	Significance
Columnar epithelium			
Intraepithelial neutrophils	89	54	0.0007
Focal loss of epithelial cells	66	50	NS
Reactive endocervical cells	75	33	0.0004
Intraluminal neutrophils	66	19	0.0001
Squamous epithelium			
Intraepithelial neutrophils	63	30	NS
Spongiosis	26	10	NS
Epithelial edema	78	56	NS
Deep tissue changes			
Extent of inflammation			
0	6	7	NS
1	2	26	NS
2	18	33	NS
3	75	33	0.0008
Well-formed germinal centers	34	17	NS
Granulation tissue	87	59	0.008
Necrotic ulceration	25	4	0.02

Modified from Kiviat et al. Hum Pathol 1990; 21:831, with permission.
NS = not significant at the p ≤ 0.01.

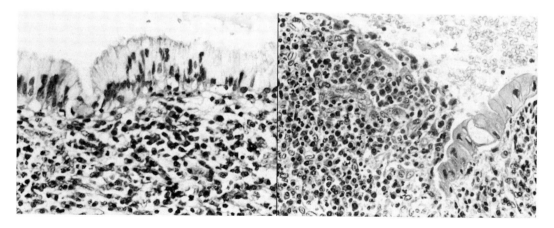

Fig. 5-18. Chronic cervicitis with formation of lymphoid follicles.

sections. Immunohistochemical stains may be used to demonstrate the pathogens.

Granulomatous cervicitis is a feature of tuberculosis that may involve any part of the female genital tract (Nogales-Ortiz et al., 1979). Granulomas are not diagnostic of tuberculosis, however, and may occur in sarcoidosis and other granulomatous diseases. Frequently, cervical granulomas of tuberculosis are overshadowed by dense lymphocytic infiltrates. This probably reflects the peripheral location of the cervix to the main nidus of inflammation, which is most often in the fallopian tubes (Nogales-Ortiz et al., 1979) or the endometrium (Bazaz-Malik et al., 1983).

Syphilis may cause cervical ulceration or endocervicitis. Primary chancre occurs presumably in the cervix in almost one third of all patients, but there are no reliable recent reports documenting these claims from the older literature. As in other syphilitic lesions, perivascular infiltrates of lymphocytes and plasma cells predominate and occasionally giant cells may be found (Tchertkoff and Ober, 1966).

Endometritis

Endometritis is inflammation of the endometrium that occurs in acute and chronic forms. Endometritis may be isolated, but more often it is associated with salpingitis and cervicitis and is just one feature of PID (Kiviat et al., 1990b). The conditions predisposing to endometritis are listed in the box at right.

The endometrial biopsy is essential for the diagnosis, which is typically made by combining the histopathologic and bacteriologic data. Diagnostic histopathologic findings include the following:

1. *Dense infiltrates of polymorphonuclear leukocytes.* These infiltrates are typically found in the superficial layers of the endometrium, extending into the lumen and permeating the epithelial layers of the glands or surface lining (Fig. 5-19). Scattered polymorphonuclear leukocytes are normally found in the endometrium, and the infiltrates become prominent toward the end of the menstrual cycle (Poropatich et al., 1987). Thus, leukocytic infiltrates should be interpreted judiciously and in conjunction with other findings, most notably the presence or absence of tissue destruction and the presence or absence of plasma cells. Epithelial cells should also be evaluated to determine whether the endometrium shows normal cyclicity and whether there is coordinated menstrual cycle–related maturation of stromal and epithelial components.
2. *Abscesses.* Localized suppuration with tissue destruction is a reliable sign of endometritis. Unfortunately, abscesses are common.
3. *Plasma cell infiltrates.* Infiltrates of plasma cells and even scattered plasma cells in the endometrial stroma are good evidence of endometritis. In con-

Conditions predisposing to endometritis not related to PID

Postpartum period
Abortion
Intrauterine procedures
    Curettage
    Aspiration biopsy
    Hysteroscopy
    Hysterography
Foreign body
    Intrauterine contraceptive device
    Sundry objects, parasites
Necrotic tissue
    Endometrial hemorrhagic infarct
    Polyp
    Endometrial cancer
    Myometrial leiomyoma
Uterine prolapse
Traumatic or iatrogenic cervical stenosis
Systemic infection
    Sepsis
    Tuberculosis

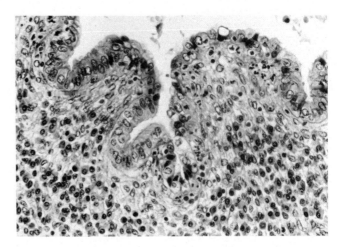

Fig. 5-19. Acute endometritis.

trast to lymphocytes, histiocytes, and mast cells that normally occur in the endometrium, plasma cells are not normally found and their presence indicates inflammation.
4. *Eosinophils.* These cells are not found normally in the endometrium and are signs of inflammation. However, inflammations dominated by eosinophils are uncommon (Miko et al., 1988).
5. *Foamy macrophages.* Dense infiltrates of foamy macrophages in the endometrium are found in so-called xanthomatous endometritis.
6. *Malacoplakia.* Infiltrates composed of von Hansemann histiocytes that show intracytoplasmic calcific

inclusions or Michaelis-Gutmann bodies are similar to those seen in malacoplakia of other organs (Damjanov and Katz, 1981).

7. *Granulomas*. Aggregates of epithelioid cells, lymphocytes, and giant cells with or without caseating necrosis are characteristic of tuberculosis and other granulomatous disorders (Nogales-Ortiz et al., 1979; Falk et al., 1980).

Endometritis is associated with numerous other histologic changes reviewed by Clement (1991) and presented in the box at right. Although these histologic findings are not specific and do not suffice for the diagnosis of endometritis, they provide additional evidence that the endometrium is pathologically altered (Fig. 5-20).

Histologic diagnosis of endometritis is typically made on about 3% to 10% of all endometrial biopsies and surgically removed uteri examined by the pathologist (Clement, 1991). Endometritis may be an isolated finding, but more often it is a part of PID and is associated with salpingitis and cervicitis (Rotterdam, 1978). Thus, endometrial biopsy is useful for documenting PID.

Several morphologic findings in the endometrial biopsy strongly correlate with inflammation involving the fallopian tubes and are thus good predictors of salpingitis (Paavonen et al., 1985 and 1987; Kiviat et al., 1990b). Paavonen et al. (1985) diagnosed salpingitis by laparoscopy in 89% of patients with histologic evidence of endometritis, compared with an incidence of salpingitis of 33% in those without evidence of endometritis. The extent of plasma cellular infiltration of the endometrium correlated with the severity of salpingitis (Paavonen et al., 1987).

The following histologic findings in endometrial biopsies predict the coexistence of salpingitis according to Kiviat et al. (1990b):

1. Presence of neutrophils in the surface epithelial layer of the endometrium
2. Neutrophils within glandular lumina
3. Dense subepithelial stromal lymphocytic infiltrates
4. Stromal plasma cells
5. Lymphoid germinal centers containing transformed lymphocytes

The best predictor of salpingitis was finding in the same high-power field (X400) five or more polymorphonuclear leukocytes within the surface epithelium together with one or more plasma cells in the stroma observed at medium-power magnification (X120).

Infertility is the major complication of endometritis. The inflamed endometrium does not respond appropriately to hormonal stimulation and cannot provide the adequate environment for the implantation of the blastocyst. Furthermore, the inflammatory cells damage the tissue and secrete various bioactive substances that are cytotoxic to spermatozoa as well as the embryo.

> **Nonspecific histologic changes in endometritis**
>
> *Stromal changes*
>
> Aggregates of lymphocytes
> Lymphoid follicles with germinal centers showing activation of lymphocytes
> Hemosiderin-laden macrophages
> Superficial stromal edema
> Periglandular palisading of stromal cells
> Fibrosis with an increased density of fibroblasts
> Stromal necrosis
> Intrasinusoidal thrombi
>
> *Epithelial changes*
>
> Out-of-date appearance of glands (glandulo-stromal discordance)
> Marked variation size, shape, and cells lining the glands
> Inactive epithelium—atrophic, eosinophilic cytoplasm
> Metaplasia, squamous, or morule formation
> Proliferative foci—mitoses, stratification of epithelium
> Nuclear changes—clearing of the chromatin, prominent nucleoli

Data from Clement PB. In Kraus FT, Damjanov I, Kaufman N (Eds). Pathology of Reproductive Failure. Baltimore, Williams & Wilkins, 1991, © Williams & Wilkins, 1991. Used by permission.

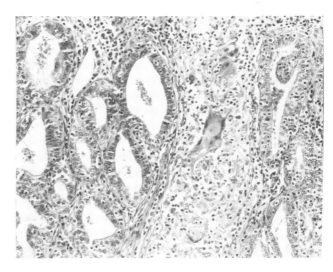

Fig. 5-20. Chronic endometritis. Heterogenous stromal infiltrate surrounds glands that show crowding and cannot be dated.

Salpingitis and the pelvic inflammatory disease

Salpingitis denotes inflammation of the fallopian tubes. However, since salpingitis represents the principal sign of PID, these two conditions are often considered under the same heading or as synonyms.

PID is a major health problem (reviewed by Cates et al., 1990). About 17% of all American women reported in 1988 that they had been treated for PID. It has been estimated that 420,000 women required treatment for PID in 1990 (Cates et al., 1990). From 1979 to 1988 a mean of 180,000 women aged 15 to 44 years were hospitalized

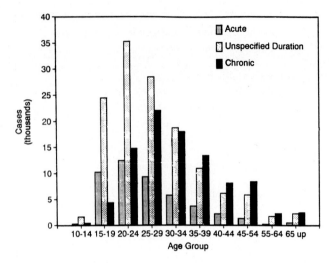

Fig. 5-21. Average annual number of hospitalizations for PID in the United States from 1979 to 1988. (From Rolfs et al., 1992, with permission.)

Factors contributing to changes in the pattern of infectious causes of infertility

1. Sexual behavior
   Promiscuity
   Bisexuality
2. Contraception
   Legalized abortion
   Oral contraceptives
   Intrauterine contraceptive devices
   Barrier methods
3. Microbial flora
   Sexually transmitted diseases
   Polymicrobial infection
   Systemic pathogens
4. Treatment modalities
   Antibiotics—sensitivity, resistance
   Gynecologic surgery
   Postpartum care
5. Cultural and social factors
   Vaginal douching
   Menstrual tampons

Parameters of sexual behavior of potential importance for epidemiology of pelvic inflammatory disease

Coitus-related behavioral variables

Duration of coitus
Frequency of coitus
Activities during coitus
Douching after coitus
Timing during menstrual cycle
Time since last coitus
Age at first coitus
Coitus in the presence of genital infections
Use of coitally dependent contraceptive methods
Concomitant alcohol or drug use

Sexual partner–related variables

Number of recent partners
Number of lifetime partners
Prostitution
Sexual preference
Duration of relationships
Knowledge of partners' sexual behavior
Method of choosing partners
Concurrent versus sequential partners
Sexual behavior of the partners (e.g., number of partners, prostitution, sexual preference)

Variables that may influence the development of PID

Gender
Age
Marital status
Race or ethnicity
Socioeconomic status
Pregnancy history
History of sexually transmitted diseases
Current and past contraceptive methods
Use of vaginal douching
Use of medications that may affect sexual behavior
Debilitating health problems

Modified from Lee et al. with permission from The American College of Obstetricians and Gynecologists, Obstet Gynecol 1991; 77:425.

---

each year for acute PID (3.03 of 1000); 94,000 were hospitalized for chronic PID (0.90 of 1000); and nearly 400,000 (7.2 of 1000) had visited physicians' offices for PID (Rolfs et al., 1992).

Women of all ages are hospitalized for PID, although most are typically in the reproductive years (Fig. 5-21). According to the estimates of the Centers for Disease Control, the total economic cost of PID was more than $4 billion for 1990 (Rolfs et al., 1992).

Pathogenesis. The pathogenesis of PID has been changing under the influence of many societal and medical factors (box above). In the vast majority of cases salpingi-

tis and PID develop from ascending infections (Paavonen et al., 1987). The pathogens gain access to the fallopian tubes by entering the uterus through the cervix and by ascending along the endometrial mucosa. Lymphatic and hematogeneous spread and transperitoneal spread of infections account for less than 1% of all cases. PID closely reflects the sexual mores of society. Various behavioral and social risk factors for PID are listed in the box above.

Etiology. PID is typically a polymicrobial disease most often caused by *C. trachomatis, N. gonorrhoeae,* and mixed aerobic and anaerobic bacteria (Cates et al., 1990; Walters and Gibbs, 1990).

C. trachomatis is the most common sexually transmitted pathogen (Martin, 1990), which accounts for 50% of

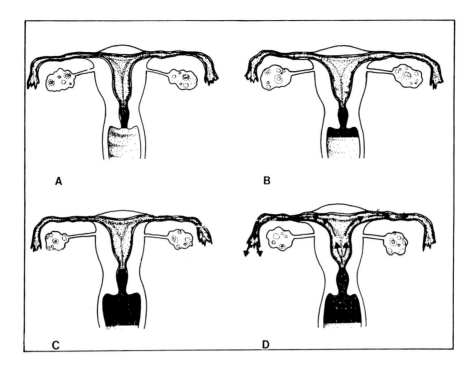

Fig. 5-22. Pathogenesis of PID caused by mixed infection. The initial events are cervicitis or bacterial vaginosis, which predisposes to ascending infection of the uterus and fallopian tubes. (From Wasserheit JN. Pelvic inflammatory disease and infertility. Md State Med J 1987; 36(1):58–63, with permission.)

all PID (Weström, 1980; Paavonen, 1989) and a considerable number of infertility problems in women (Sweet, 1987; Sellors et al., 1988). Approximately 20% of chlamydial infections result in long-term complications, such as tubal occlusion and pelvic adhesions (Winkler and Crum, 1987; Brunham et al., 1988). Up to three fourths of all chlamydial infections of the female genital tract may be asymptomatic (Handsfield et al., 1986). The infection is almost never limited to the fallopian tubes, and the pathogen can be isolated from the cervix, endometrium, or the pelvic aspirates (Stacey et al., 1990).

Gonorrhea is the most common reported communicable disease in the United States (Judson, 1990). From 1966 to 1976 the number of cases of gonorrhea increased 13% per year until 1975, when approximately 1 million cases were reported (McNeeley, 1989). In 1986 there were approximately 900,000 cases, but estimates are that only half of all treated cases are reported (McNeeley, 1989). The highest incidence has been registered in young nonwhite urban dwellers of low socioeconomic status (Barnes and Holmes, 1984). However, since *N. gonorrhoeae* cannot always be isolated from chronic PID lesions, the number of PID cases caused by this sexually transmitted pathogen cannot be determined precisely.

Mycoplasma (M. hominis, M. genitalium, U. urealyticum) frequently can be isolated from the cervix and endometrium and less often from the fallopian tubes of women with PID (Risi and Sanders, 1989). The pathogenetic role of these microorganisms in genital infections is controver-

sial (Gump et al., 1985). Generally, *Mycoplasma* is thought to be of limited significance as a primary cause of major pathologic changes in the female genital tract (Clement, 1991). However, it cannot be excluded that it might increase the virulence and the pathogenecity of other microbes and promote polymicrobial infection.

Anaerobic and aerobic bacteria that colonize the lower female genital tract play an important role in the pathogenesis of PID (Clement, 1991). Bacteria such as *E. coli, P. aeruginosa,* and *H. influenzae* are commonly isolated from PID lesions.

Wasserheit (1987) has proposed a four-step sequence of events leading to polymicrobial PID (Fig. 5-22). According to this view, an initial cervical inflammation caused by *C. trachomatis* or *N. gonorrhoeae* or some other pathogen could change the cervical microenvironment by increasing the vaginal pH, by depleting oxygen, and by generating new metabolic by-products. Anoxic conditions and alkaline favor overgrowth of anaerobes, which subsequently spread into the deeper parts of the endocervix and the uterine cavity and the fallopian tubes. Menstrual bleeding seems to facilitate the spread of *N. gonorrhoeae* and *C. trachomatis* (Sweet et al., 1985), whereas other pathogens ascend independently of the menstrual cycle.

Clinical findings. According to Sweet (1987), the clinical diagnosis of PID is based on symptoms, gynecologic findings, and laboratory data in the box on p. 120. These criteria, however, are not generally accepted. Furthermore, salpingitis may be "atypical" or clinically "silent"

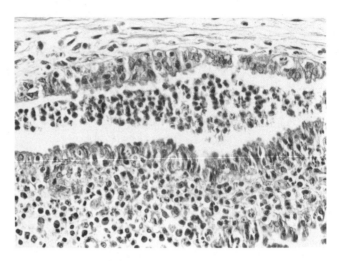

Fig. 5-23. Acute salpingitis.

(Patton et al., 1989). Laparoscopy is diagnostically useful (Method, 1988). Additional clinical data may be found in excellent monographs by Parish and Gschnait (1989) and by MacLean (1990) and in the multiauthored textbook *Sexually Transmitted Diseases,* edited by Holmes et al. (1990).

Pathologic findings. The gross morphology and the histologic findings vary depending on the cause of salpingitis, its duration, and other extenuating circumstances (Weström, 1980 and 1987). On the basis of the duration of symptoms and the gross and histologic findings, it is customary to recognize for didactic purposes and systematization an *acute* and a *chronic* form of the disease. Histologically, salpingitis may be classified as *serous, suppurative,* or *granulomatous.* On the basis of pathogenesis, salpingitis may be classified as *primary,* if acquired through ascending infection, or *secondary,* if related to some other infection of the pelvic organs. Etiologically, salpingitis may be classified according to the bacteriologic findings. Epidemiologically, salpingitis may be a *sexually acquired* disease or an *iatrogenic, endogenous,* or *spontaneous* infection. The distinction between these various forms of salpingitis is rarely possible in practice.

Acute salpingitis. Acute salpingitis begins as an exudative inflammation of the mucosa. On gross examination the fallopian tubes appear swollen and congested and have a narrowed lumen. Pus may be expressed from the fimbrial end. The serosal surface may be covered with a fibrinous exudate. Histologically, the mucosal folds appear edematous and are infiltrated predominantly with polymorphonuclear leukocytes (Fig. 5-23). Initially, the inflammatory cells occupy the stromal spaces. Subsequently, the leukocytes invade the mucosal epithelium and migrate into the lumen of the tube. Ulceration of the mucosa and the exu-

date in the lumen causes adhesions between the folds and complete obliteration of the lumen. The inflammation also spreads into the muscularis and to the serosa. Abscesses form inside the wall of the fallopian tube and are frequently interconnected or confluent with one another.

Chronic salpingitis. Unresolved acute salpingitis or recurrent attacks of acute inflammation lead to chronic salpingitis. The inflammatory lesions may be limited to the fallopian tube, but more often, the inflammation spreads to adjacent pelvic organs. Chronic salpingitis may present morphologically in several forms:

1. Obliteration of the lumen with minimal distortion of the fallopian tube
2. Occlusion of the fimbrial end of the tube
3. Fibrosis with deformity and increased tortuosity of the fallopian tube
4. Perisalpingian connective tissue adhesions distorting the fallopian tube
5. Pyosalpinx
6. Hydrosalpinx

All these forms of salpingitis are associated with histologic findings typical of chronic inflammation. These include infiltrates of lymphocytes, macrophages, and plasma cells and extensive fibrosis (Fig. 5-24). Foci of persistent suppuration are common. Granulomas (Fig. 5-25) are found in tuberculosis (Nogales-Ortiz et al., 1979) or fungal diseases, such but also may occur in Crohn's disease (Brooks and Wheeler, 1977).

Acute and chronic inflammation of the fallopian tubes may spread to the ovary and into the pelvis, leading to the formation of *tubo-ovarian abscesses.* Peritonitis limited to the pelvis or even generalized peritonitis and systemic sepsis are rare complications. *Fitz-Hugh-Curtis syndrome,* characterized by perihepatic adhesions, is a complication resulting from peritoneal spread of the inflammation.

Infertility is one of the major sequelae of salpingitis and PID, especially if the disease is bilateral. Destruction of

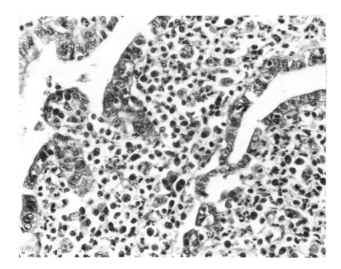

Fig. 5-24. Chronic salpingitis.

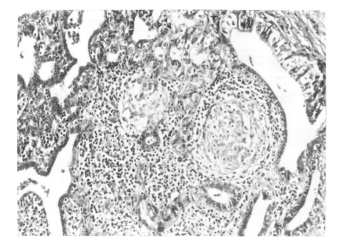

Fig. 5-25. Chronic salpingitis with granuloma.

the normal mucosa, obliteration of the lumen of the fallopian tubes, loss of normal peristalsis, or distortion of the tube by peritubal adhesions interferes with the passage of spermatozoa, the oocyte, and the zygote. Chronic salpingitis is also considered the major risk factor of extrauterine pregnancy.

REFERENCES

Aitchison M, Mufti GR, Farrel J, Paterson PJ, Scott R: Granulomatous orchitis. Review of 15 cases. Br J Urol 1990; 66:312.

Aktar M, Ashraf M, Mackey DM: Lepromatous leprosy presenting as orchitis. Am J Clin Pathol 1980; 73:712.

Amenta PS, Gonick P, Katz SM: Sarcoidosis of testis and epididymis. Urology 1981; 17:616.

Barnes RC, Holmes KK: Epidemiology of gonorrhea: Current perspectives. Epidemiol Rev 1984; 6:1.

Bazaz-Malik G, Maheshwari B, Lal N: Tuberculous endometritis: a clinicopathological study of 1000 cases. Br J. Obstet Gynecol 1983; 90:84.

Berger RE: Acute epididymitis: Etiology and therapy. Semin Urol 1991; 9:28.

Berger RE, Alexander ER, Harnisch JP, Paulsen CA, Monda GD, Ansell J, Holmes KK: Etiology, manifestations and therapy of acute epididymitis: Prospective study of 50 cases. Urology 1979; 121:750.

Berger RE, Holmes KK: Infection and male infertility. In Male Reproductive Dysfunction: Diagnosis and Management of Hypogonadism Infertility and Impotence, edited by Santen RJ, Swerdloff RS, New York, Marcel Dekker, 1986, p 407.

Blandy JP: Urethral stricture. Postgrad Med J 1980; 56:383.

Boström K: Chronic inflammation of human accessory sex glands ducts: Effect on the morphology of the spermatozoa. Scand J Urol Nephrol 1971; 5:233.

Brooks JJ, Wheeler JE: Granulomatous salpingitis secondary to Crohn's disease. Obstet Gynecol 1977; 49(Suppl):31S.

Brunham RC, Binns B, Guijon F, Danforth D, Kasseim ML, Rand F, McDowell J, Rayner E: Etiology and outcome of acute pelvic inflammatory disease. J Infect Dis 1988; 158:510.

Brunham RC, Paavonen J, Stevens CE, Kiviat N, Kuo C, Critchlow CW, Holmes KK: Mucopurulent cervicitis: The ignored counterpart in women of urethritis in men. N Engl J Med 1984; 311:1.

Cates W Jr, Rolfs RT Jr, Aral SO: Sexually transmitted diseases, pelvic inflammatory disease, and infertility: An epidemiologic update. Epidemiol Rev 1990; 12:199.

Clark WR, Lieber MM: Genital filariasis in Minnesota. Urology 1986; 28:518.

Clement PB: Pathology of gamete and zygote transport: Cervical, endometrial, myometrial, and tubal factors in infertility. In Pathology of Reproductive Failure, edited by Kraus FT, Damjanov I, Kaufman N, Baltimore, Williams & Wilkins, 1991, p 140.

Colpi GM: Inflammatory pathology of the genital tract and male infertility. Acta Eur Fertil 1989; 20:125.

Comhaire FH, de Kretser D, Farley TMM, Rowe PJ: Towards more objectivity in diagnosis and management of male infertility. Int J Androl 1987; 7(Suppl):1.

Damjanov I, Katz SM: Malakoplakia. Pathol Annu 1981; 16:103.

Dao AH, Adkins RB: Bilateral gummatous orchitis. South Med J 1980; 73:954.

Das S, Tuerk D, Amar AD, Sommer J: Surgery of male genital lymphedema. J Urol 1983; 129:1240.

dePaepe ME, Vuletin JC, Lee MH, Rojas-Corona RR, Waxman M: Testicular atrophy in homosexual AIDS patients: An immune-mediated phenomenon? Hum Pathol 1989; 20:572.

dePaepe ME, Waxman M: Testicular atrophy in AIDS: A study of 57 autopsy cases. Hum Pathol 1989; 20:210.

Dubey NK, Tavadia HB, Hehir M: Malacoplakia: A case involving the epididymis and a case involving a bladder complicated by calculi. J Urol 1988; 139:359.

Duckek M, Winblad B: Tuberculosis of the spermatic cord. Case report. Scand J Urol Nephrol 1974; 8:65.

Eickenberg HU, Amin M, Lich R Jr: Blastomycosis of the genitourinary tract. J Urol 1975; 113:650.

Ekwere PD: Filaria orchitis: A cause of male infertility in the tropics. Case report from Nigeria. Cent Afr J Med 1989; 35:456.

Elbadawi A, Khuri FJ, Crockett AT: Polypoid granulomatous and sclerosing endophlebitis of spermatic cord. New pathologic type of schistosomal funiculitis. Urology 1979; 13:309.

Epstein JI, Hutchins GM: Granulomatous prostatitis: Distinction among allergic, nonspecific, and posttransurethral resection lesions. Hum Pathol 1984; 15:818.

Fahmy NW, Honore LH, Cumming DC: Subacute focal endometritis. Association with cervical colonization with *Ureaplasma urealyticum*, pelvic pathology and endometrial maturation. J Reprod Med 1987; 32:685.

Falk V, Ludvikson K, Agren G: Genital tuberculosis in women. Am J Obstet Gynecol 1980; 138:974.

Ferrie BG, Rundle JSH: Tuberculous epididymo-orchitis: A review of 20 cases. Br J Urol 1983; 55:437.

Fox CW Jr, Vaccaro JA, Kiesling VJ Jr, Belville WD: Seminal vesicle abscess: The use of computerized coaxial tomography for diagnosis and therapy. J Urol 1988; 139:384.

Freij L, Norby R, Olsson B: A small outbreak of Coxsackie B5 infection with two cases of cardiac involvement and orchitis followed by testicular atrophy. Acta Med Scand 1970; 187:177.

Gall AE: The histopathology of mumps orchitis. Am J Pathol 1947; 23:637.

George VK, Russell GL, Harrison BDW, Green NA: Tuberculous epididymo-orchitis following intravesical BCG. Br J Urol 1991; 66:101.

Gerstenhaber BJ, Green ZR, Sachs LL: Epididymal sarcoidosis: A report of two cases and a review of the literature. Yale J Biol Med 1977; 50:669.

Gorelick JI, Senterfit LB, Vaughan ED, Jr: Quantitative bacterial tissue culture from 209 prostatectomy specimens: findings and implications. J Urol 1988; 139:57

Gottesman JE: Coccidiodomycosis of prostate and epididymis with urethrocutaneous fistula. Urology 1974; 4:311.

Greenberg SH, Lipshultz LI, Wein AJ: Experience with 425 subfertile male patients. J Urol 1978; 119:507.

Greenfield SP: Type B Hemophilus influenzal epididymo-orchitis in the prepubertal boy. J Urol 1986; 136:1311.

Gump DW, Gibson M, Ashikaga T: Lack of association between genital mycoplasmas and infertility. N Engl J Med 1985; 310:937.

Halim A, Vaezzadeh K: Hydatid disease of the genitourinary tract. Br J Urol 1980; 52:75.

Handsfield HH, Jasman LL, Roberts PL, Hanson VW, Kothenbeutel RL, Stamm WE: Criteria for selective screening for *Chlamydia trachomatis* infection in women attending family planning clinics. JAMA 1986; 255:1730.

Hanid TK: Infectious mononucleosis complicated by hydrocele. BMJ 1977; 2:706.

Hedinger CE, Dhom G: Pathologie des nidnulichen genitale, Berlin, Springer, 1991.

Hermansen MC, Chusid MJ, Sty JR: Bacterial epididymo-orchitis in children and adolescents. Clin Pediatr 1980; 19:812.

Hillier SL: Relationship of bacteriologic characteristics to semen indices in men attending an infertility clinic. Obstet Gynecol 1990; 75:800.

Holmes KK, Maedh P-A, Sparling PF, Wiesner PJ, Cates W Jr, Lemon SM, Stam WE (Eds): Sexually Transmitted Diseases, 2nd ed. New York, McGraw-Hill, 1990.

Honoré LH, Coleman GU: Solitary epididymal schistosomiasis. Canad J Surg 1975; 18:479.

Houston W: Bilhaziasis of the testis. Br J Urol 1964; 36:220.

Judson FN: Gonorrhea. Med Clin North Am 1990; 74:1353.

Kahn RI, Mcaninch J: Granulomatous disease of the testis. J Urol 1980; 123:868.

Katz BP, Caine JA, Jones RB: Diagnosis of mucopurulent cervicitis among women at risk for *Chlamydia trachomatis* infection. Sex Transm Dis 1989; 16:103.

Kauffman CA, Slama TG, Wheat LJ: *Histoplasma capsulatum* epididymitis. J Urol 1981; 125:434.

Kawamura N, Murakami Y, Okada K: Three cases of malakoplakia of prostate. Urology 1980; 15:77.

Kirk D, Gingell JC, Feneley RC: Infarction of the testis: A complication of epididymitis. Br J Urol 1982; 54:311.

Kiviat MD, Shurtleff D, Ansell JS: Urinary reflux via vas deferens. Unusual cause of epididymitis in infancy. J Pediatr 1972; 80:476.

Kiviat NB, Paavonen J, Wolner-Hanssen P, Critchlow CW, Stamm WE, Douglas J, et al.: Histopathology of culdocervical infection caused by *Chlamydia trachomatis*, herpes simplex virus, *Trichomonas vaginalis*, and *Neisseria gonorrhoeae*. Hum Pathol 1990; 21:831a.

Kiviat NB, Wolner-Hanssen P, Eschenbach DA, Paavonen JA, Bell TA, Critchlow CW, et al.: Endometrial histopathology in patients with culture-proven upper genital tract infection and laparoscopically diagnosed acute salpingitis. Am J Surg Pathol 1990; 14:167b.

Klein FA, Vick CW, Schneider V: Bilateral granulomatous orchitis: Manifestation of idiopathic systemic granulomatosis. J Urol 1985; 134:762.

Lee NC, Rubin GL, Grimes DA: Measures of sexual behavior and the risk of pelvic inflammatory disease. Obstet Gynecol 1991; 77:425.

Lees MM: Infection and male infertility. In Clinical Infection in Obstetrics and Gynecology, edited by MacLean AB. Oxford, England, Blackwell, 1990, p 287.

MacLean AB (Ed): Clinical Infection in Obstetrics and Gynecology. Oxford, England, Blackwell, 1990.

Manson AL: Mumps orchitis. Urology 1990; 36:355.

Martin DH: Chlamydial infections. Med Clin North Am 1990; 74:1367.

McCarthy JM, McLoughlin MG, Shackleton CR, Cameron EC, Yeung CK, Jones EC, Keown PA: Cytomegalovirus epididymitis following renal transplantation. J Urol 1991; 146:417.

McClure J: A case of malacoplakia of the epididymis associated with trauma. J Urol 1980; 124:934.

McConnell EM: The histopathology of the epididymis in a group of cases of azoospermia with normal testicular function. Br J Urol 1981; 53:173.

McNeeley SG Jr: Gonococcal infections in women. Obstet Gynecol Clin North Am 1989; 16:467.

Megalli M, Gursel E, Lattimer JK: Reflux of urine into the ejaculatory ducts as a cause of recurring epididymitis in children. J Urol 1972; 108:978.

Melekos ME, Asbach HW: Epididymitis: Aspects concerning etiology and treatment. J Urol 1987; 138:83.

Method MW: Laparoscopy in the diagnosis of pelvic inflammation disease: Selection criteria. J Reprod Med 1988; 33:901.

Miko TL, Lampe LG, Thomazy VA, Molnar P, Endes P: Eosinophilic endomyometritis associated with diagnostic curettage. Pathology 1988; 7:162.

Mikuz G, Damjanov I: Inflammation of the testis, epididymis, peritesticular membranes and scrotum. Pathol Annu 1982; 17:101.

Mittemeyer BT, Lennox KW, Borski AA: Epididymitis: A review of 610 cases. J Urol 1966; 95:390.

Monroe M: Granulomatous orchitis due to *Histoplasma capsulatum* and masquerading as a sperm granuloma. J Clin Pathol 1974; 27:929.

Murphy WM; Urological Pathology, Philadelphia, WB Saunders, 1989.

Murray JJ, Clark CA, Lands RH, Heim CR, Burnett LS: Reactivation blastomycosis presenting as a tubo-ovarian abscess. Obstet Gynecol 1984; 64:828.

Nahoum CRD: Inflammation and infection. In Treatment of Male Infertility, edited by Bain J, Schill W-B, Schwarzstein L. Berlin, Springer, 1982, p 5.

Naveh Y, Friedman A: Orchitis associated with adenoviral infections. Am J Dis Child 1975; 129:257.

Nilsson S, Obrant KO, Persson PS: Changes in the testis parenchyma caused by acute nonspecific epididymitis. Fertil Steril 1968; 19:748.

Nistal M, Paniagua R: Testicular and Epididymal Pathology. New York, Thieme-Stratton, 1984.

Nistal M, Santana A, Paniagua R, Palacios J: Testicular toxoplasmosis in two men with acquired immunodeficiency syndrome (AIDS). Arch Pathol Lab Med 1986; 1:10:744.

Nogales-Ortiz F, Tarancon I, Nogales FF: The pathology of female genital tract tuberculosis: A 31-year study of 1436 cases. Obstet Gynecol 1979; 53:422.

Paavonen J: *Chlamydia trachomatis*: A major threat to reproduction. Hum Reprod 1989; 4:111.

Paavonen J, Kiviat N, Brunham RC, Stevens CE, Kuo C, Stamm WE, et al: Prevalence and manifestations of endometritis among women with cervicitis. Am J Obstet Gynecol 1985; 152:280.

Paavonen J, Teisala K, Heinonen PK, Aine R, Laine S, Lebtinen M, et al.: Microbiological and histopathological findings in acute pelvic inflammatory disease. Br J Obstet Gynaecol 1987; 94:454.

Parish LC, Gschnait F (Eds): Sexually Transmitted Diseases: A Guide for Clinicians. New York, Springer-Verlag, 1989.

Patton DL, Moore DE, Spadoni LR, Soules MR, Halbert SA, Wang S: A comparison of the fallopian tube's response to overt and silent salpingitis. Obstet Gynecol 1989; 73:622.

Persaud V, Rao A: Gumma of the testis. Br J Urol 1977; 49:142.

Petersen RO: Urologic Pathology, 2 ed, Philadelphia, JB Lippincott, 1992.

Poropatich C, Rojas M, Silverberg SG: Polymorphonuclear leukocytes in the endometrium during the normal menstrual cycle. Int J Gynecol Pathol 1987; 6:2300.

Priebe CJ, Holahan JA, Ziring PR: Abnormalities of the vas deferens and epididymis in cryptorchid boys with congenital rubella. J Pediatr Surg 1979; 14:834.

Raghavaiah NV: Epididymal calcifications in genital filariasis. Urology 1981; 18:78.

Reeve HR, Weinerth JL, Peterson LJ: Tuberculosis of epididymis and testicle presenting as hydrocele. Urology 1974; 4:329.

Reisman EM, Colquitt LA IV, Childers J, Preminger GM: Brucella orchitis: A rare cause of testicular enlargement. J Urol 1990; 143:821.

Riggs S, Sanford JP: Viral orchitis. N Engl J Med 1962; 266:990.

Rinaudo P, Damjanov I, Stoesser B: Malacoplakia of testis. Int Urol Nephrol 1977; 9:249.

Risi GF Jr, Sanders CV: The genital mycoplasmas. Obstet Gynecol Clin North Am 1989; 16:611.

Rolfs RT, Galaid EI, Zaidi AA: Pelvic inflammatory disease: Trends in hospitalizations and office visits, 1979 through 1988. Am J Obstet Gynecol 1992; 166:983.

Ross JC, Gow JG, St Hill CA: Tuberculous epididymitis. A review of 170 patients. Br J Urol 1961; 48:663.

Rotterdam H: Chronic endometritis. A clinicopathologic study. Pathol Annu 1978; 13:209.

Rowland A: Infertility therapy: Effect of innovations and increasing experience. J Reprod Med 1980; 25:42.

Scarselli G, Noci I, Tantinig C: Chronic prostato-vesiculitis and sperm cell mobility in male infertility. Acta Urol Fertil 1978; 9:7.

Scott MB, Cosgrove MD: Salmonella infection and the genitourinary system. J Urol 1977; 118:64.

Sellors JV, Mahany JB, Chernesky MA, Rath DJ: Tubal factor infertility: An association with prior chlamydial infection and asymptomatic salpingitis. Fertil Steril 1988; 43:451.

Sherris JD, Fox G: Infertility and sexually transmitted disease: A public health challenge. Popul Rep 1983; 11:L113.

Siegel A, Snyder H, Duckett JW: Epididymitis in infants and boys: Underlying urogenital anomalies and efficacy of imaging modalities. J Urol 1987; 138:1100.

Simon GL, Worthington MG: An unusual case of pleural, epididymal and sternoclavicular tuberculosis. J Infect 1982; 4:259.

Stacey C, Munday P, Thomas B, Gilchrist C, Taylor-Robinson D, Beard R: Chlamydia trachomatis in the fallopian tubes of women without laparoscopic evidence of salpingitis. Lancet 1990; 336:960.

Stein AL, Miller DB: Tuberculous epididymoorchitis: A case report. J Urol 1983; 129:613.

Steinhauser K, Wurster K: Die Nebenhoden Tuberkulose in Wandel der Zeit. Urologe [A] 1975; 14:6.

Sulak PJ, Hayslip CC, Letterie GS, Woodward JE, Cuddington CC, Klein TA: Histology of proximal tubal occlusion. Fertil Steril 1987; 48:437.

Sweet RL: Pelvic inflammatory disease in infertility in women. Infect Dis Clin North Am 1987; 1:199.

Sweet RL: Pelvic inflammatory disease. Sex Trans Dis 1985; 13:192.

Sweet RL, Blankford-Doyle M, Robbie MO, Schacter J: The occurrence of chlamydial and gonococcal salpingitis during menstrual cycle. JAMA 1985; 255:2062.

Tchertkoff V, Ober WB: Primary chancre of cervix uteri. NY State J Med 1966; 66:121.

Templeton A: Pelvic infection and female infertility. In Clinical Infection in Obstetrics and Gynecology, edited by MacLean AB. Oxford, England, 1990, Blackwell, p 274.

Thind P, Gerstenberg TC, Bilde T: Is micturition disorder a pathogenic factor in acute epididymitis? An evaluation of simultaneous bladder pressure and urine flow in men with previous epididymitis. J Urol 1990; 143:323.

Thomas D, Simpson K, Ostojic H, Kaul A: Bacteremic epididymo-orchitis due to Hemophilus influenzae type B. J Urol 1981; 126:832.

Wah RM, Anderson DJ, Hill JA: Asymptomatic cervicovaginal leukocytosis in infertile women. Fertil Steril 1990; 54:445.

Walters MD, Gibbs RS: A randomized comparison of gentamicin, clindamycin and cefoxitin-doxycycline in the treatment of acute pelvic inflammatory disease. Obstet Gynecol 1990; 75:867.

Wasserheit JN: Pelvic inflammatory disease and infertility. Md Med J 1987; 36:58.

Watson RA: Gonorrhea and acute epididymitis. Milit Med 1979; 144:785.

Watson RA, Gangai MP, Skinsnes OK: Genitourinary leprosy. Urol Int 1974; 29:312.

Weinstein LW, Carcillo J, Scott SJ, Simon GL: Paratyphoid orchitis. Diagn Microbiol Infect Dis 1983; 1:163.

Welliver RC, Cherry JD: Aseptic meningitis and orchitis associated with echovirus 6 infection. J Pediatr 1978; 92:239.

Werner CA: Mumps, orchitis and testicular atrophy. Ann Intern Med 1950; 32:1066.

Weström L: Incidence, prevalence and trends of acute pelvic inflammatory disease and its consequences in industrialized countries. Am J Obstet Gynecol 1980; 138:880.

Weström L: Pelvic inflammatory disease: Bacteriology and sequelae. Contraception 1987; 36:111.

Wheeler JS Jr, Culkin DJ, O'Connell J, Winters G: Nocardia epididymoorchitis in an immunosuppressed patient. J Urol 1986; 136:1314.

Wiener LB, Richl PA, Baum M: Xanthogranulomatous epididymitis: A case report. J Urol 1987; 138:621.

Williams CB, Litvak AS, McRoberts JW: Epididymitis in infancy. J Urol 1979; 121:125.

Winblad B: Male genital tuberculosis—the possibility of lymphatic spread. A case report. Acta Pathol Microbiol Scand 1975; 83:425.

Windslow RC, Funkhouser JW: Sarcoidosis of the female reproductive organs. Obstet Gynecol 1968; 32:285.

Winkler B, Crum CP: Chlamydia trachomatis infection of the female genital tract. Pathogenic and clinicopathologic correlations. Pathol Annu 1987; 22:193.

Wolin LH: On the etiology of epididymitis. J Urol 1971; 105:531.

Wong T-W, Straus FH II, Warner NE: Testicular biopsy in the study of male infertility. II. Posttesticular causes of infertility. Arch Pathol 1973; 95:160.

Yoshikawa Y, Truong LD, Fraire AE, Kim H-S: The spectrum of histopathology of the testis in acquired immunodeficiency syndrome. Mod Pathol 1989; 2:233.

Chapter 6

PHYSICAL, CHEMICAL, IMMUNE, AND IATROGENIC CAUSES OF INFERTILITY

Traumatic lesions of the male reproductive organs
    Torsion of the testis and its appendages
Lesions related to surgery
    Vasectomy
Autoimmune disorders
    Autoimmune orchitis
    Vasculitis
    Amyloidosis
Effects of chemotherapy on the testis
Radiation-induced changes
Varicocele
Trauma of the female genital organs
Postpartum and postabortion lesions
Tubal sterilization
Contraceptive devices
Effects of chemotherapy on the ovary
Radiation injury
Autoimmune lesions of the female reproductive organs
    Sarcoidosis
    Crohn's disease
    Autoimmune oophoritis

Physical, chemical, immunologic, and iatrogenic causes of infertility account for a small number of cases of involuntary infertility. The pathology of these conditions is discussed in terms of pathogenesis, morphology, and clinicopathologic presentations. The morphologic changes related to vasectomy and tubal ligation, two popular contraceptive methods currently in use (Peterson et al., 1990), are highlighted, especially because patients voluntarily sterilized may request that the procedure be reversed and the fertility restored.

TRAUMATIC LESIONS OF THE MALE REPRODUCTIVE ORGANS

Traumatic lesions are caused by mechanical force applied directly or indirectly to genital organs. The trauma may be localized or systemic.

Direct trauma to the external genitalia may inflict minor or major lesions, which range from *avulsion* of the penis and the entire scrotum to partial *amputation* or blunt injury of one or more organs without an open wound or major mutilation. These lesions may result in infertility.

Unilateral or bilateral *rupture* of the body of the penis represents a major surgical emergency discussed in detail in clinical papers (McConnell et al., 1982). *Laceration* of the testes with rupture of the tunica albuginea may cause irreversible damage and require orchidectomy (Schuster, 1982). Testicular rupture may result in *hematocele* (McDermott et al., 1988; Vaccaro et al., 1988). *Hemorrhagic suffusion* of the entire scrotum, external or internal scrotal hematomas, or penile hematomas have been described in blunt trauma after motor vehicle accidents, bicycle and sports injuries, and other forms of physical injury.

Reproductive function of the traumatized person depends primarily on the nature and extent of the injury, the interval between the trauma and treatment, and the nature of postoperative complications (Cass, 1988). Even a unilateral injury may cause infertility, presumably because a systemic reaction to tissue necrosis and the associated release of cytotoxic substances or an immune response to testicular antigens occurs (Tarter and Kogan, 1988).

Testicular hemorrhage is a common complication of blunt trauma, but it may follow even minor traumatization in everyday life or during sexual intercourse. Clinically significant testicular hemorrhage, however, is not limited to adult life. Torsion of the testis, hemorrhage, and infarction are rare but are well-known and documented obstetric

125

Causes of testicular hemorrhage and infarction

1. Trauma
2. Torsion
3. Hematologic disorders
     Coagulopathy
     Polycythemia
     Leukemia
     Sickle cell anemia
4. Compression of blood vessels
     Tumors
     Hernia
5. Thromboembolism
     Thrombosis of the vena cava, renal vein, and sper-
         matic vein
     Arterial emboli (e.g., endocarditis)
6. Vasculitis
     Allergic vasculitis
     Polyarteritis nodosa
     Buerger's disease
     Henoch-Schönlein purpura

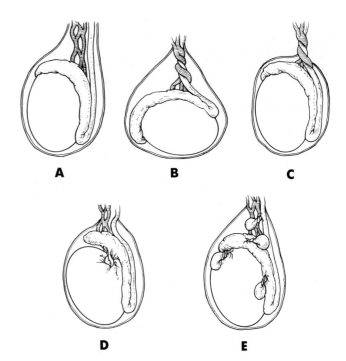

Fig. 6-1. Schematic presentation of the torsion of the testis and related intrascrotal structures. **A,** Normal testis. **B,** Intravaginal torsion. **C,** Extravaginal torsion. **D,** Torsion of the epididymotesticular junction. **E,** Torsion of peretesticular vestigeal structures. (From Leape LL. In Ascheraft KW (Ed). Pediatric Urology. Philadelphia, WB Saunders, 1990, with permission.)

complications in the neonate (Burge, 1987). Other causes of testicular hemorrhage and infarction that should be considered in the differential diagnosis of testicular trauma are listed in the box above.

Torsion of the testis and its appendages

Torsion of the testis is an imprecise but generally accepted term for torsion of the spermatic cord, resulting in an ischemic injury of the testis. Testicular appendages, such as the appendix testis (the hydatid of Morgagni), paradidymis, appendix epididymis, and vas aberrans, may rotate at their site of attachment and undergo torsion as well (Leape, 1990).

Incidence, etiology, and pathogenesis. Intrascrotal torsion of the testis occurs most often in the peripubertal period (Williamson, 1976). A second incidental peak occurs in the neonatal period (Das and Singer, 1990). Testicular torsion is rare in men over 30 (Dennis et al., 1987) but occasionally occurs in older men (Alfert and Canning, 1987). Familial cases have been reported (Collins and Broecker, 1989). Intrauterine torsion of the spermatic cord occasionally is diagnosed in newborn boys, and it is considered to be the cause of anorchia (Aynsley-Green et al., 1976).

Torsion of testicular and epididymal appendages accounts for a significant number of clinical emergencies known as acute scrotum (Skoglund et al., 1970 a, b; Melekos et al., 1988). According to some reports, torsion of the appendages is more common than testicular torsion itself (McCombe and Scobie, 1988). The consequences of appendiceal torsion are not as serious as torsion of the testis and are easily repaired surgically.

The etiology of testicular torsion conjecturally is related to trauma, which, however, cannot always be documented. The left testis has a longer spermatic cord and is therefore affected twice more often than the right testis. This suggests that the increased mobility of the testis or its inadequate fixation could predispose to torsion. Cryptorchid and retractile testes are also more prone to torsion (Nistal and Paniagua, 1984). The abnormal insertion of the tunica vaginalis testis may also predispose to torsion, and since the condition is usually bilateral, it has been recommended that repair of the torsion should always be combined with an orchiopexy of the contralateral testis (Leape, 1990).

Surgeons recognize four forms of intrascrotal torsions (Leape, 1990):

1. Intravaginal torsion of the spermatic cord
2. Extravaginal torsion of the spermatic cord
3. Intravaginal torsion of the epididymotesticular junction
4. Torsion of the appendages of the testis and epididymis (Fig. 6-1)

Intravaginal torsion is associated with a high reflection of the tunica vaginalis, resulting in the so-called bell-clapper deformity. This deformity prevents the proper posterior fixation of the epididymis and testis to the scrotal wall, allowing the testis to remain mobile. This is the most common form of torsion in peripubertal boys. *Extravaginal torsion* typically occurs in neonates and boys with incompletely descended or retractile testes who have an open processus vaginalis (Attalah et al., 1976). The torsion occurs near the inguinal canal or in the upper scrotum. *Torsions of the epididymotesticular junction* usually are related to congenital hypermobility of the epididymis or abnormalities of its size and shape. Torsions of the embryonic *vestigeal structures* appended to the testis and epididymis are typically intravaginal. The appendix testis, which is found in more than 90% of males, is most often affected; the vas aberrans is the least frequently affected (Virdi et al., 1990).

The symptoms and consequences of torsion depend on the location of the torsion and the extent and duration of interruption of blood flow (Leape, 1990). Four complete rotations of the spermatic cord produce irreversible damage within 2 hours. One rotation produces no obvious changes for up to 12 hours, although all affected testes subsequently show atrophy (Thomas and Williamson, 1983).

Pathologic findings. Torsion of the spermatic cord leads to strangulation of the blood vessels. Since the veins have much thinner walls than the arteries and are therefore more easily compressed, marked venous congestion and extravasation of blood from the capillaries predominate. If the blood flow is not restored, a hemorrhagic infarct evolves with massive necrosis of the entire testis. Mikuz (1985) has graded the severity of histologic lesions as follows:

1. Mild injury marked by interstitial edema that typically is found during the first 4 hours
2. Interstitial hemorrhages with early signs of seminiferous tubule necrosis 4 to 12 hours after torsion.
3. Hemorrhagic infarct, which typically occurs if the torsion is not relieved within 12 hours of its onset

The final outcome of testicular torsion depends on the extent of torsion and the duration of ischemia (Nistal et al., 1992). Long-term follow-up data are generally discouraging (Leape, 1990). Thomas and Williamson (1983) have shown that the degree of atrophy is directly proportional to the duration of ischemia. With early intervention the results are somewhat better, but even short-term ischemia can apparently have a detrimental outcome.

Patients in whom torsion of the testis is corrected surgically have abnormal spermiograms if the affected testis is left in the scrotum (Thomas and Williamson, 1983). The fact that a significant number of patients whose twisted testis has undergone atrophy show atrophic changes in the contralateral testis favors unilateral resection of the ischemic testis as a treatment of choice (Bartsch et al., 1980). Early orchidectomy of the affected testis has been shown to preserve the normal function of the contralateral testis.

The mechanism of the adverse effects of the damaged testis remaining in situ on the contralateral testis is not fully understood (Anderson and Williamson, 1986; Hadziselimovic et al., 1986 b; Fisch et al., 1988; Tarter and Kogan, 1988). The most popular theory, in part supported by experimental data, is based on the assumption that the damaged testis evokes an autoimmune reaction and that the antibodies or immune cells adversely affect spermatogenesis in the contralateral testis. Other hypotheses that postulate the effect of damaged tissue reactants on the hypothalamic-pituitary-testis axis or direct toxic effect on the contralateral testis are even less documented.

From the therapeutic point of view, it remains uncertain whether early correction of the torsion can prevent the damage to the contralateral testis. Some authorities claim that orchidectomy should always be performed even if the period between the torsion and surgical intervention has been less than 4 hours (Leape, 1990). Others favor preservation of the testes exposed to ischemia for short invervals and recommend resection of the irreversibly damaged organ (Mizrahi and Shtamler, 1992).

LESIONS RELATED TO SURGERY

Lesions of the testis and epididymis may evolve as uncommon complications of surgical procedures in the inguinal canal and scrotum. These lesions most often follow childhood hernia repair, which may be complicated by ipsilateral testicular atrophy.

Acute infarction of the testis from inadvertent transection of the testicular artery and scrotal spread of infection from contaminated wounds are uncommon medical mishaps. Such surgical sequelae are typically unilateral and have no significant impact on male fertility.

Unilateral orchidectomy for testicular tumors has no significant effect on previously fertile men unless it is combined with chemotherapy and radiation therapy (Javadpour, 1986). Treatment of an advanced testicular tumor may require more radical surgery, which has mutilating consequences. Dissection of retroperitoneal lymph nodes may cause lymphedema of the scrotum, varicocele, and obstruction of the seminal ducts or retrograde ejaculation, thus impairing fertility. Transection of penile nerves and removal of autonomic ganglia may cause impotence.

Transurethral or suprapubic resection of the prostate may be associated with minor or major complications that could affect male reproductive function (Mebust et al., 1989). These complications include protracted erection or impotence, inability to ejaculate, retrograde ejaculation, and obstruction of the ejaculatory duct.

Vasectomy

The World Health Organization estimates that more than 40 million men have been vasectomized so far (Thomas, 1987). Every year between 500,000 and 750,000

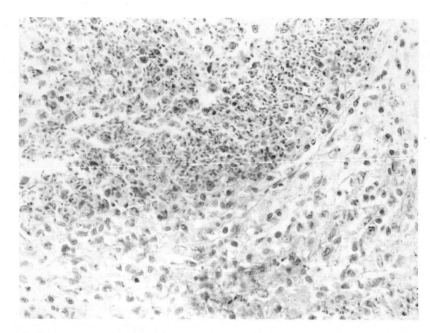

Fig. 6-2. Early sperm granuloma. The dilated duct is filled with spermatozoa. The epithelium of epididymis has disappeared and the stroma is infiltrated with numerous macrophages.

American men undergo voluntary vasectomy (Lipshultz and Benson, 1980). This most efficient, inexpensive, and simple approach to contraception has few complications, which can be related to:

1. Technical problems during surgery
2. Healing of the wound
3. Late sequelae of vas transection

Acute surgical complications of vasectomy are rare since this procedure is relatively simple (Alderman, 1988). Minor complications occur in 2% to 4% of patients and include hematoma, infection, scrotal pain, and epididymitis (Leader et al., 1974). Contraceptive failures have been reported to range from 0.1% to 2% (Peterson et al., 1990). These failures are related to faulty transection or ligation of the vas deferens, recanalization of the vas, or unrecognized anomalies such as a duplicated vas deferens.

Inadequate healing in an infected field may cause adhesions between the vas deferens and skin, formation of a fistula, or abscess formation at the site of ligature. Even without infection one may have adhesions between the stump of the transected vas deferens and the skin. Recanalization of the vas occurs in 0.2% to 0.5% of cases.

Sperm granulomas develop in 40% to 50% of cases. Granulomas represent a reaction to the extravasation of sperm from the caudal aspects of the transected vas into the connective tissue (Taxy et al., 1981). The lesions typically are nodular and measure 2 to 20 mm in diameter, although on occasion larger nodules measuring up to 4 cm may appear. Histologically, the nodules are composed of lymphocytes, histiocytes, and remnants of spermatozoa in-

terposed between smooth muscle cells in the wall of the epididymis (Fig. 6-2). Sperm granulomas are four times more common after surgical ligation of the vas deferens than fulguration (Nistal and Paniagua, 1984). Suture granulomas, which are unavoidable after ligation, probably contribute to the formation of sperm granulomas (Taxy et al., 1981).

Sperm granulomas may occur without vasectomy or apparent trauma (Glassy and Mostofi, 1956). Such granulomas usually are associated with an obstructive lesion of the epididymis.

Vasitis nodosa is a sign of abortive regeneration of the transected vas deferens that occurs in two thirds of vasectomized men (Taxy et al., 1981). The lesion evolves as a result of a proliferation of ductal cells from the lumen of the proximally obstructed end of the vas deferens. The epithelial cells form a meshwork of anastomosing channels filled with spermatozoa (Fig. 6-3). The newly formed ductules may extend through the entire thickness of the vas deferens and into the surrounding soft tissue or adjacent nerves (Goldman and Azzopardi, 1983; Zimmerman et al., 1983).

Vasitis nodosa has been described in men who have had no vasectomy. In such cases the lesion probably is a consequence of unrecognized infection, congenital defects of the epididymis, or aberrant ducts or diverticula (Olson, 1971).

It has been hypothesized that sperm granulomas may augment the autoimmune reaction to sperm (Alexander and Schmidt, 1977) and could adversely affect fertility in men who undergo vasovasostomy for reversal of vasec-

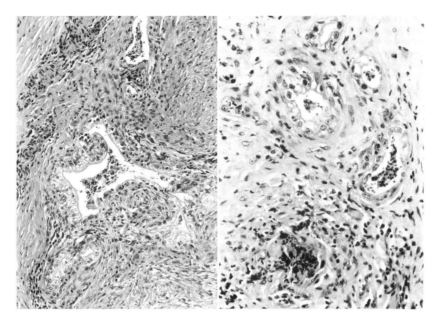

Fig. 6-3. Vasitis nodosa. The branching ductules contain spermatozoa and are surrounded by inflammatory cells.

tomy. A correlation between autoantibodies and testicular endocrine abnormalities also has been noted (Fisch et al., 1989). However, Taxy et al. (1981) found no differences in the reproductive potential of men who had vasectomy reversal with granulomas and those who did not have granulomatous lesions.

Late sequelae of vasectomy include testicular changes that result from retrograde pressure caused by the transection of the vas and by autoimmune phenomena related to sperm antigens. These testes show tubular dilatation, hypospermatogenesis, and maturation arrest (Gupta et al., 1975). Hellema and Rümke (1978) found sperm agglutinating antibodies in 73% of patients, sperm immobilizing antibodies in 42%, and antinuclear antibodies in 29% of patients 1 year after vasectomy. The significance of these autoantibodies is unknown, and their effects on fertility in men who have undergone vasectomy reversal remain controversial (Fuchs and Alexander, 1983).

Vasovasostomy is an efficient procedure for reversal of voluntary infertility of vasectomized men. Microsurgical recanalization can be achieved in most cases (Engelmann et al., 1990). However, only one half of these men will become fertile.

AUTOIMMUNE DISORDERS
Autoimmune orchitis

Autoimmune granulomatous orchitis can be produced in rabbits and other laboratory animals by autologous immunization with sperm or testicular tissue (Tung and Lu, 1991). After immunization with sperm-related antigens, these experimental animals develop interstitial orchitis and hypospermatogenesis. Although it is plausible that humans

develop similar lesions, such allergic orchitis rarely is encountered in clinical practice (Salomon et al., 1982; Lehmann et al., 1987).

Human autoimmune orchitis results presumably from immunization with sperm antigens. Indirect support for this hypothesis is found in the fact that these patients often have antisperm antibodies (Lehmann et al., 1987). Autoimmunity to sperm antigens theoretically could develop after trauma and infarction or following vasectomy, but none of these conditions seems to be associated with an increased incidence of autoimmune orchitis. Furthermore, orchitis is rarely a feature of other systemic autoimmune diseases. Thus, the autoimmune etiology of granulomatous orchitis remains inadequately documented in most cases and its pathogenesis is poorly understood.

Histologically, granulomatous orchitis presents as concentric peritubular infiltrates of cells that in later stages completely obliterate the tubules and nonselectively destroy germ cells, Sertoli cells, and Leydig cells. The infiltrates consist of lymphocytes, plasma cells, histiocytes, and occasional multinucleated giant cells (Fig. 6-4). In chronic disease there is marked tubular destruction and fibrosis. In contrast to sperm granulomas of the epididymis, sperm phagocytosis is not a prominent finding.

The morphologic features of granulomatous orchitis may resemble those of malacoplakia, and it is quite possible that they represent the same disease. The so-called lymphocytic interstitial orchitis (Agarwal et al., 1990) probably is a variant of the same disease (Mikuz and Damjanov, 1982).

Before a testicular lesion is labeled idiopathic or autoimmune granulomatous orchitis, it is important to ex-

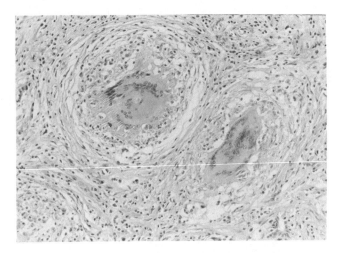

Fig. 6-4. Granulomatous orchitis of unknown etiology with prominent giant cells.

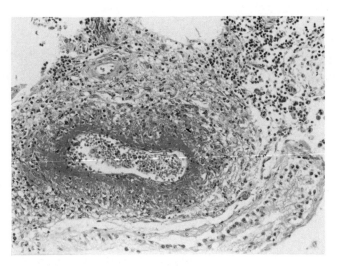

Fig. 6-5. Polyarteritis nodosa involving the testis.

clude viral, bacterial, and other identifiable causes of orchitis that may produce the same morphologic picture. Immunofluorescence and electron microscopy studies have demonstrated deposits of immunoglobulins and complement along the tubular basement membranes (Salomon et al., 1982). Additional electron microscopic findings have demonstrated basement membrane abnormalities reminiscent of immune complex nephritis (Salomon and Hedinger, 1982). Lehmann et al. (1987) found immune deposits inside the tubules along the tubular basement membranes and in the interstitial spaces. These findings implicate antibodies in the pathogenesis of orchitis. The various patterns of deposition of immunoglobulin and complement are not diagnostic. Therefore, the usefulness of immunohistochemical staining for the diagnosis of autoimmune orchitis remains questionable.

Vasculitis

Testicular lesions are found on autopsy in 60% to 80% of autopsied cases of systemic polyarteritis nodosa (Fig. 6-5). Occasionally, these testicular lesions are the initial presentation of the disease, but only exceptionally. Vasculitis is limited to the testis (Shurbaji and Epstein, 1988) and epididymis (McLean and Burnett, 1983). Other systemic diseases such as Henoch-Schönlein purpura (Mikuz et al., 1979), systemic lupus erythematosus (Kuehn et al., 1989), and hypersensitivity vasculitis (Baer et al., 1989) may involve the testis and epididymis and cause infarcts, hemorrhage, and inflammation.

Amyloidosis

Amyloidosis is a rare cause of hypogonadism (Handelsman et al., 1983). On the other hand, the testis and epididymis are not spared from amyloid deposits in systemic amyloidosis (Nistal et al., 1989) or in senile amyloidosis (Ishii et al., 1983), albeit such lesions rarely present clinical problems.

Amyloidosis of the seminal vesicles is common in older men, and autopsy findings indicate that at least one third of all men older than 75 years have this form of isolated senile amyloidosis (Pitkanen et al., 1983). These deposits of amyloid in the lamina propria cause a thickening of the entire wall of the seminal vesicles. There usually are no related clinical symptoms. Systemic amyloidosis may also involve the seminal vesicles. In contrast to senile amyloidosis, the deposits of systemic amyloidosis are not limited to the lamina propria but also appear in the small blood vessels and the muscular layer of the glands (Hedinger and Dhom, 1991).

EFFECTS OF CHEMOTHERAPY ON THE TESTIS

Chemotherapy with cytotoxic drugs adversely affects testicular germ cells, but the final outcome depends on the age of the patient, the duration of therapy, and the combination of drugs given (Averette et al., 1990). The chemotherapeutic regimen of choice for treatment of Hodgkin's disease and lymphoma combines nitrogen mustard, vincristine (Oncovin), procarbazine, and prednisone (MOPP). MOPP induces azoospermia and permanent depletion of germ cells from the seminiferous tubules (Waxman et al., 1982; Whitehead et al., 1982). Treatment of Hodgkin's disease with cyclophosphamide, vincristine, procarbazine, and prednisone (COPP) leads to irreversible sterility as well (Charak et al., 1990). These drugs given before puberty or during puberty apparently damage not only the germ cells but the Leydig cells as well (Bramswig et al., 1990). The most widely used treatment regimen for testicular cancer includes bleomycin, *cis*-platinum, and vinblastine sulfate. This triad also is cytotoxic, but 75% of patients regain fertility within 18 months after treatment (Lange et al., 1982). Similar treatment protocols containing doxorubicin also cause reversible testicular changes (Drasga et al., 1983).

The reproductive potential of men treated for childhood

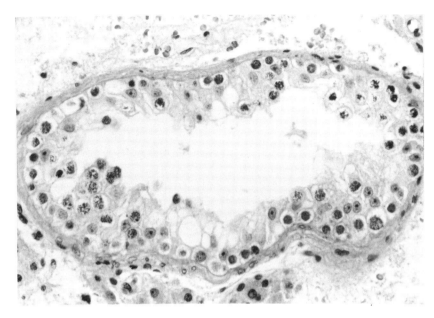

Fig. 6-6. Radiation induced depletion of germ cells in the seminiferous tubule showing maturation arrest.

malignancy can be predicted by the measurements of serum follicle-stimulating hormone (FSH) and testicular size, which correlate with the extent of cytotoxic injury of the testis (Siimes and Rautonen, 1990). Thus, testicular biopsy is rarely performed.

RADIATION-INDUCED CHANGES

Radiation-induced testicular injury is dose dependent (Lushbaugh and Casarett, 1976). The sensitivity of testicular cells to radiation varies; spermatogonia are the most sensitive cells and as they mature within the seminiferous tubules their sensitivity decreases; Sertoli and Leydig cells are relatively resistant (Clarke and Resnick, 1978). Even small doses of radiation (in the range of 10 rads) may damage spermatogonia (Lushbaugh and Casarett, 1976), but recovery is relatively quick. In general, the duration of the recovery period is directly proportional to the total dose of radiation received (Hahn et al., 1982) and varies from 9 to 18 months for doses less than 100 rads to 5 years for high doses in the range of 400 to 600 rads (Lushbaugh and Casarett, 1976).

The morphology of irradiated testes depends on the duration and dose of radiation and the time that has elapsed between the irradiation and the histologic examination. Radiation-induced necrosis of germinal epithelium occurs quickly and results in a depletion of germ cells (Fig. 6-6). Spermatogenic arrest persists for a variable length of time. Irradiated tubules are populated with Sertoli cells and scattered germ cells, have a narrower lumen than nonirradiated tubules, and show thickening of the lamina propria (Fig. 6-7). Interstitial fibrosis and vascular changes are seen in more pronounced lesions.

VARICOCELE

A varicocele is a tortuous dilatation of the testicular veins resulting in stagnation of venous blood in the pampiniform plexus (Fig. 6-8). Dubin and Amelar (1970) grade varicoceles as follows:

1. Small varicocele—Less than 1 cm in diameter
2. Moderate varicocele—1 to 2 cm in diameter
3. Large varicocele—Measures more than 2 cm in diameter and is readily discernible even without palpation or Valsalva's maneuver

Steeno et al. (1976) recognize three degrees of varicocele and an additional group of clinically suspect cases as follows:

1. Normal
   No distended veins
   No reflux on Valsalva's maneuver
   Symmetric testicular volume
   Symmetric testicular consistency
2. Clinical suspected varicocele
   Distended vein, less than 1 cm
   No reflux on Valsalva's maneuver
   Asymmetric testicular volume
   Asymmetric testicular consistency
3. Grade I varicocele
   Palpable scrotal varicosity of less than 1 cm in diameter and with reflux during Valsalva's maneuver
4. Grade II varicocele
   Pronounced varicocele mass with a diameter of 1 to 2 cm

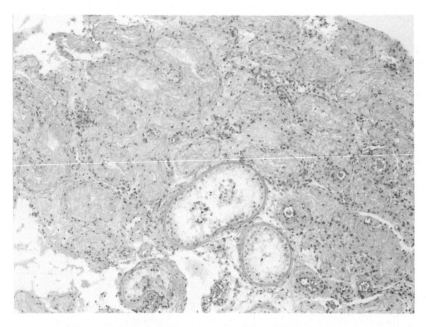

Fig. 6-7. Tubular hyalinization and atrophy from irradiation.

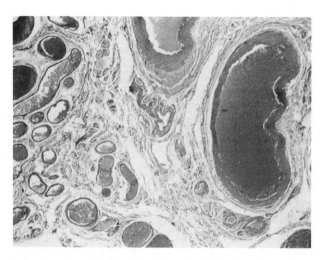

Fig. 6-8. Varicocele. The resected scrotal tissue contains numerous dilated vessels engorged with blood.

5. Grade III varicocele
   Venous mass fills the hemiscrotum, is easily visible at a distance, and has a diameter greater than 2 cm at the time of positive-pressure reflux

Incidence, etiology, and pathogenesis. Varicocele may be found in as many as 25% of all adult males (Nistal and Paniagua, 1984), most of whom have normal fertility. According to data published from several centers, reviewed by Pryor and Howards (1987), varicocele is more common among infertile men, of whom 19% to 39% show some degree of scrotal varicosity. The left side is affected in at least 70% of cases; 10% to 20% of cases are bilateral; a varicocele confined to the right side is found in less than

10% of cases. Overall, varicocele is considered to be the most common cause of male infertility (Dubin and Amelar, 1971; Greenberg et al., 1978).

The etiology and pathogenesis of varicocele remain enigmatic. Various theories proposed to explain the pathogenesis of varicocele have been summarized recently by Nagler and Zippe (1991). Essentially, these hypotheses postulate abnormal venous outflow from the scrotum. The fact that most varicoceles develop on the left side has been ascribed to the anatomic connection between the internal spermatic veins and the major abdominal veins (Fig. 6-9). In contrast to the right internal spermatic vein, which is confluent at an acute angle with the inferior vena cava, the left internal spermatic vein drains perpendicularly into the left renal vein, which may hinder the venous return on the left side. The left internal spermatic vein is also 8 to 10 cm longer than the right vein. The right-angle insertion and the longer course of the left internal spermatic vein predispose to venous blood stagnation and backflow of the renal vein into the scrotum. Furthermore, the left renal vein may be compressed between the superior mesenteric artery and the aorta, which results in the so-called nutcracker phenomenon, thus hemodynamically creating a milieu for varicocele formation. Finally, the left internal spermatic vein does not have valves, another predisposition for varicosities.

Varicocele has an adverse effect on fertility in males. A considerable number of males with varicocele are infertile and show sperm abnormalities. Varicocelectomy results in an improved quality of semen. Pryor and Howards (1987) have reviewed data from a dozen studies that report improved semen in 50% to 80% of treated infertile men and a subsequent fertilization in 24% to 39% of cases.

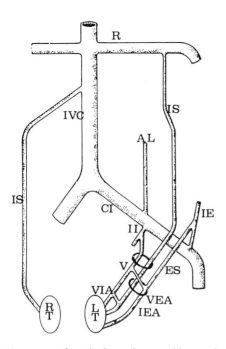

Fig. 6-9. Anatomy of testicular veins provides a clue for the preferential appearance of varicocele on the left side. Abbreviations: IVC, inferior vena cava; R, renal vein; IS, internal spermatic vein; AL, ascending lumbar vein; CI, common iliac vein; II, internal iliac vein; IE, inferior epigastric vein; ES, external spermatic vein; V, vasal vein; F, femoral vein; T, testis; VIA, vasal vein-internal spermatic vein anastomosis; VEA, vasal vein-external spermatic vein anastomosis; IEA, internal spermatic vein-external spermatic vein ansastomosis. (Modified from Glezerman M, Jecht EW (Eds). Varicocele and Male Infertility II. Berlin, Springer Verlag, 1984, with permission.)

Although varicocele usually occurs unilaterally, it may affect both testes. Internal communications of the left and right pampiniform plexus contribute to this phenomenon (Nagler and Zippe, 1991).

Several hypotheses have been put forward to explain the adverse influence of varicocele on spermatogenesis, but none of these has been proved beyond reasonable doubt. Working theories include the following:

1. *Hyperthermia theory.* The pampiniform plexus has a countercurrent cooling effect on the testicular arterial blood flow, and the stagnation of venous blood could contribute to elevating the temperature in the scrotum. Since spermatogenesis requires that the scrotal temperature be lower than the systemic temperature, the relative hyperthermia of venous stasis could adversely affect spermatogenesis.
2. *Reflux of renal and adrenal venous blood into the testis.* It has been postulated that blood from the kidney and the adrenals contains metabolic degradation products that could be toxic to spermatogenic cells. Similarly, adrenaline, biogenic amines, prostaglandins, and cortisol, which are released from the kidney and adrenals, may have adverse effects on the normal metabolism of testicular cells.
3. *Altered testicular steroidogenesis.* Venous stagnation, which would contribute to a slower outflow of testosterone, theoretically could inhibit the availability of testosterone and affect the negative feedback exerted by testosterone and inhibin on hypothalamic and pituitary release of regulatory hormones. A considerable number of patients with varicocele have an exaggerated response to the injection of luteinizing hormone–releasing hormone indicative of a testicular hormonal defect (Kass et al., 1989).
4. *Hypoxia.* Venous congestion could cause ischemic changes and slow the metabolism of steroidogenic and spermatogenic cells in the testis.
5. *Mechanical compression.* Dilated venous plexuses theoretically could compress other structures in the scrotum and cause edema. There is no evidence that this is of functional significance.

None of these hypotheses has been accepted unequivocally, although clearly each has merit.

Pathologic findings. Dilated veins can be seen on scrotal examination. Testicular biopsy, which is rarely performed these days, usually shows disturbed spermatogenesis (Agger and Johnsen, 1978; McFadden and Mehan, 1978). Both testes usually are affected, indicating that the lesions are not restricted to the testis with the varicocele (Terquem and Dadoune, 1981). The lesions appear to be progressive and lead to testicular atrophy (Lipshultz and Corriere, 1977).

The common histopathologic changes include:

1. Peritubular sclerosis, tubular atrophy, and hyalinization
2. Decreased spermatogenesis with maturation arrest, which may be mild and focal or severe, presenting as the Sertoli-cell–only syndrome
3. Degeneration of the adluminal Sertoli cells
4. Leydig cell hyperplasia
5. Small blood vessel changes such as hyalinization and fibrosis
6. Interstitial fibrosis

None of the changes described in the testes of patients with varicocele is diagnostic of this condition. Decreased spermatogenesis varies from one patient to another in the same way the sperm parameters vary among affected individuals (Dubin and Amelar, 1975). Varicocelectomy generally improves the quality of sperm produced; reversible changes in the testis will improve or at least not continue to progress.

According to Comhaire (1988), the prognosis for patients with varicocele depends on several variables such as the degree of venous stasis serum, FSH levels, the number of motile spermatozoa in the ejaculate, testicular volume, and the presence or absence of other factors that could influence fertility. These prognostic factors are presented in Table 6-1.

Table 6-1. Prognostic factors in the treatment of varicocele

	Estimated probability of success (%)
1. Good prognosis (>50% overall success rate)	
Grade II–III varicocele, FSH <2 ng/ml	80
Secondary infertility	78
No other factors in the man or woman	65
Motile sperm count before treatment >2 million/ml	62
Total testicular volume >28 ml	60
2. Reasonable prognosis (20%–50% overall success rate)	
Total testicular volume >28 ml, FSH > 2ng/ml	40
Grade II–III varicocele, total testicular volume >28 ml	30
Other factor in the female partner	30
Motile sperm count before treatment <0.5 million/ml	30
3. Poor prognosis (<20% overall success rate)	
Simultaneous male accessory gland infection	12
Grade I or subclinical varicocele total testicular volume <28 ml	8
FSH >6 ng/ml	0
Simultaneous sperm antibodies	0

Modified from Comhaire FH. In Barrat CLR, Cooke ID (Eds). Advances in Clinical Andrology. Lancaster, UK, MTP Press, Kluwer Academic, 1988, with permission.

TRAUMA OF THE FEMALE GENITAL ORGANS

Traumatic injuries of the female genitalia are not uncommon; however, these injuries generally have no serious impact on female reproductive potential. Straddle injuries predominate in children and young adults (Perlmutter, 1980). Motor vehicle accidents, assaults, accidental injuries, and firearm injuries may cause varying degrees of mutilation, rupture, or penetrating wounds. Sexual abuse during childhood may lead to vaginal occlusion, presumably because the premenarchal vaginal epithelium is more susceptible to injury and healing tends to cause scarring (Muram and Gale, 1990).

POSTPARTUM AND POSTABORTION LESIONS

The most important complications of pregnancy and abortion for future reproductive function are intrauterine adhesions. Conversely, most intrauterine adhesions are related to gynecologic procedures on a gravid uterus. Other causes of intrauterine adhesions are listed in Table 6-2.

Typically, these adhesions cause abnormal menstrual blood flow, primarily amenorrhea and hypomenorrhea,

Table 6-2. Causes of intrauterine adhesions

Predisposing condition	Percentage
Procedures associated with pregnancy	
Curettage after abortion	66.7
Postpartum curettage	21.50
Cesarean section	2.0
Hydatidiform mole	0.60
Procedures unrelated to pregnancy	
Myomectomy	1.3
Diagnostic curettage	1.2
Cervical biopsy or polypectomy	0.5
Curettage for menorrhagia	0.4
Infection	
Tuberculosis	4.0

Adapted from Schenker JG, Margalioth EJ. Fertil Steril 1982; 37:593. Reproduced with permission of the publisher, The American Fertility Society.

which are found in more than 75% of affected women (Siegler et al, 1990). Cyclic abdominal pain at the time of expected menses is common. The diagnosis of intrauterine adhesions cannot be excluded even in women who have cyclic, painless menses with a normal discharge of blood.

A history of curettage for an incomplete spontaneous abortion, elective termination of pregnancy, or postpartum interventions, coupled with amenorrhea, are typical presentations. The final diagnosis can be made only by hysteroscopy or hysterosalpingography. The curettage may not provide a diagnosis but may cure the symptoms.

On the basis of hysteroscopic findings, intrauterine adhesions may be classified into three groups based on the degree of occlusion of the uterine cavity, especially the lower segment and fundal areas (Siegler et al., 1990). Findings are classified as minimal, moderate, or severe if the adhesions occupy less than one fourth, one half, or more than three fourths of the uterine cavity, respectively. These hysteroscopic findings correlate with hysterographic findings. The American Fertility Society has adopted a hysteroscopic classification, taking into account the extent to which the cavity which is occupied by the adhesions, the type of adhesions, and the menstrual pattern.

According to Hamou et al. (1983), three types of intrauterine adhesions can be recognized and are classified as mild, moderate, or severe:
1. White endometrial adhesions with glandular and vascular patterns similar to the adjacent endometrium—These can be easily dissected.
2. Fibrous synechiae that appear as thin, transparent, poorly vascularized strands—These usually are found in the central part of the cavity or the isthmus.
3. Myometrial adhesions—These contract the uterine cavity and cannot be lysed readily.

Gynecologic surgery may be complicated by infection from endogenous or exogenous sources. The vagina and

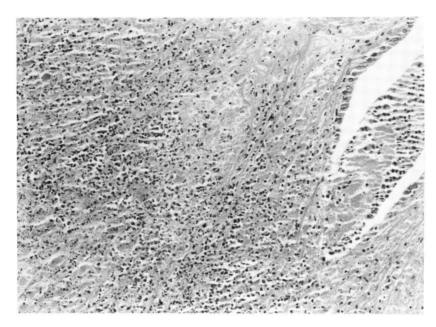

Fig. 6-10. Endometrial necrosis following a septic abortion.

cervix contain a wide variety of aerobic and anaerobic bacteria, some of which may become pathogenic and colonize the wounds (Fig. 6-10). Bacteria from the urinary tract are another common source of infection. All infections have clear, obvious implications for reduced fertility. They have been reviewed by Kitchener and Kingdom (1990) and are listed in the box at right.

TUBAL STERILIZATION

According to Peterson et al. (1986), more than 60 million women have undergone tubal sterilization; it remains one of the safest and most reliable contraceptive methods. Since 1978 a group called Collaborative Review of Sterilization (CREST) has been collecting data from 12 hospitals and outpatient surgical facilities in six U.S. cities; the registry contains follow-up data on thousands of women who have undergone tubal sterilization. This multicenter, multivariant analysis indicates that tubal sterilization is safe and has few serious complications in comparison to other surgical procedures or most other methods of contraception. The risk of pregnancy with postpartum tubal ligation is 1 in 300; with laparoscopic tubal sterilization the failure rate is 1 in 100 (Peterson et al., 1986). The procedure has a fatality rate of 4 per 100,000 procedures; unintended major surgery is required in 1.1% of procedures; rehospitalization is necessary in 0.5% of cases; and febrile morbidity occurs in 0.2% of cases. The rate of one or more complications is 1.7. Tubal and pelvic adhesions are the most common complications. Comparative results have been reported with unipolar and bipolar coagulation, use of Silastic bands, and other procedures, although each of these procedures has its own advantages and disadvan-

> **Infections after gynecologic surgery**
>
> **Wound infection**
> External
> Internal
>
> **Necrotic tissue infection**
> Postpartum endometrium
> Postabortion endometrium
> Tissue traumatized by surgery
> Surgery for repair of trauma
> Necrotic tumors
>
> **Infection of fluid collection**
> Hematoma
> Vault hematoma
> Lymphocyst after radical pelvic surgery
>
> **Pelvic cellulitis**
> Pelvic thrombophlebitis
> Necrotizing fasciitis
> Septicemia

tages. Reversal of sterilization may be most readily accomplished after Silastic band insertion. Microsurgery and tubo-tubal anastomosis are used with high efficiency for restoring fertility in patients who had electrocoagulated fallopian tubes.

CONTRACEPTIVE DEVICES

Women using the Dalkon shield contraceptive intrauterine device (IUD) are at an increased risk to develop pelvic

Effects of common cytotoxic drugs on reproductive function of the ovary

Definite effect

Chlorambucil
Cyclophosphamide
L-Phenylalanine mustard
Nitrogen mustard
Busulfan
Procarbazine

Probable effect

Doxorubicin
Vinblastine
Cytosine arabinoside
Cisplatin
Nitrosoureas
Etoposide

Negligible effect

Methotrexate
Fluorouracil
Mercaptopurine
Vincristine

Modified from Gradishar WJ, Schilsky RL. Semin Oncol 1989; 16:425, with permission.

inflammatory disease (PID). The tubal factor infertility risk was 3.3 to 6.8 times higher in these women (Cramer et al., 1985; Daling et al., 1985) than in those who never used an IUD. However, hormone-containing and copper IUDs do not increase the risk (Editorial, 1992). Monogamous women or those who have only one sexual partner and use an IUD do not seem to be at a higher risk for developing PID (Lee et al., 1988). The use of oral contraceptives is not associated with an increased incidence of PID or subsequent tubal factor infertility (Washington et al., 1985). Barrier methods of contraception actually decrease the risk of PID.

EFFECTS OF CHEMOTHERAPY ON THE OVARY

Cytotoxic drugs affect the ovaries in a dose- and time-dependent manner (Rivkees and Crawford, 1988). Germ cells and granulosa cells of growing follicles are the primary targets of chemotherapeutic agents, although there is evidence that other components of the ovary may be affected as well (Marcello et al., 1990). The structural and functional changes induced by chemotherapy may be explained in terms of direct cytotoxicity, resulting in follicle depletion; and in terms of ischemia related to microvascular injury leading to replacement of the functioning, hormonally active sex cord cells with fibrous tissue.

Older women, who have fewer ovarian follicles remaining, obviously are more susceptible to chemotherapy (Verp, 1983). Infertility and premature ovarian failure develop in a considerable number of women treated with drugs listed in the box above.

Alkylating agents have the highest toxicity. The typical treatment of Hodgkin's disease causes signs of ovarian dysfunction, including amenorrhea, and progressive ovarian failure in as many as 80% of women (Chapman, 1982). Most women who develop amenorrhea do not resume normal menstrual activity after treatment.

Combination therapy—chemotherapy combined with radiation—causes more pronounced damage than the use of one therapy alone (Byrne et al., 1992; Fig. 6-11).

Single-agent chemotherapy with some cytotoxic drugs such as methotrexate and actinomycin D, which are used for the treatment of trophoblastic disease, carries almost no risk to reproductive function. Low-dose cyclophosphamide administered for juvenile nephrotic syndrome does not seriously affect gonadal function in most instances (Pennisi et al., 1975).

Fertility was preserved to some extent in women taking oral contraceptives during chemotherapy (King et al., 1985), suggesting that the nonovulating ovary is less susceptible to injury. On the other hand, even prepubertal children treated with multidrug regimens for acute leukemia have severe germ cell damage (Quigley et al., 1989). Apparently some germ cell injury is unavoidable. Although direct comparisons between children and adults are not feasible, it seems that the reproductive sequelae of chemotherapy in prepubertal children are less deleterious than in older women (Verp, 1983; Young and Scully, 1991).

The histologic features of acute drug-induced injury include necrosis, hemorrhage, and involution of the follicles (Marcello et al., 1990). Subsequently, the histologic pattern corresponds to that of the quiescent ovary, in which there are no follicles beyond the primordial follicles. Finally, the ovary undergoes fibrosis and hyalinization of blood vessels with some evidence of periovarian fibrosis and capsular thickening.

RADIATION INJURY

The effects of external radiation on the ovaries have been reviewed recently by Gradishar and Schilsky (1989) and Young and Scully (1991). Ovarian cells show differential sensitivity to irradiation. This is, in part, age related and also reflects the functional or proliferative status of each cell type. The highest sensitivity is demonstrated in mitotic oogonia and granulosa cells of the proliferative follicles. Theoretically, by suppressing the normal menstrual cycle with oral contraceptives or antagonists of gonadotropin-releasing hormone, one could diminish the injury from irradiation or chemotherapy (Chapman and Sutclife, 1981).

Radiation injury to the ovary differs in several aspects from an equivalent injury to the tesis, although the calculations made by Wallace et al. (1989) indicate that in principle the male and female germ cells are equally sensitive to external radiation. The different effects of radiation on the male and female gonads reflect the basic differences in

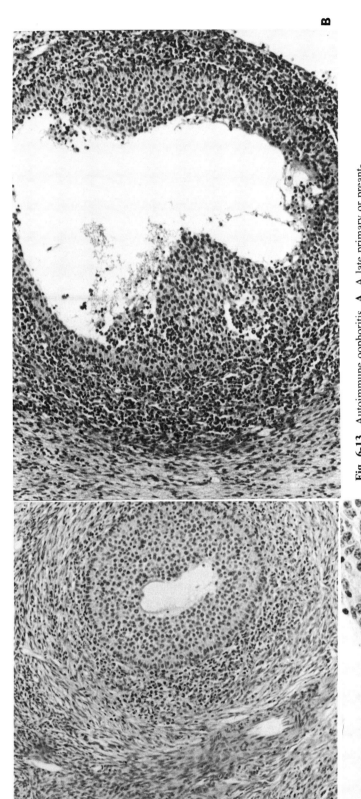

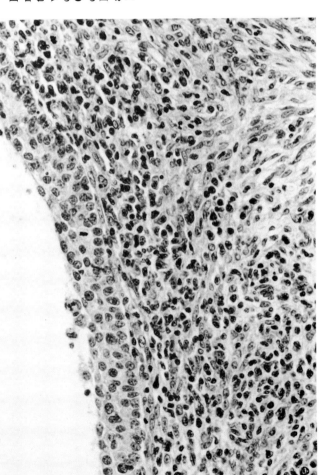

Fig. 6-13. Autoimmune oophoritis. **A,** A late primary or preantral follicle shows inflammation in the theca layer, with sparing of the granulosa. The small primordial follicle on the left is not involved. **B,** An antral follicle shows an infiltrate of mononuclear cells in the granulosa and theca layer adjacent to the cumulus. **C,** The theca interna of a large cyst is infiltrated with lymphocytes and plasma cells while the granulosa layer is spaced. (From Bannatyne P, Russell P, Shearman RP. Autoimmune oophoritis: a clinicopathologic assessment of 12 cases. Int J Gynecol Pathol 1990; 9:191, with permission.)

Crohn's disease

Crohn's disease is a granulomatous disease of the intestinal tract that may extend into the adjacent organs, forming fistulas and adhesions (Donaldson, 1978). Tubo-ovarian abscesses may develop and mimic sexually acquired PID. Granulomatous salpingitis and oophoritis have also been described (Wlodarski and Trainer, 1975; Brooks and Wheeler, 1977). These noncaseating granulomas are not pathognomonic, and the diagnosis is made by excluding infectious granulomatous diseases and by demonstrating gastrointestinal involvement.

Autoimmune oophoritis

Oophoritis can be produced experimentally in mice by neonatal thymectomy or by immunizing the animals with zona pellucida antigens (Tung and Lu, 1991). Animals vaccinated with a zona pellucida glycoprotein develop antibodies with contraceptive properties (Millar et al., 1989). Binding of these antibodies to the zona pellucida ovaries can be demonstrated by immunfluorescence techniques.

In view of these experimental data, there is little doubt that some cases of premature ovarian failure are probably caused by autoimmune mechanisms. The best evidence is that in some cases of ovarian failure patients have antiovarian antibodies (Damewood et al., 1986; Alper and Garner, 1987; Luborsky et al., 1990), antibodies to adrenal and steroidal cells (Ahonen et al., 1987; Lonsdale et al., 1991), or antibodies to luteinizing hormone or human chorionic gonadotropin receptor (Moncayo et al., 1989). In some cases, ovarian failure is part of a pluriglandular endocrine autoimmune disease and is most likely antibody mediated. However, ovarian failure does not develop in all women who have circulating antiovarian antibodies. Furthermore, autoantibodies are often induced during harvesting of oocytes for in vitro fertilization without serious consequences (Barbarino-Monnier, 1991). Finally, there are many patients with histologically documented oophoritis who did not have antiovarian antibodies (Russell et al., 1982).

In contrast to experimental autoimmune oophoritis, caused by antibodies to zona pellucida, antibodies detected in humans react not with the zona pellucida but with granulosa and follicular cells (Tung and Lu, 1991). The cell-mediated immunity apparently plays an important role, which remains to be elucidated further.

Lonsdale et al. (1991) reviewed 17 previously published, histologically documented cases of autoimmune oophoritis, and Bannatyne et al. (1990) reported 12 new cases (Fig. 6-13). Histologically, all these cases are remarkably similar to each other.

According to Lonsdale et al. (1991), infiltrates of lymphocytes and plasma cells appear first around the preantral follicles. The primary follicles are not affected in more advanced stages of the disease, and the infiltrates obliterate the follicles, destroying the theca interna and externa, while the granulosa cells remain relatively intact unless they are luteinized. Cystic transformation of the affected follicles is found in approximately one third of all cases.

Immunophenotyping performed on two cases studied by Lonsdale et al. (1991) disclosed that the infiltrates consist predominantly of T-lymphocytes, only a few scattered B cells, and a few macrophages. These data suggest that in autoimmune oophoritis the destruction of ovarian follicles is mediated by T cells. Antibodies that develop may contribute to the ovarian lesions but also could be a secondary epiphenomenon of limited pathogenetic significance.

REFERENCES

Abercrombie GF: Thrombo-angiitis obliterans of the spermatic cord. Br J Surg 1965; 52:632.

Agarwal V, Li JKH, Bard R: Lymphocytic orchitis: A case report. Hum Pathol 1990; 21:1080.

Agger P, Johnsen S: Quantitative evaluation of testicular biopsies in varicocele. Fertil Steril 1978; 29:52.

Ahonen P, Miettinen A, Perheentupa J: Adrenal and steroidal cell antibodies in patients with autoimmune polyglandular disease type I and risk of adrenocortical and ovarian failure. J Clin Endocrinol Metab 1987; 64:494.

Aiman J, Smetek C: Premature ovarian failure. Obstet Gynecol 1985; 66:9.

Alderman PM: The lurking sperm. A review of failures in 8,879 vasectomies performed by one physician. JAMA 1988; 259:3142.

Alexander NJ, Schmidt SS: Incidence of antisperm antibody levels and granulomas in men. Fertil Steril 1977; 28:655.

Alfert HJ, Canning DA: Testicular torsion in a 62-year-old man. J Urol 1987; 138:149.

Alper MM, Garner PR: Circulating antiovarian antibodies in premature ovarian failure. Obstet Gynecol 1987; 70:144.

Anderson JB, Williamson RCN: The fate of the human testes following unilateral torsion of the spermatic cord. Br J Urol 1986; 58:698.

Andres TL, Trainer TD, Lapenas DJ: Small vessel alterations in the testes of infertile men with varicocele. Am J Clin Pathol 1981; 76:378.

Atallah MW, Ippolito JJ, Rubin BW: Intrauterine bilateral torsion of the spermatic cord. J Urol 1976; 116:128.

Averette HE, Boike GM, Jarrell MA: Effects of cancer chemotherapy on gonadal function and reproductive capacity. CA 1990; 40:199.

Aynsley-Green A, Zachmann M, Illig R, Rampini S, Prader A: Congenital bilateral anorchia in childhood: A clinical, endocrine and therapeutic evaluation of twenty-one cases. Clin Endocrinol (Oxf) 1976; 5:381.

Azar N, Guillevin L, Huong Du LTH, Herreman G, Meyrier A, Godeau P: Symptomatic urogenital manifestations of polyarteritis nodosa and Churg-Strauss angiitis: Analysis of 8 of 165 patients. J Urol 1989; 142:136.

Baer HM, Gerber WL, Kendall AR, Locke JL, Putong PB: Segmental infarct of the testis due to hypersensitivity angiitis. J Urol 1989; 142:125.

Baker TG: Radiosensitivity of mammalian oocytes with particular reference to the human female. Am J Obstet Gynecol 1971; 110:746.

Bannatyne P, Russell P, Shearman RP: Autoimmune oophoritis: A clinicopathologic assessment of 12 cases. Int J Gynecol Pathol 1990; 9:191.

Barbarino-Monnier P, Gobert B, Guillet-Rosso F, Bene MC, Landes P, Faure G: Antiovary antibodies, repeated attempts, and outcome of in vitro fertilization. Fertil Steril 1991; 56:928.

Barratt CL, Bolton AE, Cooke ID: Functional significance of white blood cells in the male and female reproductive tract. Hum Reprod 1990; 5:639.

Bartsch G, Frank S, Marberger H, Mikuz G: Testicular torsion: Late results with special regard to fertility and endocrine function. J Urol 1980; 124:375.

Bramswig JH, Heimes U, Heiermann E, Schlegel W, Nieschlag E, Schellong G: The effects of different cumulative doses of chemotherapy on testicular function. Results in 75 patients treated for Hodgkin's disease during childhood or adolescence. Cancer 1990; 65:1298.

Brooks JJ, Wheeler JE: Granulomatous salpingitis secondary to Crohn's disease. Obstet Gynecol 1977; 49:31s.

Bumpers PM Jr, Hulbert WC Jr, Jimenez JF: Arteriovenous malformation of the spermatic cord. J Urol 1989; 141:103.

Burge DM: Neonatal testicular torsion and infarction: Aetiology and management. Br J Urol 1987; 59:70.

Byrne J, Fears TR, Gail MH, Pec D, Connelly RR, Austin DF et al.: Early menopause in long-term survivors of cancer during adolescence. Am J Obstet Gynecol 1992; 166:788.

Cass AS: Value of early operation in blunt testicular contusion and hematocele. J Urol 1988; 139:746.

Chalvardjian A: Sarcoidosis of the female genital tract. Am J Obstet Gynecol 1978; 132:78.

Chapman RM: Effects of cytotoxic therapy on sexuality and gonadal function. Semin Oncol 1982; 9:84.

Chapman RM, Sutcliffe SB: Protection of ovarian function by oral contraceptives in women receiving chemotherapy for Hodgkin's disease. Blood 1981; 58:849.

Chapman S: The acute scrotum: A complication of cardiac catherization. Br J Radiol 1988; 61:162.

Charak BS, Gupta R, Mandrekar P, Sheth NA, Banavali SD, Saikia TK, et al.: Testicular dysfunction after cyclophosphamide-vincristine-procarbazine-prednisolone chemotherapy for advanced Hodgkin's disease. A long-term follow-up study. Cancer 1990; 65:1903.

Clark SJ, Resnick MI: Infertility following radiation and chemotherapy. Urol Clin North Am 1978; 5:531.

Collins K, Broecker BH: Familial torsion of the spermatic cord. J Urol 1989; 141:128.

Comhaire FH: Varicocele and its treatment. In Advances in Clinical Andrology, edited by Barratt CLR, Cooke ID. Lancaster, UK, MTP Press, Kluwer Academic, 1988, p 49.

Cramer DW, Schiff I, Schoenbaum SC, Gibson M, Belisle S, Albrecht B et al.: Tubal infertility and the intrauterine device. N Engl J Med 1985; 312:941.

Cust MP, Whitehead MI, Powles R, Hunter M, Miliken S: Consequences and treatment of ovarian failure after total body irradiation for leukemia. BMJ 1989; 299:1494.

Daling JR, Weiss NS, Metch BJ, Chow WH, Soderstrom RM, Moore DE, et al.: Primary tubal infertility in relation to the use of an intrauterine device. N Engl J Med 1985; 312:937.

Damewood MD, Grochow LB: Prospects for fertility after chemotherapy or radiation for neoplastic disease. Fertil Steril 1986; 45:443.

Damewood MD, Zacur HA, Hoffman GJ, Rock JA: Circulating antiovarian antibodies in premature ovarian failure. Obstet Gynecol 1986; 68:850.

Das S, Singer A: Controversies of perinatal torsion of the spermatic cord: A review, survey and recommendations. J Urol 1990; 143:231.

Dennis MJ, Fahim SF, Doyle PT: Testicular torsion in older men. BMJ 1987; 294:1680.

Donaldson LB: Crohn's Disease. "Its gynecologic aspect". Am J Obstet Gynecol 1978; 131:196.

Drasga RE, Einhorn LH, Williams SD, Patel DN, Stevens EE: Fertility after chemotherapy for testicular cancer. J Clin Oncol 1983; 1:179.

Dubin L, Amelar RD: Etiologic factors in 1294 consecutive cases of male infertility. Fertil Steril 1971; 22:469.

Dubin L, Amelar RD: Varicocele size and results of varicocelectomy in selected subfertile men with varicocele. Fertil Steril 1970; 21:606.

Dubin L, Amelar RD: Varicocelectomy as therapy in male infertility: A study of 504 cases. Fertil Steril 1975; 26:217.

Editorial: Does infection occur with modern intrauterine devices? Lancet 1992; 339:783.

Engelmann UH, Schramek P, Tomamichel G, Deindl F, Senge T: Vasectomy reversal in central Europe: Results of questionnaire of urologists in Austria, Germany and Switzerland. J Urol 1990; 143:64.

Fajardo LF, Berthrong M: Radiation injury in surgical pathology. Part I. Am J Surg Pathol 1978; 2:159.

Fisch H, Laor E, BarChama N, Witkin SS, Tolia BM, Reid RE: Detection of testicular endocrine abnormalities and their correlation with serum antisperm antibodies in men following vasectomy. J Urol 1989; 141:1129.

Fisch H, Laor E, Reid RE, Tolia BM, Freed SZ: Gonadal dysfunction after testicular torsion: Luteinizing hormone and follicle-stimulating hormone response to gonadotropin releasing hormone. J Urol 1988; 139:961.

Fuchs EF, Alexander NJ: Immunologic considerations before and after vasostomy. Fertil Steril 1983; 40:497.

Glassy FJ, Mostofi FK: Spermatic granulomas of the epididymis. Am J Clin Pathol 1956; 26:1303.

Glezerman M, Jecht EW (Eds): Varicocele and Male Infertility. II. Berlin, Springer-Verlag, 1984.

Goldman RL, Azzopardi JG: Benign neural invasion in vasitis nodosa. Histopathology 1982; 6:309.

Gradishar WJ, Schilsky RL: Effects of cancer treatment on the reproductive system. Crit Rev Oncol Hematol 1988; 8:153.

Gradishar WJ, Schilsky RL: Ovarian function following radiation and chemotherapy for cancer. Semin Oncol 1989; 16:425.

Greenberg SH, Lipshultz LI, Wein AJ: Experience with 425 subfertile male patients. J Urol 1978; 119:507.

Gupta AS, Kothari LK, Bapna R: Surgical sterilization by vasectomy and its effect on the structure and function of the testis in man. Br J Surg 1975; 62:59.

Hadziselimovic F, Herzog B, Leibundgut R, Jenny P, Buser M: Testicular and vascular changes in children and adults with varicocele. J Urol 1989; 142:583.

Hadziselimovic F, Leibundgut B, Da Rugna D, Buser MW: The value of testicular biopsy in patients with varicocele. J Urol 1986a; 135:707.

Hadziselimovic F, Snyder H, Duckett J, Howard S: Testicular histology in children with unilateral testicular torsion. J Urol 1986b; 136:208.

Hahn EW, Feingold SM, Simpson L, Batata M: Recovery from aspermia induced by low-dose radiation in seminoma patients. Cancer 1982; 50:337.

Hamou J, Salat-Baroux J, Siegler AM: Diagnosis and treatment of intrauterine adhesions by microhysteroscopy. Fertil Steril 1983; 39:321.

Handelsman DJ, Yue DK, Turtle JR: Hypogonadism and massive testicular infiltration due to amyloidosis. J Urol 1983; 129:610.

Hedinger CE, Dhom G: Pathologie des männlichen Genitale. Berlin, Springer-Verlag, 1991.

Hellema HWJ, Rümke P: Sperm autoantibodies as a consequence of vasectomy. I. Within one year post-operation. Clin Exp Immunol 1978; 31:18.

Himelstein-Braw R, Peters H, Faber M: Morphological study of the ovaries of leukaemic children. Br J Cancer 1978; 38:82.

Ishii T, Hosoda Y, Ikegami N, Shimada H: Senile amyloid deposition. J Pathol 1983; 139:1.

Jarow JP, Budin RE, Dym M, Zirkin BR, Noren S, Marshall FF: Quantitative pathologic changes in the human testis after vasectomy. A controlled study. N Engl J Med 1985; 313:1252.

Javadpour N (Ed): Principles and Management of Testicular Cancer. New York, Thieme, 1986.

Jecht EW, Zeitler E: Varicocele and Male Infertility. Berlin, Springer-Verlag, 1982.

Jones MA, Sharp GH, Trainer TD: The adolescent varicocele. A histopathologic study of 13 testicular biopsies. Am J Clin Pathol 1988; 89:321.

Jones WR: Immunology and infertility. In Progress in infertility, ed 3. Edited by Behrman SJ, Kistner RW, Patton GW, Boston, 1988, Little, Brown, p 751.

Kalash SS, Young JD Jr: Fracture of penis: Controversy of surgical versus conservative treatment. Urology 1984; 24:21.

Kaplan GW: Complications of circumcision. Urol Clin North Am 1983; 10:543.

Kass EJ, Freitas JE, Bour JB: Adolescent varicocele: Objective indications for treatment. J Urol 1989; 142:579.

Kedia KR, Markland C, Fraley EE: Sexual function after high retroperitoneal lymphadenectomy. Urol Clin Am 1977; 4:523.

King DJ, Ratcliffe MA, Dawson AA, Bennett B, Macgregor JE, Klopper AI: Fertility in young men and women after treatment for lymphoma: A study of a population. J Clin Pathol 1985; 38:1247.

Kitchener HC, Kingdom JCP: Sepsis in gynaecological surgery. In MacLean AB, ed: Clinical infections in obstetrics and gynecology, Oxford, 1990, Blackwell, p 313.

Koraitim M, Khalil R: Preservation of urosexual functions after radical cystectomy. Urology, 1992; 39:117.

Kuehn MW, Oellinger R, Kustin G, Merkel KH: Primary testicular manifestations of systemic lupus erythematosus. Eur Urol 1989; 16:72.

Kupeli S, Safak M, Yaman S: Vas deferens calculus. J Urol 1989; 141:378.

Kutteh WH, Blackwell RE, Gore H, Kutteh CC, Carr BR, Mestecky J: Secretory immune system of the female reproductive tract: II. Local immune system in normal and infected fallopian tube. Fertil Steril 1990; 54:51.

Lange PH, Narayan P, Vogelzang NJ, Shafer RB, Kennedy BJ, Fraley EE: Return of fertility after treatment for nonseminomatous testicular cancers: changing concepts. J Urol 1982; 129:1131.

Leader AJ, Axelrad SD, Frankowski R, Mumford SD: Complications of 2,711 vasectomies. J Urol 1974; 111:365.

Leape LL: Testicular torsion. In Pediatric Urology, edited by Aschcraft KW. Philadelphia, WB Saunders, 1990, p 429.

Lee NC, Rubin GL, Borucki R: The intrauterine device and pelvic inflammatory disease revisited. New results from the Women's Health Study. Obstet Gynecol 1988; 72:1.

Lehmann D, Temminck D, Da Rugna D, Leibundgut B, Sulmoni A, Müller AJ: Role of immunological factors in male infertility: Immunohistochemical and serological evidence. Lab Invest 1987; 57:21.

Lipshultz LI, Benson GS: Vasectomy 1980. Urol Clin Am 1980; 7:89.

Lipshultz LI, Corriere JN Jr: Progressive testicular atrophy in the varicocele patient. J Urol 1977; 117:175.

Lonsdale RN, Roberts PF, Trowell JE: Autoimmune oophoritis associated with polycystic ovaries. Histopathology 1991; 19:77.

Luborsky JL, Visintin I, Boyers S, Asari T, Caldwell B, DeCherney A: Ovarian antibodies detected by immobilized antigen immunoassay in patients with premature ovarian failure. J Clin Endocrinol Metab 1990; 70:69.

Lushbaugh CC, Casarett GW: The effects of gonadal irradiation in chemical radiation therapy: A review. Cancer 1976; 37:1111.

Marcello MF, Nuciforo G, Romeo R, Di Dino G, Russo I, Russo A, Palumbo G, Schiliro G: Structural and ultrastructural study of the ovary in childhood leukemia after successful treatment. Cancer 1990; 66:2099.

McCombe AW, Scobie WG: Torsion of scrotal contents in children. Br J Urol 1988; 61:148.

McConnell JD, Peters PC, Lewis SE: Testicular rupture in blunt scrotal trauma: A view of 15 cases with recent application of testicular scanning. J Urol 1982; 128:309.

MacDermott JP, Gray BK, Stewart PAH: Traumatic rupture of the testis. Br J Urol 1988; 62:179.

McFadden MR, Mehan DJ: Testicular biopsies in 101 cases of varicocele. J Urol 1978; 119:372.

McLean NR, Burnett RA: Polyarteritis nodosa of epididymis. Urology 1983; 21:70.

Mebust WK, Holtgrewe HL, Cockett AT, Peters DC: Transurethral prostatectomy: Immediate and postoperative complications. A cooperative study of 13 participating institutions evaluating 3,885 patients. J Urol 1989; 141:243.

Melekos MD, Ashback HW, Markou SA: Etiology of acute scrotum in 100 boys with regard to age distribution. J Urol 1988; 139:1023.

Mikuz G: Testicular torsion: Simple grading for histological evaluation of tissue damage. Appl Pathol 1985; 3:134.

Mikuz G, Damjanov I: Inflammation of the testis, epididymis, peritesticular membranes and scrotum. Pathol Annu 1982; 17:101.

Mikuz G, Hofstädter F, Hager J: Testis involvement in Schönlein-Henoch purpura. Pathol Res Pract 1979; 165:323.

Millar SE, Chamow SM, Baur A, Oliver C, Robey F, Dean J: Vaccination with a synthetic zona pellucida peptide produces long-term contraception in female mice. Science 1989; 246:935.

Mizrahi S, Shtamler B: Surgical approach and outcome in torsion of testis. Urology 1992; 39:52.

Moncayo H, Moncayo R, Benz R, Wolf A, Lauritzen C: Ovarian failure and autoimmunity. Detection of autoantibodies directed against both the unoccupied luteinizing hormone/human chorionic gonadotropin receptor and the hormone-receptor complex of bovine corpus luteum. J Clin Invest 1989; 84:1857.

Muram D, Gale CL: Acquired vaginal occlusion. Adolesc Pediatr Gynecol 1990; 3:141.

Nagler HM, Zippe CD: Varicocele: Current concepts and treatment. In Infertility in the Male, 2nd ed. edited by Lipschultz LI, Howard SS. St Louis, Mosby-Year Book, 1991, p 313.

Nicosia SV, Matus-Ridley M, Meadows AT: Gonadal effects of cancer therapy in girls. Cancer 1985; 55:2364.

Nistal M, Martinez C, Paniagua R: Primary testicular lesions in the twisted testis. Fertil Steril 1992; 57:381.

Nistal M, Paniagua R: Testicular and Epididymal Pathology. New York, Thieme, 1984.

Nistal M, Santamaria L, Codesal J, Paniagua R: Secondary amyloidosis of the testis: An electron microscopic and histochemical study. Appl Pathol 1989; 7:2.

Olson AL: Vasitis nodosa. Am J Clin Pathol 1971; 55:364.

Pennisi AJ, Grushkin CM, Lieberman E: Gonadal function in children with nephrosis treated with cyclophosphamide. Am J Dis Child 1975; 129:315.

Perlmutter AD: Injuries to the genitalia. Dial Pediatr Urol 1980; 3:2.

Peters H, Byskov AG, Himelstein-Braw R, Faber M: Follicular growth: The basic event in the mouse and human ovary. J Reprod Fertil 1975; 45:559.

Peterson HB, Grubb GS, DeStefano F, Rubin GL: Complications of tubal sterilization. In The Fallopian Tube: Basic Studies and Clinical Contributions, edited by Siegler AM. Mount Kisco, New York, Futura 1986, p 329.

Peterson HB, Huber DH, Belker AM: Vasectomy: An appraisal for the obstetrician-gynecologist. Obstet Gynecol 1990; 76:568.

Pitkanen P, Westermark P, Cornwell GG 3d, Murdoch W: Amyloid of the seminal vesicles. A distinctive and common localized form of senile amyloidosis. Am J Pathol 1983; 110:64.

Pryor JL, Howards SS: Varicocele. Urol Clin North Am 1987; 14:499.

Pugh RCB, Hanely GH: Spontaneous recanalisation of the divided vas deferens. Br J Urol 1969; 41:340.

Quigley C, Cowell C, Jimenez M, Burger H, Kirk J, Bergin M, et al : Normal or early development of puberty despite gonadal damage in children treated for acute lymphoblastic leukemia. N Engl J Med 1989; 321:143.

Rabinowe SL, Ravnikar VA, Dib SA, George KL, Dluhy RG: Premature menopause: Monoclonal antibody defined T lymphocyte abnormalities and antiovarian antibodies. Fertil Steril 1989; 51:450.

Rivkees SA, Crawford JD: The relationship of gonadal activity and chemotherapy-induced gonadal damage. JAMA 1988; 259:2123.

Russell P, Bannatyne P, Shearman RP, Fraser IS, Corbett P: Premature hypergonadotropic ovarian failure: Clinicopathological study of 19 cases. Int J Gynecol Pathol 1982; 1:185.

Salomon F, Hedinger CE: Abnormal basement membrane structures of seminiferous tubules in infertile men. Lab Invest 1982; 47:543.

Salomon F, Saremeslani P, Jakob M, Hedinger CE: Immune complex orchitis in infertile men. Immunoelectron microscopy of abnormal basement membrane structures. Lab Invest 1982; 47:555.

Sandvei R, Bang G: Sarcoidosis of the uterus. Acta Obstet Gynecol Scand 1991; 70:165.

Schenker JG, Margalioth EJ: Intrauterine adhesions: An updated appraisal. Fertil Steril 1982; 37:593.

Schlappack OK, Kratzik C, Schmidt W, Spona J, Schuster E: Response of the seminiferous epithelium to scattered radiation in seminoma patients. Cancer 1988; 62:1487.

Schuster G: Traumatic rupture of the testicle and a review of the literature. J Urol 1982; 127:1194.

Shurbaji MS, Epstein JI: Testicular vasculitis: Implications for systemic disease. Hum Pathol 1988; 19:186.

Siegler AM, Valle RF, Lindemann HJ, Mencaglia L: Therapeutic Hysteroscopy: Indications and Techniques. St. Louis, Mosby–Year Book, 1990.

Siimes MA, Rautonen J: Small testicles with impaired production of sperm in adult male survivors of childhood malignancies. Cancer 1990; 65:1303.

Skoglund RW, McRoberts JW, Ragde H: Torsion of testicular appendages; presentation of 43 new cases and a collective review. J Urol 1970a; 104:598.

Skoglund RW, McRoberts JW, Ragde H: Torsion of the spermatic cord: A review of the literature and an analysis of 70 new cases. J Urol 1970b; 104:604.

Steeno O, Knops J, Declerck L, Adimoelja A, van de Voorde H: Prevention of fertility disorders by detection and treatment of varicocele at school and college age. Andrologia 1976; 8:47.

Tarter TH, Kogan SJ: Contralateral testicular disease after unilateral testicular injury: Current concepts. Semin Urol 1988; 6:120.

Taxy JB, Marshall FF, Ehrlichman RJ: Vasectomy: Subclinical pathologic changes. Am J Surg Pathol 1981; 5:767.

Terquem A, Dadoune JR: Morphologic findings in varicocele: An ultrastructural study of 30 bilateral testicular biopsies. Int J Androl 1981; 4:515.

Thomas AJ: Vasectomy and vasovasostomy. In Andrology, edited by Pryor JP, Lipschultz LI. London, Butterworth, 1987, p 305.

Thomas AJ Jr, Timmons JW, Perlmutter AD: Progressive penile amputation. Tourniquet injury secondary to hair. Urology 1977; 9:42.

Thomas WE, Williamson RC: Diagnosis and outcome of testicular torsion. Br J Surg 1983; 70:213.

Tung KSK, Lu CY: Immunologic basis of reproductive failure. In Pathology of Reproductive Failure, edited by Kraus FT, Damjanov I, Kaufman N. Baltimore, Williams & Wilkins, 1991, p 308.

Urwin GH, Kehoe N, Dundas S, Fox M: Testicular infarction in a patient with sickle cell trait. Br J Urol 1986; 58:340.

Vaccaro JA, Davis R, Belville WD, Kiesling VJ: Traumatic hematocele: Association with rupture of the testicle. J Urol 1986; 136:1217.

Verp MS: Environmental causes of ovarian failure. Semin Reprod Endocrinol 1983; 1:101.

Virdi JS, Conway W, Kelly DG: Torsion of the vas aberrans. Br J Urol 1990; 61:435.

Wallace WH, Shalet SM, Hendry JH, Moris-Jones PH, Gattamaneni HR: Ovarian failure following abdominal irradiation in childhood: The radio-sensitivity of the human oocyte. Br J Radiol 1989; 62:995.

Washington AE, Gove S, Schachter J, Sweet RL: Oral contraceptives, Chlamydia trachomatis infection, and pelvic inflammatory disease. A word of caution about protection. JAMA 1985; 253:2246.

Waxman JH, Terry YA, Wrigley PFM, Malpas JS, Rees LH, Besser GM, et al.: Gonadal function in Hodgkin's disease: Long term follow-up of chemotherapy. BMJ 1982; 285:1612.

Whitehead E, Shalet SM, Blackledge G, Todd I, Crowther D, Beardwell CG: The effects of Hodgkin's disease and combination chemotherapy on gonadal function in the adult male. Cancer 1982; 49:418.

Williamson RCN: Torsion of the testis and allied conditions. Br J Surg 1976; 63:465.

Wlodarski FM, Trainer TD: Granulomatous oophoritis and salpingitis associated with Crohn's disease of the appendix. Am J Obstet Gynecol 1975; 122:527.

Young RH, Scully RE: Ovarian pathology of infertility. In Kraus FT, Damjanov I, Kaufman N, editors: Pathology of reproductive failure, Baltimore, 1991, Williams & Wilkins, p 104.

Zimmerman KG, Johnson PC, Paplanus SH: Nerve invasion by benign proliferating ductules in vasitis nodosa. Cancer 1983; 51:2066.

Chapter 7

INFERTILITY DUE TO
ENDOCRINE DISORDERS

The female and male reproductive functions are critically dependent on an intact and fully integrated hypothalamic-pituitary-gonadal axis, which acts as the central regulator and coordinator of complex endocrine and paracrine effector and feedback mechanisms. *Congenital* and genetic pre-pubertal lesions of the hypothalamus and the pituitary, as discussed in Chapter 3, may interfere with normal gonadal development and cause hypogonadotropic hypogonadism. *Acquired* lesions in the same anatomic location may have similar effects, especially in prepubertal individuals. *Post-pubertal* lesions suppress spermatogenesis in males and inhibit ovulation and disrupt the normal menstrual cycle in females. The complex endocrine disorders that result from disturbances of the hypothalamic-pituitary-gonadal axis have been discussed in great detail in clinical textbooks of endocrinology (Speroff et al., 1989; Yen and Jaffe, 1991; Wilson and Foster, 1992), and this chapter is limited to the pathology of lesions associated with infertility.

HYPOTHALAMIC AND PITUITARY LESIONS

Hypothalamic and pituitary diseases that affect reproductive functions in males and females can be *functional*—i.e., without a recognizable morphologic substrate—or *organic*—i.e., caused by a morphologically visible and pathologically defined lesion. Morphologically identifiable lesions account for infertility in less than 1% of all males seeking treatment. Functional disturbances involving the hypothalamic-pituitary-gonadal axis also are rare in males but more common in females. Central disturbances of ovulation are the cause of reproductive problems in approximately 25% to 30% of all women treated for infertility (Speroff et al., 1989).

Etiologic classification of hypogonadotropic hypogonadism

Tumors

Craniopharyngioma
Glioma of hypothalamus
Pituitary adenoma
Meningioma
Histiocytosis X
Metastases

Circulatory disturbances

Pituitary apoplexy
Aneurysm
Hemorrhages of the base of the brain

Inflammation

Encephalitis
Hypophysitis
Autoimmune disorders
Sarcoidosis
AIDS

Genetic and developmental syndromes

Kallmann's syndrome
Prader-Willi syndrome
Laurence-Moon syndrome
Bardet-Biedl syndrome

Psychosomatic disorders

Anorexia nervosa
Bulimia
Emotional distress

Systemic diseases

Hemochromatosis
Liver disease
Kidney disease

Miscellaneous causes

Athletics
Drugs
Irradiation
Trauma

Idiopathic functional disorders

Features of hypogonadotropic hypogonadism

Occurrence

PRIMARY
1. Sporadic
2. Familial
(male > female)
SECONDARY
1. Hypothalamic
2. Pituitary

Clinical forms

1. Complex syndrome—associated anomalies
2. Isolated hypogonadism—delayed or no puberty
MALES
Small testes
Micropenis
Scrotal hypoplasia
Eunuchoid body
    proportions
FEMALES
Primary amenorrhea
Lack of breasts and pubic and axillary hair

Laboratory findings

Low LH, FSH, or both

Therapy

1. Gn-RH (pulsatile)
2. Substitution pituitary or sex hormone therapy (if Gn-RH is ineffectual)

2. Measurement of androgens and/or estrogens in urine
3. Radiologic examination of the base of the skull to assess the pituitary and hypothalamus anatomically
4. Gynecologic and andrologic evaluation
5. Measurement of plasma and/or urine concentration of sex steroids
6. Systemic physical examination
7. Biopsy of identifiable lesions
8. Chromosomal and genetic analysis

On the basis of these data, one can usually determine whether the patient has an organic or a functional disease.

Various causes of hypogonadotropic hypogonadism are listed in the box at left. The symptoms of various hypothalamic and pituitary lesions depend primarily on the nature and duration of the disease. The symptoms may be indicative of multihormonal disturbances or a selective hormonal deficiency such as isolated gonadotropin deficiency (Yeh et al., 1989) or excess such as hyperprolactinemia (Thorner et al., 1992). Symptoms also are sex and age dependent. Features of hypogonadotropic hypogonadism are listed in the box above.

Hypogonadotropic hypogonadism in males. Congenital or acquired lesions of the hypothalamic and pituitary regions affect profoundly the development of gonads and

Hypogonadotropic hypogonadism

Low levels of gonadotropin in the blood are indicative of central lesions, and it is incumbent on the clinician to determine whether the cause of that deficiency resides in the hypothalamus or the pituitary. A typical work-up includes:

1. Measurement of plasma gonadotropins (luteinizing hormone [LH] and follicle-stimulating hormone [FSH])

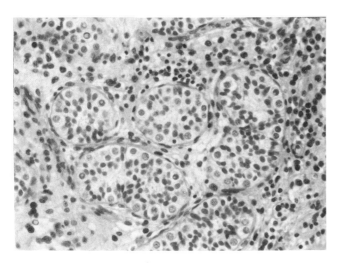

Fig. 7-1. Hypogonadotropic hypogonadism. The seminiferous tubules are immature.

secondary sexual characteristics. Typical of this condition are patients with Prader-Willi syndrome, who appear eunuchoid and have hypoplastic genitalia characterized by micropenis, cryptorchidism, and a small scrotum. This triad is found in more than 90% of patients with the syndrome (Butler et al., 1986). The testes never develop fully and remain small. The seminiferous tubules of such testes are lined by immature Sertoli cells with round nuclei and small or absent nucleoli (Fig. 7-1). There are few germ cells, and no evidence of spermatogenesis can be seen. The interstitial spaces contain a normal complement of Leydig's cells; these, however, usually lack the typical features of fully functional adult Leydig's cells. Other hypothalamic and pituitary lesions produce the same developmental arrests. Destruction of hypothalamic centers in adult males usually results in a loss of libido and hypospermatogenesis.

The pulsatile administration of gonadotropin-releasing hormone (Gn-RH) has been used successfully in patients with Gn-RH deficiency caused by genetic diseases, radiation injury of the brain, and pituitary tumors (reviewed by Conn and Crowley, 1991). Mimicking the normal pulsatile release of Gn-RH, this treatment stimulates the episodic secretion of gonadotropins and results in testicular growth, normalization of sex hormone secretion, and initiation and maintenance of spermatogenesis.

Hypogonadotropic hypogonadism in females. As in males, hypothalamic lesions profoundly affect the gonads (Santoro et al., 1986). Primary hypothalamic lesions in females are associated with sexual infantilism, which usually becomes evident only after puberty. Such women do not enter menarche and do not develop normal female secondary sexual characteristics. Secondary amenorrhea develops in women with acquired hypothalamic and secondary hypothalamic lesions. Amenorrhea has successfully been treated with pulsatile administration of Gn-RH (Conn and Crowley, 1991).

Table 7-1. Classification and relative frequency of pituitary adenomas

Tumor type	Frequency (%)
Growth hormone cell adenoma	16
Prolactinoma	27
Corticotropic adenoma	15
Thyrotropic adenoma	1
Gonadotropic adenoma	4
Nonfunctioning (null cell) adenoma	25
Plurihormonal adenoma	12
TOTAL	100

Modified from Kovacs K, Horvath E. In Gondos B, Riddick G (Eds). Pathology of Infertility. New York, © Thieme Medical Publishers, 1987, with permission.

Selective deficiency of gonadotropic hormones. This deficiency occurs in several congenital syndromes that affect either the hypothalamus or the pituitary. For no obvious reasons, males are more often affected than females. Kallmann's syndrome, or hypogonadotropic hypogonadism with anosmia, which develops as a result of congenital malformations of the olfactory bulbs and the interrupted migration of luteinizing hormone–releasing hormone (LH-RH) neurons (Schwanzel-Fukuda et al., 1989), is probably the most common of these conditions. It is characterized by a selective deficiency of LH-RH and LH.

Congenital deficiency of LH is associated with the so-called fertile eunuch syndrome (Smals et al., 1978). Congenital deficiency of FSH also has been described (Rabin et al., 1972). A congenital form of adrenal hypoplasia that usually is lethal in childhood and occurs in an X-linked form in males seems to result from a related defect in pituitary gonadotropic cells (Kikuchi et al., 1987). Typically, hypogonadism in these boys is associated with a cytomegalic form of adrenal hypoplasia in which the adrenal cortical cells appear enlarged and vacuolated. The patients lack mineralocorticoids and glucocorticoids and do not respond to Gn-RH (Kikuchi et al., 1987). Some cases could be of hypothalamic origin as well (Kruse et al., 1984).

Pituitary tumors

Pituitary tumors cause a variety of hormonal abnormalities, most of which interfere with normal reproductive functions. These include symptoms related to an excess of specific pituitary hormones found in patients with functioning tumors; symptoms related to a deficiency of pituitary hormones found in nonfunctioning tumors; and a combination of excess of one hormone and deficiency of another in patients who have a functioning pituitary tumor that compresses the remaining pituitary and causes atrophy or disappearance of normal cells.

Pituitary tumors can be divided into several groups corresponding to cell types of the normal anterior lobe of the pituitary (Table 7-1). Approximately 12% of tumors are composed of several cells types and are plurihormonal; 25% of the tumors are nonfunctional, i.e., composed of "null" cells that do not correspond to any of the well-characterized cells in the adult pituitary gland (Kovacs and Horvath, 1987). All of these tumors can cause anovulation and amenorrhea in females and hypogonadism and hypospermatogenesis in males.

The large nonfunctioning tumors cause symptoms by compressing adjacent structures. These tumors may compress the normal pituitary and cause atrophy of gonadotrophs; compress the pituitary stalk and thus prevent the influx of Gn-RH through the portal circulation into the pituitary; or even compress the hypothalamus and destroy the Gn-RH neurons. However, not all cases can be explained in terms of tumor mass effect as evidenced by some cases of hypogonadism caused by small tumors composed of nonfunctioning cells or corticotropin-producing adenomas typical of Cushing's disease (Kovacs and Horvath, 1987).

Reproductive dysfunctions are most often caused by adenomas composed of prolactin and gonadotropin-producing cells. These tumors may cause infertility in males as well as in females.

Prolactinomas are the most common pituitary tumors, and they occur as either macroscopic or microscopic adenomas. Microadenomas are found in one fourth of all pituitaries examined at autopsy, and approximately 40% of these are composed of prolactin-producing cells (Burrow et al., 1981). However, most of these tumors either are asymptomatic or do not cause significant elevation of plasma prolactin and thus have no clinical effects.

Hyperprolactinemia presents in women as the amenorrhea-galactorrhea syndrome, oligomenorrhea, or other menstrual abnormalities. The effect of elevated levels of prolactin on the ovary is not fully understood. Theoretically, it could be due to an abnormal release of Gn-RH; inhibition of pulsatile release of Gn-RH; disturbance in the secretion of LH and FSH; an abnormal ratio of LH to FSH; or a direct inhibitory action of prolactin on granulosa cells (Archer, 1988).

Galactorrhea occurs in 30% to 80% of cases (Thorner et al., 1992). It is less common in women with long-standing amenorrhea than in those with recent onset. This probably reflects the decreasing output of estrogen from inactive ovaries that invariably occurs in long-standing amenorrhea. Infertility associated with prolactinomas may be treated successfully either medically or surgically (Thorner et al., 1992).

Hyperprolactinemia in males causes varying degrees of hypogonadism and hypospermatogenesis (Carter et al., 1978). Cohen et al. (1984) found decreased libido in 83% of patients, adiposity in 69%, apathy in 63%, and headaches in 63% of patients with prolactinomas. These symptoms are reversible and disappear upon removal of the pituitary tumor or with medical treatment of hyperprolactinemia. The effects of hyperprolactinemia on the male gonad are not fully understood but are most likely secondary to the abnormal release of Gn-RH from the hypothalamus

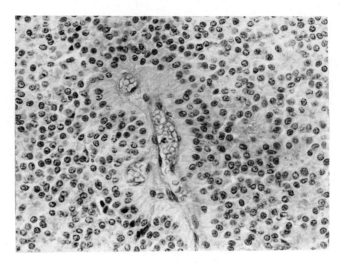

Fig. 7-2. Prolactinoma.

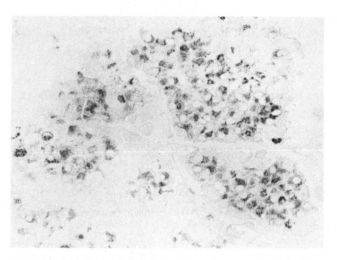

Fig. 7-3. Immunohistochemistry of prolactinoma shows perinuclear reactivity of tumor cells with antibody to prolactin.

and gonadotropic hormones from the pituitary (Thorner et al., 1992).

The pathology of prolactinomas has been reviewed extensively (Horvath and Kovacs, 1986; Kovacs and Horvath, 1987; Thorner et al., 1992). In standard tissue sections stained with hematoxylin and eosin, most tumors appear as solid adenomas composed of cells with a chromophobic or slightly eosinophilic cytoplasm (Fig. 7-2). A few tumors show papillary features and are composed of large acidophilic cells. Immunohistochemically, the cells are immunoreactive with antibodies to prolactin. Typically, the immunoreactivity is limited to the perinuclear Golgi's zone (Fig. 7-3) but may present as diffuse cytoplasmic staining in densely granulated tumors. Microscopic calcospherites and intracellular and extracellular amyloid may be useful for the diagnosis but are found only in a small fraction of all tumors. Secondary changes such as necrosis, calcifications, amyloid deposition, and fibrosis are found in tumors of patients who received prolonged

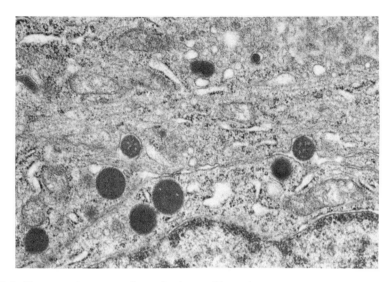

Fig. 7-4. Electron microscopy of a prolactinoma illustrating exocytosis of secretory granules.

medical treatment (Thorner et al., 1992). Malignant prolactinomas are extremely rare (U and Johnson, 1984)

By electron microscopy one can distinguish two types of prolactinomas (Horvath and Kovacs, 1986), the more common, sparsely granulated variant and the rare, densely granulated variant. The sparsely granulated tumors have a moderate number of neurosecretory granules that measure 120 to 300 nm in diameter and are scattered throughout the cytoplasm. Typically, the granules accumulate along the cell membrane and are extruded into the extracellular space (Fig. 7-4). Exocytosis is seen in densely granulated prolactinoma cells as well; this is an important diagnostic finding because the densely granulated prolactinoma cells, in all other respects, are indistinguishable from growth hormone–secreting adenomas, which include the prominent large neuroendocrine granules measuring 400 to 700 nm in diameter. The electron microscopic evidence of activity of tumor cells does not correlate with the hormonal findings. Moreover, there are no clinical differences in the presentation of sparsely or densely granulated prolactinomas.

Gonadotropin-producing adenomas are rare and account for 4% to 5% of pituitary tumors (Kovacs and Horvath, 1987). They may produce LH or FSH, or the alpha or beta chain of LH or FSH, or both. FSH is the most common product. However, the diagnosis is rarely made because most tumors occur in older patients who already have elevated levels of gonadotropins in the plasma (Snyder, 1985, 1987).

The vast majority of gonadotropic tumors are removed because of the visual symptoms related to the compression of the optic chiasm by the tumor (Snyder, 1985). Hypogonadism may evolve, and if it does, it usually is mild and rarely of major clinical significance. The definitive diagnosis, unsuspected clinically in most cases, was made immunohistochemically.

The histologic features of gonadotropic adenomas are not pathognomonic, and the diagnosis cannot be made without immunohistochemical and electron microscopic examination. For reasons that are not fully understood, gonadotropic adenomas in males show stronger and more consistent immunoreactivity with antibodies to FSH and LH than gonadotropic adenomas in females. By electron microscopy, the male tumors do not show typical or diagnostic features. Most cells are elongated and appear polarized because of an eccentric location of the nucleus. The degree of cytoplasmic differentiation varies from one case to another. Some tumors have abundant organelles and granules, and some may be indistinguishable from so-called null cell adenomas (Horvath and Kovacs, 1986). Nevertheless, most tumors contain sparse, nondescript neuroendocrine granules averaging 200 nm in diameter. Gonadotropic adenomas in females are sparsely granulated and show a unique feature, the so-called honeycomb Golgi's apparatus (Kovacs and Horvath, 1987), which is composed of dilated cisterns filled with flocculent material of low density. It may be that this dilation of the Golgi's apparatus reflects an inherent defect of hormone synthesis, accounting for the lack of mature neurosecretory granules in the cytoplasm of these tumor cells and the slight elevation of gonadotropins in the plasma.

TESTICULAR TUMORS

Hormonally active testicular tumors may impair fertility. These include Leydig cell tumors, Sertoli cell tumors, and germ cell tumors that contain trophoblastic elements (Table 7-2).

Leydig cell tumors

Leydig cell tumors account for approximately 1% to 3% of all testicular tumors (Kim et al., 1985). The tumors may be hormonally active or inactive. The active tumors secrete androgens, estrogens, or a combination of various steroid hormones. Precocious sexual maturation is com-

Table 7-2. Hormonal activity of testicular tumors

Tumor	Hormone
Leydig cell tumor	Androgens
	Estrogens
Sertoli cell tumor	Estrogens
Seminoma	—
Seminoma + TRGC	hCG
Embryonal carcinoma (EC)	—
Choriocarcinoma (Ch)	hCG
Yolk sac carcinoma (YSC)	—
EC + YSC	—
EC + YSC + Ch	hCG
Teratoma (T)	—
EC + YSC + Ch + T	hCG

hCG, Human chorionic gonadotropin.
TRGC, Trophoblastic giant cells.

Table 7-3. Symptoms and hormonal changes in patients with malignant Leydig cell tumors

Symptom/finding	Frequency (%)
Testicular enlargement	81
Metastases	72
Elevation of urinary 17-ketosteroids	64
Elevation of serum and/or urinary androgens	54
Elevation of serum and/or urinary estrogen	50
Gynecomastia	19

Modified from Grem JL et al. Cancer 1986; 58:2116, with permission.

mon in prepubertal boys. Gynecomastia, loss of libido, and signs of hyperestrogenism are found in approximately 30% of adult males (Gabrilove et al., 1975).

Hormonal analysis reveals that testosterone is the major hormone produced by these tumor cells, but serum and urine elevations of estrogens, progesterone, ketosteroids, and prolactin have been documented (Bercovici et al., 1984). The features of hormonally active Leydig cell tumors were reviewed by Grem et al. (1986) and are presented in Table 7-3.

Leydig cell tumors affect spermatogenesis, but the effect depends on the age of the patient and the hormonal activity of the tumor. In prepubertal boys, spermatogenesis may be initiated precociously by local testosterone secretion. In adults spermatogenesis typically is suppressed. This is due in part both to the local and systemic excess of estrogen and androgens and to the compression of the normal parenchyma by the tumor. These changes are reversible.

Histologically, the tumors are composed of polygonal or spindle-shaped cells with well-developed granular or vacuolated or acidophilic or clear cytoplasm (Fig. 7-5). Tumor cells often contain lipofuscin. Reinke crystals are pathognomonic of Leydig cells in general but are found in only 25% to 40% of tumors (Kim et al., 1985). Ultrastruc-

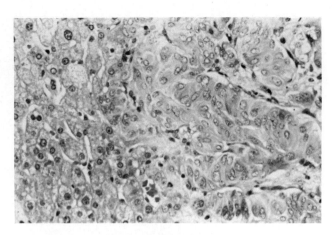

Fig. 7-5. Leydig cell tumor.

turally, the neoplastic cells resemble normal Leydig cells. These cells have prominent profiles of rough and smooth endoplasmic reticulum, mitochondria with tubulovesicular cristae, lipid droplets, and occasional Reinke crystals (Fig. 7-6).

All prebuteral Leydig cell tumors are benign, whereas 10% of tumors in adults are malignant. Histologic distinctions between benign and malignant Leydig cell tumors cannot be made with certainty unless there are metastases and obvious signs of invasion (Damjanov, 1989).

Sertoli cell tumors

Sertoli cell tumors account for less than 1% of all testicular tumors (Damjanov, 1989). Histologically, the tumors rarely occur in a pure form and usually are composed of a mixture of cells whose appearances vary (Fig. 7-7). Thus, there are spindle-shaped cells, cuboidal cells, tubule-forming cells, and cells that appear polygonal and cannot be distinguished with certainty from Leydig cells. Distinct histologic variants of Sertoli cell tumors have been described. They include tubular adenoma, lipid tubular adenoma, sex cord tumors with annular tubules, and large cell calcifying Sertoli cell tumors. All these variants can be hormonally active or inactive. Malignant Sertoli cell tumors are uncommon.

Hormonally active tumors usually secrete estrogens and cause gynecomastia and loss of libido. Hypospermatogenesis is common and is related to hyperestrinism and local compression of seminiferous tubules by the tumor mass.

Germ cell tumors

Germ cell tumors may affect spermatogenesis by compression of the normal seminiferous tubules; by extension of the tumor into the adjacent seminiferous tubules; or through the action of hormones released from various tumor cells (Fig. 7-8). Typically, these hormonal effects can be related to hypersecretion of human chorionic gonadotropin (hCG), which is elevated in the plasma of more than 80% of patients with nonseminomatous germ cell tumors

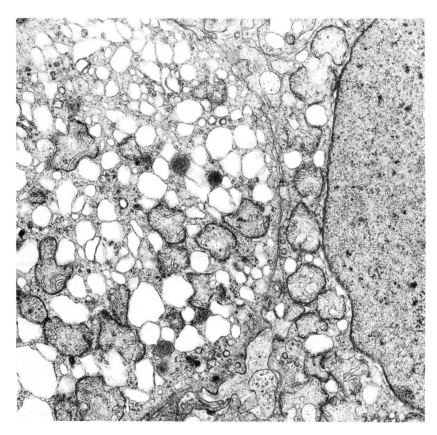

Fig. 7-6. Electron microscopy of Leydig cell tumor shows vesicular endoplasmic reticulum and mitochondria with tubulovesicular cristae.

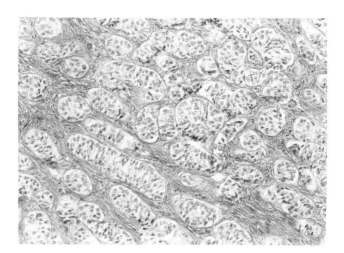

Fig. 7-7. Sertoli cell tumor.

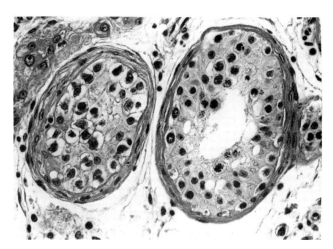

Fig. 7-8. Seminiferous tubules adjacent to a seminoma. One tubule contains tumor cell and the other shows spermatogenic maturation arrest.

and 30% to 50% of patients with seminomas (Paus et al., 1988). This placental glycoprotein hormone is synthesized by the syncytiotrophoblastic cells within the tumor. Secondary elevation of plasma levels of sex steroids and thyroid hormones is probably the cause of the hypospermatogenesis that is commonly found in these patients.

Reproductive dysfunction that is caused by testicular tumors may be reversible, but in many cases hypospermatogenesis persists even after the tumor is removed. In such cases both the tumor and the spermatogenic abnormality probably are related causally to a common preexisting lesion of germ cells (Giwercman et al., 1989).

Table 7-4. Relative ratios of benign and malignant adrenal cortical tumors causing hormonal syndromes in adults

Syndrome	Adenoma	Carcinoma
Hyperaldosteronism	+++(80%)	+
Hypercortisolism	+ (10%)	+++
Virilization	+/−	+++
Feminization	−	++++

Based on data in Gruhn and Gould (1990).

ADRENAL TUMORS

Adrenal cortical adenomas and carcinomas may present as hormonally active or inactive lesions (Gruhn and Gould, 1990). Typical syndromes caused by these tumors (i.e., hyperaldosteronism, hypercortisolism, virilization, and feminization) all interfere with the hormonal functions of the testes and ovaries and may cause infertility (Table 7-4). Adenomas secrete cortisol or aldosterone, extremely rarely secrete androgens, and almost never secrete estrogens. Approximately 50% of all carcinomas are hormonally active. Most tumors in adults that are associated with virilization are carcinomas, and essentially all tumors associated with feminization have been malignant (Page et al., 1986).

Adrenal cortical tumors are composed of polygonal cells that resemble normal adrenal cortical cells (Fig. 7-9). The distinction between benign and malignant tumors cannot be made with confidence unless the tumor is obviously malignant and shows marked anaplasia, invasive growth, and metastases. There are no histologic or electron microscopic criteria to predict whether a tumor is hormonally active or inactive.

OVARIAN TUMORS

Hormonally active neoplasms of the ovary include sex steroid–secreting sex-cord stromal tumors and hCG-secreting germ cell tumors (Table 7-5).

Sex-cord stromal tumors

Granulosa cell tumors are the most common sex-cord stromal tumors of the ovary (Czernobilsky and Czernobilsky, 1991). Most of these tumors probably produce small quantities of estrogen. The juvenile granulosa cell tumors cause clinically apparent hyperestrinism associated with isosexual precocity or menstrual irregularities (Biscotti and Hart, 1989). In general, cystic tumors produce more hormones than solid ones.

Several histologic forms of granulosa cell tumor patterns have been described that include follicular, trabecular, tubular, and solid variants (Fig. 7-10). These patterns do not correlate with hormonal activity.

Symptoms of hyperestrinism vary, depending on the age of the patient. In premenarchal girls the tumors may

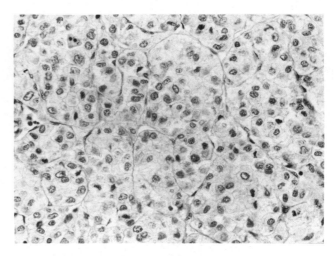

Fig. 7-9. Adrenal cortical adenoma.

Table 7-5. Hormonally active ovarian tumors

Tumor type	Hormones		
	Estrogen	Androgen	hCG
Sex-cord stromal tumors			
Granulosa cell	+	−	−
Juvenile	++	−	−
Cystic	++	−	−
Theca cell	+++	+	−
Fibroma	−	−	−
Sertoli-Leydig cell	+/−	+++	−
Lipid cell	+	++	−
Sclerosing stromal cell	+/−	−	−
Germ cell tumors			
Dysgerminoma	−	−	+/−
Embryonal carcinoma	−	−	+/−
Yolk sac carcinoma	−	−	−
Mixed germ cell tumor	−	−	+++
Choriocarcinoma	−	−	+++
Teratoma	−	−	−

Hormonal activity of tumors is indicated on a scale from − (negative) to +++ (strongly positive).

induce precocious puberty; in women of reproductive age the tumors cause changes in the menstrual cycle and dysfunctional bleeding that varies from metrorrhagia to oligomenorrhea and even amenorrhea. Infertility may be one of the complications. The uterus usually shows signs of mild cystic hyperplasia and only rarely more pronounced hyperplasia or carcinoma.

Thecomas and *fibromas* of the ovary form a group that includes hormonally active and inactive spindle cell neoplasms of the ovarian stroma (Russell and Bannatyne, 1989). Thecomas are composed of lipid-rich, luteinized cells (Fig. 7-11) and usually are hormonally active. Approximately 50% of thecomas produce estrogens and 10% are androgenic (Zhang et al., 1982). Hormonal activity of

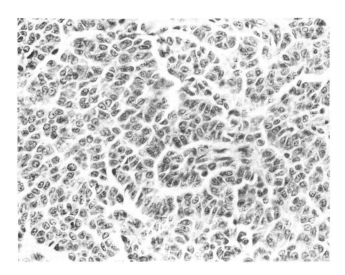

Fig. 7-10. Granulosa cell tumor.

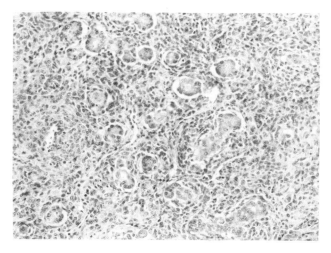

Fig. 7-12. Sertoli-Leydig cell tumor.

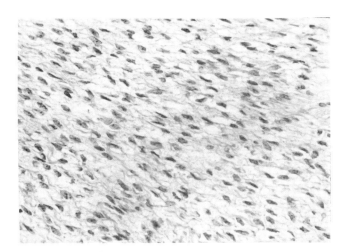

Fig. 7-11. Theca cell tumor.

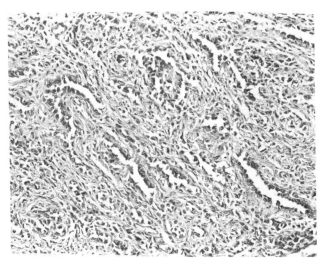

Fig. 7-13. Sertoli-Leydig cell tumor with retiform pattern.

thecomas causes menstrual disturbances during the reproductive years similar to those caused by granulosa cell tumors. However, since thecomas occur predominantly in women over 40 years of age, infertility rarely is a presenting symptom. Fibromas are usually hormonally inactive.

Sclerosing stromal cell tumor of the ovary is a benign ovarian tumor that occasionally produces hormonal symptoms (Damjanov, 1975). These tumors occur in young women and may cause menstrual abnormalities and infertility.

Sertoli-Leydig cell tumors (androblastoma or arrhenoblastoma) are the most common virilizing tumors of the ovary (Young and Scully, 1985). These tumors are rare and account for 1% of all stromal ovarian tumors (Russell and Bannatyne, 1989). However, since their incidence peaks around 25 years of age, they may cause infertility more often than some other more common tumors. Sertoli-Leydig cell tumors show a spectrum of histologic patterns that include, on the one hand, well-differentiated, biphasic

tumors composed of Sertoli cells arranged into tubules and Leydig cells in the stromal component (Fig. 7-12) and, on the other hand, poorly differentiated sarcomatoid tumors. Heterologous elements are found in more than 20% of tumors (Russell and Bannatyne, 1989). Well-differentiated tumors are benign and the poorly differentiated are usually malignant; others show varying degrees of malignancy. There is almost no correlation between the histologic pattern of Sertoli-Leydig cell tumors and their hormonal activity. However, tumors with predominantly retiform appearance (Fig. 7-13) show less pronounced androgenic activity (Young and Scully, 1982).

Lipid cell tumors are a heterogeneous group that includes several entities such as stromal luteomas, hilus cell tumors, Leydig cell tumors, and adrenocortical-type nodules (Czernobilsky and Czernobilsky, 1991). These tumors may cause symptoms of hyperestrinism or virilization and thus interfere with fertility (Shenker et al., 1989).

Germ cell tumors of the ovary

Germ cell tumors of the ovary are hormonally active only if they contain a significant number of trophoblastic cells that produce hCG. Less than 10% of dysgerminomas contain syncytiotrophoblastic cells (Zaloudek et al., 1981). Pure embryonal carcinomas do not secrete hCG. However, the primitive stem cells of these tumors often differentiate into trophoblastic cells or yolk sac cells, and therefore, the levels of hCG and alpha-fetoprotein often appear raised in the plasma. Mixed germ cell tumors almost invariably contain trophoblastic cells that produce hCG. Benign and immature teratomas are, on the other hand, hormonally inactive. The highest levels of plasma hCG are found in patients with choriocarcinomas.

POLYCYSTIC OVARY SYNDROME

The syndrome of polycystic bilateral ovarian enlargement, amenorrhea, hirsutism, infertility, and obesity was described by Stein and Leventhal (1935). Subsequent studies have shown that the Stein-Leventhal syndrome is not a single entity and that the same pathologic and clinical findings can result from several endocrine disturbances. Interestingly, not all the patients described in the original report had every feature of the syndrome. Polycystic ovaries were considered to be invariably present until ultrasonographic studies became available and showed that a significant number of women with all the clinical signs of the syndrome did not have polycystic ovaries (Ardaens et al., 1991). Polycystic ovaries could thus be either a symptom or the common denominator of several interrelated disorders. The term *polycystic ovary syndrome* (POS) is used for the clinical syndrome of persistent anovulation found in these patients. Until the highly controversial pathogenesis of this syndrome is better understood, the definition will remain elusive (Editorial, *Lancet,* 1990).

Prevalence and pathogenesis

POS is considered a common disorder, but there are no generally acceptable data on its prevalence (Adams et al., 1986). This is in part due to a lack of minimal criteria for the diagnosis; lack of diagnostic endocrine findings; and lack of correlation between the clinical findings and the ovarian pathology.

The reported prevalence of POS depends on the diagnostic approach used. On laparotomy of unselected gynecologic patients, polycystic ovaries are found in 1.4% of all women and 0.6% to 4.3% of infertile women (Goldzieher and Elkind-Hirsch, 1988). Many women with polycystic ovaries are asymptomatic (Polson et al., 1988), and only 50% of women with POS diagnosed by ultrasonography have elevated serum testosterone and/or LH (Conway et al., 1989). Hirsutism, which is one of the more common symptoms, affects approximately 10% of American women (Coney, 1984), and although some of these women could have POS, most of them seem to have no

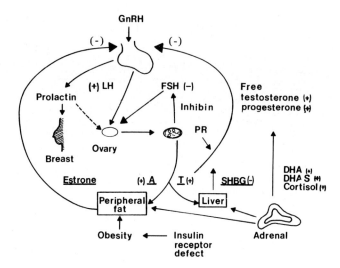

Fig. 7-14. Pathogenesis of the polycystic ovary syndrome illustrating the multifactorial nature of the syndrome and various aspects of dysregulation of the hypothalamo-pituitary-ovarian-adrenal axis. GnRH, Gonadotropin releasing hormone; LH, Luteotropic hormone; FSH, Follicle stimulating hormone; PR, Progesterone; A, Androgens; DHA, Dehydroepiandrosterone; DHAS, Dehydroepiandrosterone sulfate; SHBG, Sex hormone binding globulin.

menstrual disorders or ovarian pathology (Ehrmann and Rosenfield, 1990). There obviously are several clinical forms, *formes frustres,* and unusual variants; some appear to be familial (Lunde et al., 1989).

The pathogenesis of POS is controversial and has been reviewed extensively (Goldzieher and Elkind-Hirsch, 1988; Barbieri, 1991; Insler and Lunenfeld, 1991). There is a consensus that POS is a multifactorial disease complex and that the symptoms can evolve because of the dysfunctions of the regulatory and secretory parts of the hypothalamic-pituitary-gonadal-adrenal axis as well as the peripheral tissues. These disturbances result in anovulation in which a "steady state of gonadotropin and sex steroid secretion" (Speroff et al., 1989) replaces the normal stimulation-feedback inhibition cycles that characterize the interplay between the hypothalamus and pituitary during the reproductive years (Fig. 7-14). The hormonal findings reflect the disappearance of the normal pulsatile release of gonadotropins from the hypothalamus; increased secretion of sex steroids from the ovary; conversion of androgens to estrone in the peripheral fat tissue; increased adrenal steroid production; and resistance of peripheral tissues to insulin or insulin like growth factors (Insler and Lunenfeld, 1991).

The vicious cycle of hormonal dysregulation could begin in any of the organs involved, and indeed several well-defined endocrine diseases such as adrenal hyperfunction, adrenal tumors, thyroid dysfunction, hyperprolactinemia, and ovarian tumors should be excluded clinically before a diagnosis of POS is made (Table 7-6). Numerous theories

Table 7-6. Differential diagnosis of polycystic ovary syndrome

---

Adrenal diseases
Tumors
Hyperplasia
    21-hydroxylase deficiency
    11β-Hydroxylase deficiency
    3β-Hydroxysteroid deficiency

Hypothalamic-pituitary diseases
Tumors
    Prolactinoma
    Corticotropic adenoma
    Gonadotropic adenoma
Functional disorders

Ovarian diseases
Tumors
    Sex-cord tumors (androgenic)
    Nonfunctioning tumors associated with stromal luteinization
Stromal hyperthecosis

Insulin resistance syndromes
    HAIR-AN syndrome

---

have been proposed to explain the pathogenesis of POS, as follows:

Mechanical barrier. It was thought originally that ovarian cysts develop because of an inherent anatomic barrier to ovulation. According to this view, a sclerotic ovarian capsule hinders the ovulatory release of ova, leading to accumulation of unruptured follicles in the ovarian cortex. This theory was the rationale for ovarian wedge resection, which was the favored treatment for many years; it was abandoned because of frequent postoperative scarring and adhesions. In most subsequent cases it became apparent that most women have no ovarian disease. Anovulation is hormonally determined, and there is no inherent primary ovarian barrier to ovulation. However, there seems to be a small group of patients with POS in whom ovulation cannot be induced hormonally and for whom a wedge resection of the ovary may be indicated (Lappohn and Bogchelman, 1989). This so-called clomiphene-resistant POS may be caused by a primary ovarian disease.

Mendelian inheritance. Familial cases of POS have been reported (Givens, 1988). However, the mode of inheritance varies among kindreds, and in most patients there is no evidence of a genetic disease.

Hypothalamic disturbances. Most patients show aberrations in the pulsatile release of LH and FSH indicative of hypothalamic dysfunction. It is generally agreed that these functional disturbances are not based on primary pathologic changes of the hypothalamus and are in most instances a consequence of some other abnormalities such as inadequate feedback inhibition (Insler and Lunenfeld,

1991). Primary dysfunction of the hypothalamus or even higher central nervous system centers cannot be excluded in some cases.

Increased production of steroid hormones in the ovary. Anovulatory ovaries produce fewer cyclic estrogens (estradiol) and more androgens (androstenedione and testosterone) than normal cyclic ovaries. Androstenedione undergoes aromatization to estrone in peripheral fat tissue (see Fig. 7-14). Testosterone down-regulates the production of sex hormone–binding globulin (SHBG) in the liver. Low SHBG results in more free estradiol in the circulation. Estrone and free estradiol act on the hypothalamus inhibiting the release of FSH and stimulating the release of LH from the pituitary. LH further stimulates the ovarian stroma and contributes even more to androgen excess and the inhibition of ovulation. This hypothesis explains many of the hormonal findings in most patients with POS (Speroff et al., 1989). However, some additional endocrine disturbances such as insulin resistance and hypersecretion of adrenal androgens cannot be fully explained with this theory.

Increased adrenal function. Abnormal adrenarche or persistent overproduction of androgens from the adrenal cortex could result in androgen excess (Insler and Lunenfeld, 1991). Aromatization of androgens into estrone in the peripheral fat tissue of obese patients with POS results in an excess of acyclic estrogens that inhibit FSH and facilitate the release of LH, which in turn stimulates ovarian androgen production. This hypothesis could explain POS in some women, but it is doubtful that adrenal dysfunction is the primary cause of most POS.

Excessive fat tissue mass. Anovulatory cycles in obese women may be related to an excess of estrone, which is formed in peripheral fat tissue from androstenedione. Estrone inhibits the release of FSH and stimulates the release of LH, which stimulates androgen production. This could lead to clinical symptoms indistinguishable from those of POS. However, since morbidly obese women may have normal menstrual cycles, one would have to postulate some other dysfunction to explain the symptoms of POS in obese women with anovulation. A recent discovery of disturbances in insulin metabolism, which are common in obese women with POS, points to a possible pathogenetic role of the receptor for insulin and insulinlike growth factors and could provide new links between obesity and POS (Barbieri, 1991).

Clinical findings

Symptoms of POS are highly variable. Goldzieher and Green (1962) reviewed more than a thousand previously published cases and calculated these percentages for various symptoms: obesity, 41%; hirsutism, 69%; virilization, 21%; amenorrhea, 51%; and infertility, 74%. This review also disclosed that 12% to 40% of these women have a biphasic basal body temperature. A corpus luteum was reported at laparotomy in 0% to 71% of cases. Thus even amenorrhea and anovulation are not constant features of POS.

On ultrasonography the cross-sectional area of the polycystic ovary is increased more than 10 cm^2; the ratio of uterine width to ovarian length is less than 1; the ovaries have an increased roundness index of more than 0.7; more than 5 follicles are present; and the stroma is hyperechogenic (Ardaens et al., 1991).

Hormonal findings are variable (Franks, 1989). Typically, patients have elevated serum levels of androgens, estrone to estradiol ratios, and high LH to FSH ratios (Barnes and Rosenfield, 1989). At least 30% of affected women have hyperprolactinemia. Dynamic testing, such as progesterone treatment and withdrawal or clomiphene treatment, induces uterine bleeding and ovulation in most women.

Pathologic findings

Hughesdon (1982) has compared the ovaries of POS with those of normal, matched controls and concluded that the ovaries of POS show:

1. Increased size, as evidenced by a twofold increase in the cross-sectional surface area
2. Normal numbers of primordial follicles
3. Double the number of ripening and subsequent atretic follicles
4. Increased thickness of the tunica by 50%
5. A threefold increase in cortical stromal thickness
6. A fivefold increase in deep cortical and medullary stroma
7. Ovarian hilus cell nests four times as frequently as in normals

On gross examination the ovaries appear symmetrically enlarged and have a smooth, white, avascular, and shiny surface (Goldzieher and Green, 1962). The tunica albuginea is thickened, measuring 0.1 to 0.9 mm in width. The cortex is widened because of numerous follicles and the cortical stromal hyperplasia (Fig. 7-15). The subtunical cortex contains prominent fibrous bands that are positioned in parallel with the ovarian surface and extend into the deeper parts of the cortex and even into the medulla. The hypercellularity of the cortical stroma is in part a consequence of cortical cell hyperplasia, the cells of which are in part derived from the thecal layers of the involuting follicles. Some of the cortical cells are luteinized, but most appear nondescript and are surrounded by variable amounts of extracellular matrix.

Ovaries of POS contain a normal number of primordial follicles, an increased number of ripening and atretic follicles, and fewer mature follicles than normal ovaries. The cystic antral follicles, measuring 2 to 10 mm in diameter, usually are prominent.

Most ovaries of POS contain 20 to 100 cystic follicles. Typically, these follicles show marked hyperplasia of the

Polycystic ovary

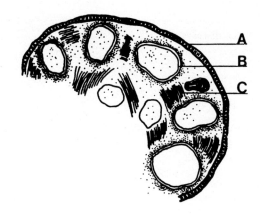

Fig. 7-15. Polycystic ovary. This diagram shows thickening of the tunica albuginea (*A*) and numerous cystic follicles which are all of approximately same size (*B*). There is also cortical stromal hyperplasia (*C*).

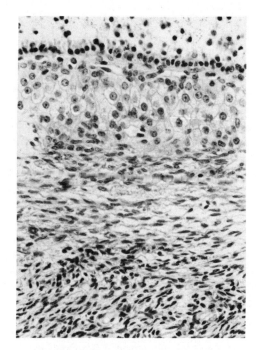

Fig. 7-16. Hyperplasia of the theca interna in the polycystic ovary.

theca interna (Fig. 7-16). Other features commonly encountered in these follicles are premature luteinization of the granulosa cells and Call-Exner bodies (Hughesdon, 1982). All these histologic findings suggest impaired maturation of follicles, but none of them is diagnostic of POS. Lappohn and Bogchelman (1989) have used the following criteria to diagnose polycystic ovaries morphologically:

1. Capsular thickening is considered to be present if the tunica albuginea exceeds 0.4 mm on three measurements.

2. Polycystic change is diagnosed if at least half of the subcapsular area consists of antral follicles and cysts. Cysts measuring 4 to 8 mm were considered small and those over 8 mm large. Cavities lined by granulosa cells that did not show signs of pyknosis were considered to be growing follicles and were not counted.
3. Activation of theca cells is determined histochemically with the 3-β-hydroxysteroid-dehydrogenase stain and is estimated to be weak, moderately strong, or strong.
4. Stromal hyperplasia is diagnosed if the stroma contains polygonal cells with well-developed pale cytoplasm and enlarged and vesicular nuclei.
5. Hyperthecosis refers to stromal cells that resemble theca lutein cells that are not connected to a corpus luteum or luteinized theca interna cells. These cells must be at least weakly positive for 3-β-Hydroxysteroid-dehydrogenase.

These pathologic changes are typically bilateral. However, symptoms of POS may occur in women with a solitary polycystic ovary or with ovaries that do not show polycystic changes. Smith et al. (1965) found normal ovaries in 40% of 301 patients with POS as well as no capsular thickening in almost half of those women who had enlarged ovaries. These reports point to the heterogeneity of the syndrome and the fact that morphologic ovarian changes are just one of the variable findings in POS in most patients and are not the primary cause of anovulation.

In response to unopposed estrogen stimulation, the endometrium of patients with POS undergoes hyperplasia and is at an increased risk for developing carcinoma (Coulam et al., 1983). Chronic hyperestrinism due to chronic anovulation carries an increased risk of 3.1 of the development of carcinoma, but the carcinomas that develop apparently are of low malignant potential and are amenable to treatment (Coulam et al., 1983).

OVARIAN STROMAL HYPERTHECOSIS

Stromal hyperthecosis is a cause of ovarian hyperestrinism that clinically may be indistinguishable from typical POS. Thus, stromal hyperthecosis may be considered to be either a form of POS without follicular cysts or a distinct clinicopathologic entity (Chang and deZiegler, 1987; Young and Scully, 1991). Since the symptoms of stromal hyperthecosis typically occur in older, postmenopausal women, it is possible that stromal hyperthecosis is a "burnt-out" form of POS. The clinical presentation includes signs of virilization, obesity, hypertension, abnormal glucose tolerance, and elevated serum testosterone levels (Young and Scully, 1991). In younger women the disease usually is less severe, and it is clinically indistinguishable from the typical POS. Occasionally, stromal hyperthecosis is associated with the HAIR-AN syndrome, which comprises hyperandrogenism, insulin resistance,

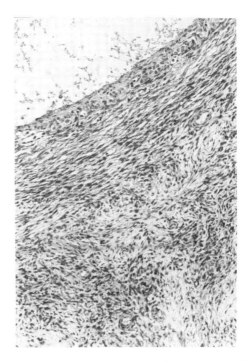

Fig. 7-17. Ovarian stromal hyperthecosis with a cortical cyst.

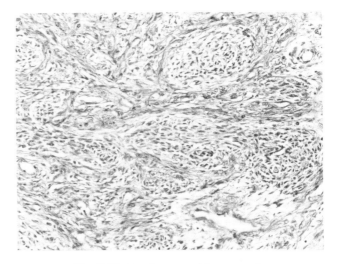

Fig. 7-18. Ovarian stromal hypertecosis.

with diabetes mellitus, and acanthosis nigricans, (Nagamani et al., 1985; Barbieri et al., 1988).

The ovaries are symmetrically enlarged and on cross section appear grayish yellow and compact with occasional subcortical cysts (Fig. 7-17). The cysts are more common in premenopausal women (Young and Scully, 1991). Histologically, the stroma appears hyperplastic and densely cellular with scattered groups of luteinized cells (Fig. 7-18). The aggregates of luteinized cells, which are filled with lipid, may occasionally form grossly visible nodules described as nodular hyperthecosis (Leedman et al., 1989) or solitary stromal luteomas (Hayes and Scully, 1987).

MASSIVE OVARIAN EDEMA AND FIBROMATOSIS

Massive edema and fibromatosis of the ovary are rare but probably interrelated disorders that affect women of reproductive age. The pathogenesis and etiology of these conditions are unknown. Oligomenorrhea or amenorrhea was reported in one fourth of all affected women (Young and Scully, 1984). Although hyperandrogenism occurs in a minority of cases and most cases show only unilateral involvement, infertility may be one of the symptoms. The ovaries are enlarged and may be either soft or firm. As in POS, the outer cortex is thickened. In massive edema of the ovary the cortex is edematous and sparsely cellular, whereas in fibromatosis the cortex appears fibrotic and hyalinized. Within this background are preserved follicles, some of which are cystically dilated and filled with fluid. The stromal cells show variable degrees of luteinization.

ENDOMETRIOSIS

Endometriosis is characterized by the appearance of normal endometrial tissue outside the uterus. Such tissue responds to hormones and undergoes cyclic changes during the menstrual cycle (Buttram, 1988). Adenomyosis, which was called endometriosis interna, does not respond to progesterone and does not undergo cyclic changes; thus it is not included under this heading.

Prevalence and pathogenesis

Endometriosis is very common among women of reproductive age. Mahmood and Templeton (1991) reviewed the data collected in several medical centers on women who had laparoscopy for infertility, abdominal pain, tubal ligation, or tubal reanastomosis and found a reported incidence of endometriosis broadly estimated from 1% to 43%. On average, endometriosis was found more frequently among women investigated for infertility (21%) than among those undergoing sterilization (6%). In all groups, prolonged use of oral contraceptives was associated with a decreased incidence of endometriosis, suggesting that a prolonged period of regular menstruation uninterrupted by hormonal contraception, or pregnancies for that matter, predisposes to endometriosis. The prevalence of endometriosis seems to increase after a woman's last childbirth, which is consistent with the hypothesis that prolonged periods without suppression of menstruation are a risk factor for endometriosis (Moen, 1991).

Several theories have been proposed to explain endometriosis and although none of these has been generally accepted, those of retrograde menstruation and metaplasia of coelomic epithelium have the most proponents (Mahmood and Templeton, 1990).

Retrograde transport of endometrial tissue. Reflux of menstrual endometrium into the fallopian tubes and the implantation of this tissue onto the peritoneum seems to be a likely mechanism of endometriosis. This theory is supported by clinical and epidemiologic findings indicating that endometriosis occurs more often in menstruating women than in those with suppressed menstruation. These data were summarized by Mahmood and Templeton (1991) as follows:

1. Prolonged periods of menstruation uninterrupted by pregnancy favor endometriosis.
2. Endometriosis is more common in women with early menarche.
3. Endometriosis is more common in women whose first gestation occurred at an early age.
4. Prolonged use of oral contraceptives is inversely proportional to the incidence of endometriosis. Use of an intrauterine device or barrier methods for contraception has no effect on the occurrence of endometriosis.
5. Tubal sterilization with electrocautery does not decrease the incidence of endometriosis, presumably because many women develop fistulas that allow the back-flow of menstrual blood and endometrial tissue into the peritoneal cavity.
6. Endometrial cells can be forced into the peritoneal cavity by carbon dioxide hysteroscopy and chromotubation, which confirms that retrograde passage of endometrial cells can occur (Ranta et al., 1990).

Retrograde flow of menstrual blood cannot be taken as an explanation for the occurrence of endometriosis in retroperitoneal sites, the umbilicus, the abdominal wall, or distant sites such as internal organs that have no contact with the peritoneal lining. Retrograde flow of menstrual blood through blood vessels and the lymphatics has been proposed for such cases (reviewed by Buttram, 1988; Mahmood and Templeton, 1990).

Metaplasia of the peritoneal surface into endometrial lining. This hypothesis has been postulated as a possible mechanism of endometriosis. It is based on the fact that the peritoneum and the lining of the müllerian ducts, which give rise to endometrium, both originate from the embryonic coelomic epithelium. Although no direct clinical observations support this theory, it is feasible that endometriomas like the endometrioid carcinomas of the ovary are of coelomic origin. Since the mesovarium is similar or identical to the rest of the peritoneal epithelium, one could assume that endometrial metaplasia could occur anywhere in the abdominal cavity. However, coelomic metaplasia cannot explain the occurrence of endometriosis in retroperitoneal organs, the umbilicus, lymph nodes, or extraabdominal sites.

Clinical findings

Symptoms of endometriosis are consistent only in their inconsistencies (Buttram, 1988). They include vague pains, dysmenorrhea, dyspareunia, and various pelvic or abdominal symptoms that vary from one patient to another. Infertility occurs often, but the exact data on the prevalence of infertility in patients with endometriosis are not available (Mahmood and Templeton, 1990). Infertile women have endometriosis ten times more often than fertile women (Guzick, 1989). Buttram (1988) considers endometriosis to be the most common cause of infertility in women over 25 and suspects that two thirds of all women with endometriosis suffer from infertility.

The effects of endometriosis on fertility remain poorly understood, and the strongest arguments for a causal relationship reportedly include a high rate of conception after the treatment of endometriosis. Other possible mechanisms contributing to infertility have been discussed by Young and Scully (1991) and include the following:

1. Mechanical hindrance to ovulation or conception
2. Down-regulation of receptors for LH
3. Luteinized, unruptured follicle syndrome
4. Abnormalities in progesterone synthesis from the corpora lutea
5. Peritoneal fluid abnormalities that have adverse effects on tubal fimbriae
6. Immune factors such as antibodies directed against endometrium
7. Peritoneal macrophages and other cytokine-secreting cells

There is no evidence that any of these hypotheses plays a crucial role in or is directly responsible for the infertility of women with endometriosis.

Pathologic findings

On gross examination, endometriosis may present may present in several forms (Clement, 1990). Laparoscopists use several descriptive terms for various forms of endometriosis (Buttram, 1988):

Implant —A small focus of endometriosis composed of glands and stroma.
Plaques —Groups of implants arranged in circular configurations with irregularly branching extensions.
Nodules —Palpable masses composed of large aggregates of endometrial tissue.
Endometrioma —Nodular lesions on the ovary.
Adhesions —Fibrous bands between organs or tissues. Adhesions are common and are considered to be part of the disease process.

On the basis of laparoscopic findings, the extent of endometriosis is graded as mild, moderate, or severe (Acosta et al., 1973) or according to the American Fertility Society classification of endometriosis (Fig. 7-19).

Assuming that most cases of endometriosis originate from retrograde menstruation, Haney (1987) proposed that the anatomic distribution of foci of endometriosis reflects four pathogenetic principles, which include:

1. The site of entry
2. The effects of gravity

3. The mobility of the transplantation site
4. Local factors that determine the survival of the graft

Endometriosis is thus common in the uterosacral ligaments adjacent to the ostia of the fallopian tubes and in the most dependent regions of the peritoneal cavity. Immobile organs such as the fixed portion of the sigmoid colon and the round ligaments are more often involved than the mobile intestines. The ovarian surface provides an unusually fertile ground for the growth of endometrial tissue (Fig. 7-20, *A*), providing evidence that the local factors may facilitate growth and thus determine the distribution of endometriosis. The most common sites of endometriosis are listed in Table 7-7 (on p. 161).

Foci of endometriosis are composed histologically of endometrial glands and stroma (Fig. 7-20). The glands and the stroma respond to hormonal stimulation and correspond to proliferative or secretory phase endometrium. Since the endometrium is shed during menstrual bleeding, there is accumulation of cellular debris and blood in the foci. This evokes an influx of macrophages that phagocytose the debris and transform the foci into lipid-laden "pseudoxanthoma" cells and/or hemosiderin-laden cells. Stromal fibrosis is common in older lesions. Fibrous adhesions are common especially between endometriotic lesions located on peritoneal surfaces that are in contact with each other. These include the posterior surface of the uterus and the sigmoid colon, the caudal surface of the ovary and the posterior ligament, or the visceral peritoneum of the bladder and the anterior uterovesical fold (Haney, 1987).

Surface implants, especially those on the ovary, resemble normal endometrium to the greatest extent. In contrast, superficial implants in other sites and those that are surrounded by adhesions tend to be fibrotic and show less obvious cyclic changes. The large "chocolate cysts" (endometriomas of the ovary) usually are filled with decomposed blood and cellular debris and lined by nondescript low cuboidal epithelium surrounded by fibrous tissue. Because of pressure atrophy, large cysts are denuded focally of epithelium. The fibrous capsule is infiltrated with macrophages and chronic inflammatory cells and usually shows few if any histologic features reminiscent of endometrial stroma. The glands and stromal cells within the foci of endometriosis respond to hormonal stimuli and may undergo hyperplasia or atrophy (Clement, 1990). Atrophy is common in postmenopausal women. Atrophy and even involution of glandular and stromal elements of endometriosis can be induced therapeutically by suppressing ovulation with oral contraceptives or Gn-RH antagonists.

LUTEAL PHASE DEFICIENCY

Luteal phase deficiency is a multifactorial syndrome characterized by inadequate maturation of the secretory endometrium (Daly, 1983). It may be caused by a defect in progesterone release from the corpus luteum or a subopti-

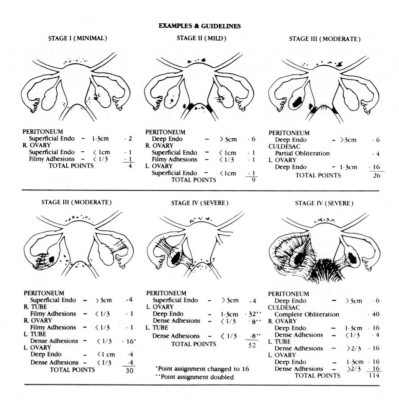

Fig. 7-19. American Fertility Society classification of endometriosis. Determination of the stage or degree of endometrial involvement is based on a weighted point system. Distribution of points has been arbitrarily determined and may require further revision or refinement as knowledge of the disease increases.

To ensure complete evaluation, inspection of the pelvis in a clockwise or counterclockwise fashion is encouraged. Number, size and location of endometrial implants, plaques, endometriomas and/or adhesions are noted. For example, five separate 0.5 cm superficial implants on the peritoneum (2.5 cm total) would be assigned 2 points. (The surface of the uterus should be considered peritoneum.) The severity of the endometriosis or adhesions should be assigned the highest score only for peritoneum, ovary, tube or cul de sac. For example, a 4 cm superficial and a 2 cm deep implant of the peritoneum should be given a score of 6 (not 8). A 4 cm deep endometrioma of the ovary associated with more than 3 cm of superficial disease should be scored 20 (not 24).

In those patients with only one adenexa, points applied to disease of the remaining tube and ovary should be multiplied by two. **Points assigned may be circled and totaled. Aggregation of points indicates stage of disease (minimal, mild, moderate, or severe).

The presence of endometriosis of the bowel, urinary tract, fallopian tube, vagina, cervix, skin etc., should be documented under "additional endometriosis." Other pathology such as tubal occlusion, leiomyomata, uterine anomaly, etc., should be documented under "associated pathology." All pathology should be depicted as specifically as possible on the sketch of pelvic organs, and means of observation (laparoscopy or laparotomy) should be noted. (Reproduced with permission of the publisher, The American Fertility Society.)

mal response of the endometrium to progesterone. Other synonymous terms include luteal phase inadequacy, luteal phase insufficiency, luteal phase defect, and inadequate corpus luteum (Wentz, 1988; McNeely and Soules, 1988).

Prevalence and pathogenesis

Luteal phase deficiency is the cause of infertility in about 5% of infertile couples (Wentz, 1988). The exact data on the prevalence of this condition are not available. However, since not all corpora lutea are equally capable of hormone production, one could assume that temporary luteal phase defects limited to a single cycle probably occur more often than suspected. Such temporary or sporadic defects are of no clinical significance. When a fully com-

petent corpus luteum develops (and that could occur without treatment), the defect is corrected and a normal pregnancy can be established.

Luteal phase deficiency may be associated with low serum progesterone, reflecting an inherent defect of the corpus luteum or inadequate endometrial response with normal serum progesterone. There are many possible causes of the luteal phase deficiency; they are listed in part in Table 7-8.

Clinical findings and diagnosis

Patients suffering from luteal phase deficiency typically are infertile or have recurrent miscarriages (Wentz, 1988). The diagnosis is based on hormonal studies and endome-

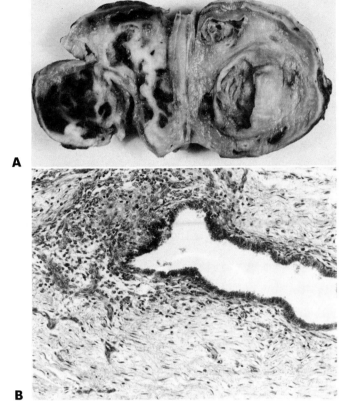

Fig. 7-20. A, Endometrioma of the ovary. **B,** Histologically, endometriosis is composed of endometrial glands and stroma.

Table 7-7. Most Common Sites of Endometriosis Observed at Laparoscopy

Anatomic site	Mean frequency (%)	Range (%)
Ovaries	60	32–80
Uterus	34	5–62
Fallopian tubes	6	2–15
Posterior cul-de-sac	25	6–44

Modified from the data collected from the literature by Haney, 1987.

Table 7-8. Etiology and pathogenesis of the luteal phase deficiency

Insufficient progesterone secretion (low serum progesterone)
1. Hypothalamic-pituitary dysfunction
    FSH release
    LH release
    Prolactin hypersecretion
2. Ovarian defect
    Reduced number of follicles
    Accelerated luteolysis
    Luteinized unruptured follicle syndrome
3. Systemic diseases
    Low body weight (e.g., banazol clomiphene)
4. Drugs
5. Status post abortion or pregnancy
6. Idiopathic

Inadequate response of the endometrium (normal serum progesterone)
1. Endometritis
2. Endometrial adhesions
3. Tumors of the uterus
4. Idiopathic

Modified from Clement, 1991.

trial biopsy (Algorithm 7-1). Because of the pulsatile secretion of progesterone, daily measurements are needed; even then, results may be misleading (McNeely and Soules, 1988). Endometrial biopsy usually provides a more definitive answer; however, even these results have serious shortcomings (reviewed by Clement, 1991).

The endometrial biopsy typically is performed within 3 days of the expected menstrual bleeding. Endometrial glands and stroma are evaluated according to the standard criteria for dating of the endometrium to determine whether both components show synchronous maturation and whether the morphologic features correspond to the day of the menstrual cycle on which the biopsy was taken. Thus, on the basis of the histologic examination, one can determine whether the endometrium is in phase or out of phase or is exhibiting glandular stromal asynchrony. Luteal phase deficiency is diagnosed if the endometrium is at least 3 days out of phase or if it shows glandular stromal asynchrony in two menstrual cycles (Fig. 7-21). Endometria that show asynchrony in the maturation of glands and stroma cannot be dated (Clement, 1991). According to Witten and Martin (1985), women who show irregular maturation and glandular stromal asynchrony respond better to clomiphene treatment, whereas progesterone is the preferred treatment for women whose endometria appear to be out of date (Algorithm 7-2).

If the patient's clinical presentation suggests luteal phase deficiency and the first biopsy does not confirm the diagnosis, another biopsy usually is performed. One third of women with suspected luteal phase deficiency and normal findings on the initial biopsy have abnormalities on the second biopsy (Wentz, 1980). If the first biopsy shows out of phase endometrium and the second biopsy is normal, some authorities advocate a third biopsy (Balasch et al., 1985).

SALPINGITIS ISTHMICA NODOSA

Salpingitis isthmica nodosa is marked by a diverticular branching of the tubular lumen and an extension of the tubal epithelium into the myosalpinx. It is also called adenomyosis of the fallopian tube or tubal diverticulosis.

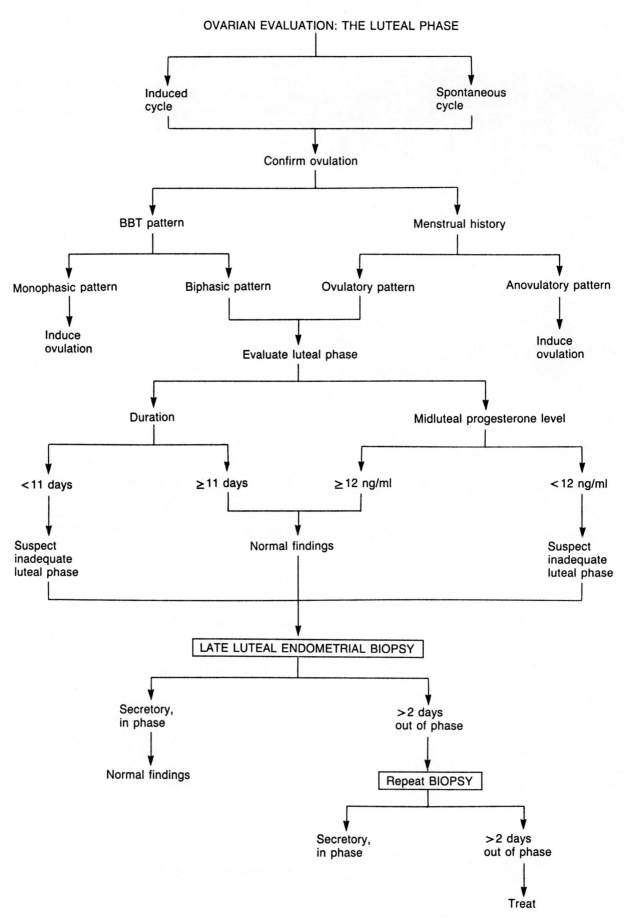

OVARIAN EVALUATION: THE LUTEAL PHASE

Algorithm 7-1. (From DeCherney et al., 1988.)

162

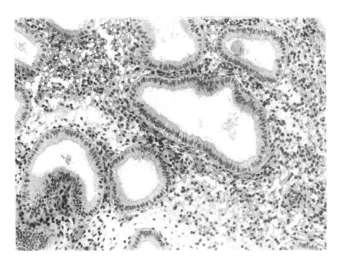

Fig. 7-21. Luteal phase deficiency evidenced in the glandular stromal asynchrony. This biopsy taken in late secretory phase shows subnuclear vacuolization of glands typical of early secretory endometrium and the stromal edema of mid secretory phase.

Etiology and pathogenesis

Salpingitis isthmica nodosa is found in 1% to 5% of all women of reproductive age (Honore, 1978). The etiology and the pathogenesis of this condition remain unclear; no theories provide an adequate explanation for the pathologic findings. The lesions probably are not congenital because they rarely are found in children. Although in most cases there are no signs of inflammation, the postinflammatory nature of some lesions cannot be excluded. Hormonal factors could play a pathogenetic role; the lesions could be hormone dependent since they usually are found during reproductive years and are extremely rare before puberty or after menopause.

Clinical findings

Salpingitis isthmica nodosa may involve one or both fallopian tubes. These lesions are associated significantly with infertility and ectopic pregnancy (Majmudar et al., 1983). Apparently, this tubal anomaly hinders the transport of gametes and embryos and could cause entrapment of embryos, thus facilitating ectopic implantation.

Pathologic findings

Salpingitis isthmica nodosa typically involves the isthmus of the fallopian tube but may extend toward the ampulla. In one third of all cases the lesion is located in the ampullary part of the fallopian tube (Majmudar et al., 1983). The lesions may cause no grossly visible changes; they may present as nodules measuring up to 2.5 cm in diameter or as a diffuse thickening of a segment of the fallopian tube (Clement, 1991). Bilateral involvement has been reported in 35% to 85% of cases.

Microscopically, the epithelium of the fallopian tubes extends into the myosalpinx and lines the glandlike spaces, diverticula, and cysts (Fig. 7-22). The cuboidal epithelium of these structures is indistinguishable from normal tubal epithelium. Some cysts are lined with flattened epithelium that has undergone atrophy due to compression. Occasionally, tubal epithelium is intermixed with uterine adenomyosis, but that is rare. Salpingitis isthmica nodosa may be associated with endosalpingiosis, i.e., tubal-type epithelial inclusions in the lymph nodes and the peritoneum.

CONSEQUENCES OF HORMONAL TREATMENT
Hormonally induced lesions of the endometrium

Hormonal treatment may produce changes in the female reproductive organs. These changes are not uncommon, but occasionally they must be considered in the differential diagnosis of lesions found in endometrial biopsies performed in patients with infertility. Additional data may be found in the comprehensive review by Deligdisch (1992).

Oral contraceptives currently in use include estrogenic and progestational compounds given in a sequence or simultaneously. Alternatively, slow-release progestational preparations may be implanted subcutaneously.

The effects of these progestational contraceptives depend on their potency, the dosage, and the host's response. The proliferation of endometrial glands is typically arrested. The glands appear inactive and are lined with low cuboidal epithelium that shows no mitotic activity (Fig. 7-23). Some abortive secretion may be seen in early stages of treatment, but later all signs of secretion usually disappear. The stroma is abundant and shows prominent decidual transformation. Often dilated, the blood vessels typically are thin walled.

Ovulation inducers such as clomiphene citrate, Gn-RH, or hCG alone or in various combinations are used for the procurement of ova for in vitro fertilization. Such therapy apparently accelerates the maturation of stroma more than it affects the endometrial glands (Navot et al., 1989, 1991), and this contributes to an asynchrony between the stroma and glands (Fig. 7-24). Stromal changes such as edema, well-developed spiral arteries, and decidual transformation correspond to days 23 and 24 of the menstrual cycle, whereas the glands show early secretory features such as subnuclear vacuoles similar to those seen in days 16 and 17. Progesterone is used to correct this asynchrony.

Hormonal replacement therapy is used in postmenopausal women and in those women who have congenitally dysfunctional ovaries or premature ovarian failure. Such therapy includes estrogens and progesterone given in a sequential or combined manner. A variety of histologic patterns can be recognized in biopsies depending on the timing of the biopsy, the duration of treatment, the hormones used, and the age of the patient (Figs. 7-25 and 7-26). The endometrial biopsy may reveal one or more patterns, which include the following:

1. Normal proliferative and/or secretory endometrium

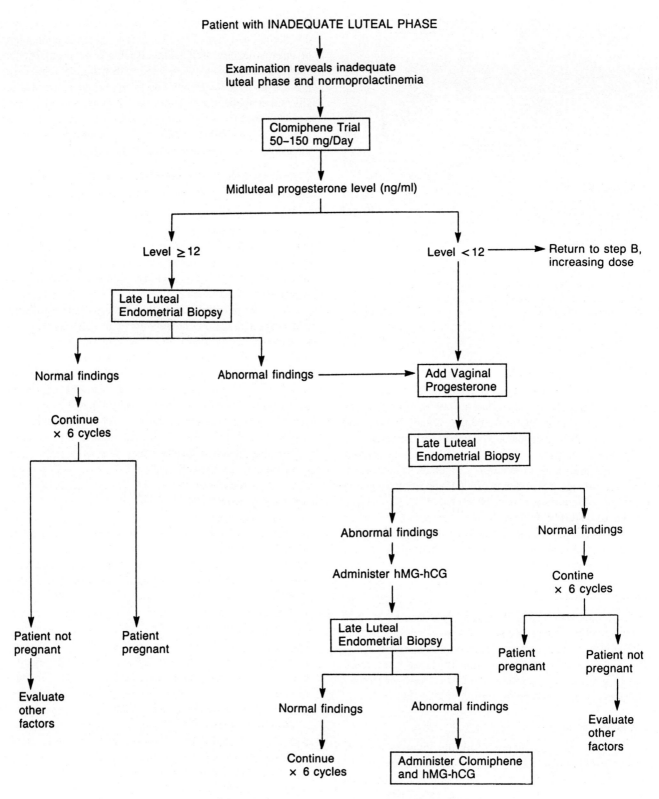

Algorithm 7-2. (From DeCherney et al., 1988.)

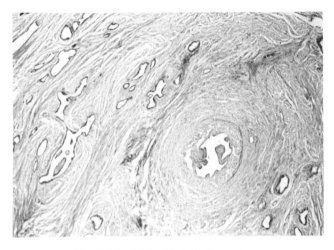

Fig. 7-22. Salpingitis isthmica nodosa.

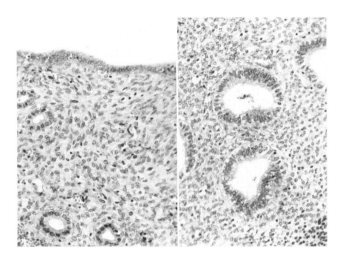

Fig. 7-23. Endometrial changes induced with oral contraceptives.

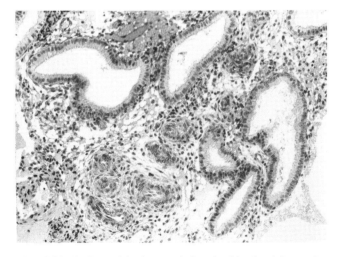

Fig. 7-24. Endometrial changes induced with clomiphene citrate.

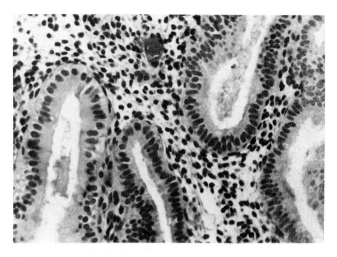

Fig. 7-25. Mixed proliferative and secretory endometrium induced by hormonal replacement therapy with estrogen and progesterone.

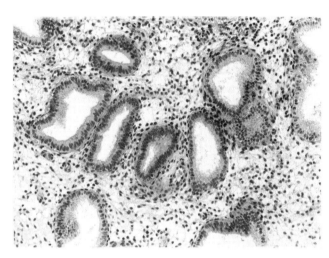

Fig. 7-26. Irregular maturation of the secretory endometrium following hormonal replacement therapy with estrogen and progesterone.

2. Mixed proliferative and secretory endometrium
3. Irregular maturation of the secretory endometrium with focal maturational differences
4. Asynchronous stromal and glandular maturation
5. Stromal hyperplasia
6. Decidual reaction
7. Glandular metaplasia into tubal, mucinous, papillary, or eosinophilic epithelium
8. Glandular atrophy
9. Global endometrial atrophy

Progesterone treatment is sometimes used for polycystic ovary syndrome, for endometrial hyperplasia in younger women, and for treatment of adenocarcinoma (Deligdisch, 1991). Short-term therapy induces secretory changes in quiescent endometrial glands and decidual transformation of the stroma.

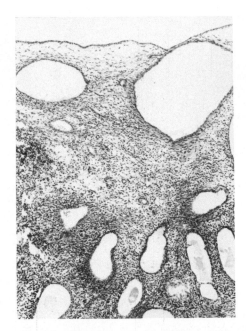

Fig. 7-27. Atrophic endometrium induced by tamoxifen.

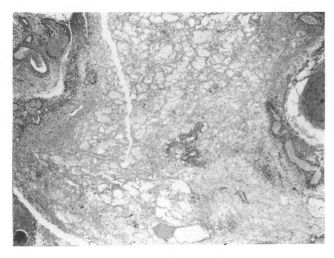

Fig. 7-28. Ovarian hyperstimulation following treatment with Gn-RH. There is massive stromal edema.

Tamoxifen, a synthetic nonsteroidal triethylene estrogen derivative, binds to estrogen receptors and thus inhibits the action of estrogen. Women being treated with tamoxifen have inactive or atrophic endometrium with occasionally weak proliferative changes (Fig. 7-27).

Hormonally induced lesions of the ovary

Ovarian hyperstimulation. The induction of ovulation with clomiphene, Gn-RH, and hCG administered in various combinations may result in the ovarian hyperstimulation syndrome, the most serious complication of such treatment (Rizk and Aboulghar, 1991).

Several grades of injury are recognized from mild to severe. In the most severe form the patient develops ascites, hydrothorax, electrolyte imbalance, hypovolemia, oliguria, and thromboembolism associated with massive ovarian enlargement. The ovary appears enlarged, soft, and edematous. Focal signs of follicular rupture and hemorrhage may be seen. Histologically, the stroma appears edematous (Fig. 7-28).

Androgen-induced ovarian lesions. Administration of androgens to adult women induces virilization. Futterweit and Deligdisch (1986) have shown that chronic administration of testosterone to women undergoing sex change produces significant changes in the ovaries (Fig. 7-29), including:

1. Multiple cystic follicles of the ovary
2. Diffuse ovarian stromal hyperplasia
3. Collagenization of the outer cortex of the ovary
4. Variable degrees of luteinization of stromal cells

Hormone-induced testicular changes. Administration of testosterone or analogs of Gn-RH induce testicular changes (Properzi et al., 1989). These include hypospermatogenesis (Fig. 7-30), disruption of the normal spermatogenic maturation, and involution of Leydig's cells variable. These effects of testosterone form the rationale for using testosterone as a male contraceptive (WHO Task Force, 1990). Similar changes are associated with hyperestrinism (Valenta, 1986).

Diethylstilbestrol-induced lesions. Intrauterine exposure to diethylstilbestrol (DES) affects the fetal genital organs and produces anatomic changes that could interfere with the reproductive functions of both females and males (Bibbo et al., 1978; Herbst et al., 1980). DES interferes with the normal development of organs derived from the müllerian ducts (Bibbo et al., 1977, 1978; Henderson et al., 1976; Driscoll and Taylor, 1980; DeCherney et al., 1981). These include:

1. Vaginal adenosis
2. Cervical deformities
3. Abnormalities of the uterine cavity such as a T-shaped uterus
4. Excessive thickness and irregular structure of the myometrium
5. Fallopian tube strictures and deformities
6. Epididymal cysts, small penis, and testicles
7. Meatal stenosis of the urethra
8. Hypospermatogenesis

Barnes et al. (1980) reviewed the outcome of pregnancies in women who were exposed to DES in utero and found an increased incidence of miscarriages, ectopic pregnancies, stillbirth, premature birth, and infertility in women both with and without visible structural defects. These findings

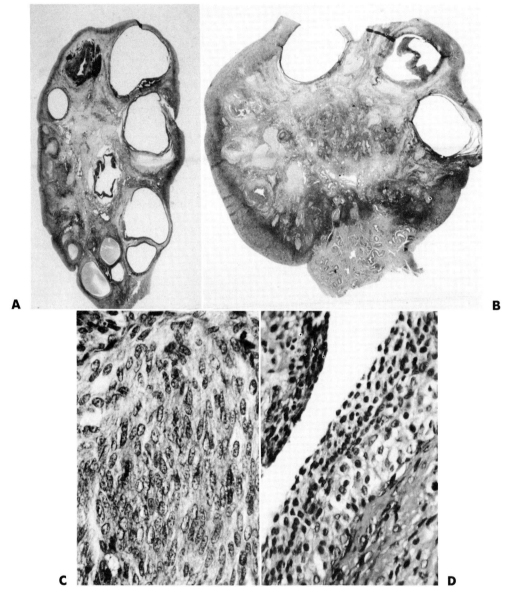

Fig. 7-29. A, Section of polycystic ovary in androgen-treated patient showing multiple cystic follicles distributed beneath a thickened collagenized external ovarian cortex. **B,** Polycystic ovary and fallopian tube in a hirsute androgen-treated patient. Note the areas of extreme capsular thickening and diffuse increase in stromal cells in both cortical and medullary zones of the ovary. **C,** Ovarian stromal hyperplasia showing dense proliferation of plump spindle-shaped cells from the same patient. **D,** Cystic follicle of androgen-treated patient lined by granulosa and prominent luteinized theca cells. (Reproduced from Futterweit W, Deligdisch L. Histopathological effects of exogenously administered testosterone in 19 female to male transsexuals. J Clin Endocrinol Metab 1986; 62:16, © The Endocrine Society, with permission. (Courtesy of Dr. L. Deligdish).

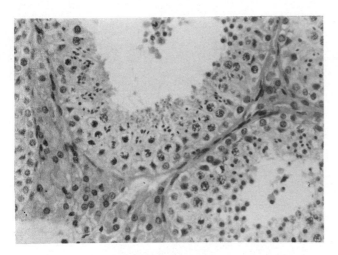

Fig. 7-30. Testosterone induced hypospermatogenesis.

corroborated by other reports (Herbst et al., 1980) indicate that a significant number of women exposed to DES will have reproductive difficulties and as many as one fourth of them will not be able to have children. The lesions in the male genital tract are not associated with reduced fertility (Bibbo et al., 1977; Henderson et al., 1976; Bibbo et al., 1978).

REFERENCES

Acosta AA, Buttram VC Jr, Besch PK, Malinak LR, Franklin RR, Vanderheyden JD: A proposed classification of pelvic endometriosis. Obstet Gynecol 1973; 42:19.

Adams J, Polson DW, Franks S: Prevalence of polycystic ovaries in women with anovulation and idiopathic hirsutism. Br Med J 1986; 293:355.

Archer DF: Hyperprolactinemia. In Progress in Infertility, 3rd ed., edited by Behrman SJ, Kistner RW, Patton GW Jr. Boston, Little, Brown, 1988, p 463.

Ardaens Y, Robert Y, Lemaitre L, Fossati P, Dewailly D: Polycystic ovarian disease: Contribution of vaginal endosonography and reassessment of ultrasonic diagnosis. Fertil Steril 1991; 55:1062.

Arnhod IJ, Mendonca BB, Bloise W, Toledo SP: Male pseudohermaphroditism resulting from Leydig cell hypoplasia. J Pediatr 1985; 106:1057.

Balasch J, Vanrell JA, Creus M, Marquez M, Gonzalez-Merlo J: The endometrial biopsy for diagnosis of luteal phase deficiency. Fertil Steril 1985; 44:699.

Barbieri RL: Polycystic ovarian disease. Annu Rev Med 1991; 42:199.

Barbieri RL, Smith S, Ryan KJ: The role of hyperinsulinemia in the pathogenesis of ovarian hyperandrogenism. Fertil Steril 1988; 50:197.

Bardin CW, Catterall JF: Testostrosterone: A major determinant of extragenital sexual dimorphism. Science 1981; 211:1285.

Barnes AB, Colton T, Gundersen J, Noller KL, Tilley BC, Strama T, et al: Fertility and outcome of pregnancy in women exposed in utero to diethylstilbestrol. N Engl J Med 1980; 302:609.

Barnes R, Rosenfield RL: The polycystic ovary syndrome: Pathogenesis and treatment. Ann Intern Med 1989; 110:386.

Bercovici JP, Nahoul K, Tater D, Charles JF, Scholler R: Hormonal profile of Leydig cell tumors with gynecomastia. J Clin Endocrinol Metab 1984; 59:625.

Berthezene F, Forest MG, Grimaud JA, Claustrat B, Mornex R: Leydig cell agenesis: A cause of male pseudohermaphroditism. N Engl J Med 1976; 295:969.

Bibbo M, Gill WB, Azizi F, Blough R, Fang V, Rosenfield RL, et al.: Follow-up study of male and female offspring of DES-exposed mothers. Obstet Gynecol 1977; 49:1.

Bibbo M, Haenszel WM, Wied GL, Hubby M, Herbst AL: A twenty-five-year follow-up study of women exposed to diethylstilbestrol during pregnancy. N Engl J Med 1978; 298:763.

Biscotti CV, Hart WR: Juvenile granulosa cell tumors of the ovary. Arch Pathol Lab Med 1989; 113:40.

Boyar RM, Finkelstein JW, Witkin M, Kapen S, Weitzman E, Hellman L: Studies of endocrine function in "isolated" gonadotropin deficiency. J Clin Endocrinol Metab 1973; 36:64.

Burrow GN, Wortzman G, Rewcastle NB, Holgate RC, Kovacs K: Microadenomas of the pituitary and abnormal sellar tomograms in an unselected autopsy series. N Engl J Med 1981; 304:156.

Butler MG, Meaney FJ, Palmer CG: Clinical and cytogenetic survey of 39 individuals with Prader-Labhart-Willi syndrome. Am J Med Genet 1986; 23:793.

Buttram VC Jr: Endometriosis. In Progress in Infertility, 3rd ed., edited by Behrman SJ, Kistner RW, Patton GW, Boston, Little, Brown, 1988, p 273.

Carter JN, Tyson JE, Tolis G, Van Vliet S, Faiman C, Friesen HG: Prolactin-secreting tumors and hypogonadism in 22 men. N Engl J Med 1978; 299:847.

Chang RJ, deZiegler D: Polycystic ovary syndrome and related abnormalities. In Pathology of Infertility: Clinical Correlations in the Male and Female, edited by Gondos B, Riddick DH, New York, Thieme, 1987, p 143.

Clement PB: Pathology of endometriosis. Pathol Annu 1990; 25:245.

Clement PB: Pathology of gamete and zygote transport: Cervical, endometrial, myometrial, and tubal factors in infertility. In Pathology of Reproductive Failure, edited by Kraus FT, Damjanov I, Kaufman N. Baltimore, Williams & Wilkins, 1991, p. 140.

Cohen LM, Greenberg DB, Murray GB: Neuropsychiatric presentation of men with pituitary tumors (the 'four A's'). Psychosomatics 1984; 25:925.

Coney P: Polycystic ovarian disease: Current concepts of pathophysiology and therapy. Fertil Steril 1984; 42:667.

Conn PM, Crowley WF Jr: Gonadotropin-releasing hormone and its analogues. N Engl J Med 1991; 324:93.

Conway GS, Honour JW, Jacobs HS: Heterogeneity of the polycystic ovary syndrome: Clinical, endocrine and ultrasound features in 556 patients. Clin Endocrinol (Oxf) 1989; 30:459.

Coulam CB, Annegers JF, Kranz JS: Chronic anovulation syndrome and associated neoplasia. Obstet Gynecol 1983; 61:403.

Czernobilsky B, Czernobilsky H: The female reproductive tract. In Functional Endocrine Pathology, vol 2, edited by Kovacs K, Asa SL. Boston, Blackwell, 1991, p 608.

Daly DC: The endometrium and the luteal phase defect. Semin Reprod Endocrinol 1983; 1:3.

Damjanov I: Tumors of the testis and epididymis. In Urological Pathology, edited by Murphy WM. Philadelphia, WB Saunders, 1989, p 314.

Damjanov I, Drobnjak P, Grizelj V, Longhino N: Sclerosing stromal tumor of the ovary. A hormonal and ultrastructural analysis. Obstet Gynecol 1975; 45:675.

DeCherney AH, Cholst I, Naftolin F: Structure and function of the fallopian tubes following exposure to diethylstilbestrol (DES) during gestation. Fertil Steril 1981; 36:741.

DeCherney AH, Polan ML, Lee RD, Boyers SP: Decision Making in Infertility. Toronto, B.C. Decker, 1988.

Deligdisch L: Hormone therapy and the endometrium. Mod Pathol 1992; (in press).

Driscoll SG, Taylor S: Effects of prenatal maternal estrogen on the male urogenital system. Obstet Gynecol 1980; 56:537.

Editorial: Polycystic ovaries—disorder or sign? Lancet 1990; 336:1099.

Ehrmann DA, Rosenfield RL: Hirsutism—beyond the steroidogenic block. N Engl J Med 1990; 323:909.

Frank S: Polycystic ovary syndrome: A changing perspective. Clin Endocrinal (Oxf) 1989; 31:87.

Futterweit W, Deligdisch L: Histopathological effects of exogenously administered testosterone in 19 female to male transsexuals. J Clin Endocrinol Metab 1986; 62:16.

Gabrilove JL, Nicolis GL, Mitty HA, Sohval AR: Feminizing interstitial cell tumor of testis: Personal observation and review of literature. Cancer 1975; 35:1184.

Givens JR: Familial polycystic ovarian disease. Endocrinol Metab Clin North Am 1988; 17:771.

Giwercman A, Bruun E, Frimodt-Moller C, Skakkebaek NE: Prevalence of carcinoma in situ and other histopathological abnormalities in testes of men with a history of cryptoorchidism. J Urol 1989; 142:998.

Goldzieher JW, Elkind-Hirsch K: Polycystic ovarian disease. In Progress in Infertility, 3rd ed., edited by Behrman SJ, Kistner RW, Patton GW. Boston, Little & Brown, 1988, p 363.

Goldzieher JW, Green JA: The polycystic ovary: I. Clinical and histologic features. J Clin Endocrinol Metab 1962; 22.325.

Gorski RA: Sexual differentiation of the endocrine brain and its control. In Brain Endocrinology, 2nd ed., edited by Motta M. New York, Raven Press, 1991, p 71.

Graham RA, Seif MW, Aplin JD, Li TC, Cooke ID, Rogers AW, Dockery P: An endometrial factor in unexplained infertility. BMJ 1990; 300:1428.

Grem JL, Robins HI, Wilson KS, Gilchrist K, Trump DL: Metastatic Leydig cell tumor of the testis. Report of three cases and a review of the literature. Cancer 1986; 58:2116.

Gruhn JG, Gould VE: The adrenal glands. In Anderson's Pathology, 9th ed., edited by Kissane JM. St. Louis, CV Mosby, 1990, p 1580.

Guzick DS: Clinical epidemiology of endometriosis and infertility. Obstet Gynecol Clin North Am 1989; 16:43.

Haney AF: Pelvic endometriosis: Etiology and pathology. In Pathology of Infertility: Clinical Correlations in the Male and Female, edited by Gondos B, Riddick DH. New York, Thieme, 1987, p 85.

Hayes MC, Scully RE: Stromal luteoma of the ovary: A clinicopathological analysis of 25 cases. Int J Gynecol Pathol 1987; 6:313.

Henderson BE, Benton B, Cosgrove M, Baptista MA, Aldrich J, Townsend D, et al.: Urogenital tract abnormalities in sons of women treated with diethylstilbestrol. Pediatrics 1976; 58:505.

Herbst AL, Bern HA (Eds): Developmental Effects of Diethylstilbestrol in Pregnancy. New York, Thieme-Stratton, 1981.

Herbst AL, Hubby MM, Blough RR, Azizi FA: A comparison of pregnancy experience in DES-exposed and DES-unexposed daughters. J Reprod Med 1980; 24:62.

Honoré LH: Salpingitis isthmica nodosa in female infertility and ectopic tubal pregnancy. Fertil Steril 1978; 29:164.

Horvath E, Kovacs K: Pathology of prolactin cell adenomas of human pituitary. Semin Diagn Pathol 1986; 3:4.

Hughesdon PE: Morphology and morphogenesis of the Stein-Leventhal ovary and of so-called "hyperthecosis." Obstet Gynecol Surv 1982; 37:59.

Insler V, Lunenfeld B: Pathophysiology of polycystic ovarian disease: New insights. Hum Reprod 1991; 6:1025.

Jackenhovel F, Khan SA, Nieschlag E: Diagnostic value of bioactive FSH in male infertility. Acta Endocrinol 1989; 121:802.

Kim I, Young RH, Scully RE: Leydig cell tumors of the testis. A clinicopathological analysis of 40 cases and review of the literature. Am J Surg Pathol 1985; 9:177.

Kikuchi K, Kaji M, Momoi T, Mikawa H, Shigematsu Y, Sudo M: Failure to induce puberty in a man with X-linked congenital adrenal hypoplasia and hypogonadotropic hypogonadism by pulsatile administration of low dose gonadotropin-releasing hormone. Acta Endocrinol 1987; 114:153.

Kovacs K, Horvath E: Hypothalamic-pituitary abnormalities in ovulatory disorders. In Pathology of Infertility: Critical Correlations in the Male and Female, edited by Gondos B, Riddick DG. New York, Thieme, 1987, p 185.

Krauss CM, Turksoy RN, Atkins L, McLaughlin C, Brown LG, Page DC: Familial premature ovarian failure due to an interstitial deletion of the long arm of the X chromosome. N Engl J Med 1987; 317:125.

Kruse K, Sippell WG, Schnakenburg KV: Hypogonadism in congenital adrenal hypoplasia: Evidence for a hypothalamic origin. J Clin Endocrinol Metab 1984; 58:12.

Lappohn RE, Bogchelman DH: The relation of fertility and ovarian histology after bilateral ovarian wedge resection. Fertil Steril 1989; 52:221.

Leedman PJ, Bierre AR, Martin FI: Virilizing nodular ovarian stromal hyperthecosis, diabetes mellitus and insulin resistance in a postmenopausal woman: Case report. Br J Obstet Gynecol 1989; 96:1095.

Lunde O, Magnus P, Sandvik L, Hoglo S: Familial clustering in the polycystic ovarian syndrome. Gynecol Obstet Invest 1989; 28:23.

Mahmood TA, Templeton A: Pathophysiology of mild endometriosis: Review of literature. Hum Reprod 1990; 5:765.

Mahmood TA, Templeton A: Prevalence and genesis of endometriosis. Hum Reprod 1991; 6:544.

Majmudar B, Henderson PH 3d, Semple E: Salpingitis isthmica nodosa: A high risk factor for tubal pregnancy. Obstet Gynecol 1983; 62:73.

McNeely MJ, Soules MR: The diagnosis of luteal phase deficiency: A critical review. Fertil Steril 1988; 50:1.

Moen MH: Is a long period without childbirth a risk factor for developing endometriosis? Hum Reprod 1991; 10:1404.

Mozaffarian GA, Higley M, Paulsen CA: Clinical studies in an adult male patient with "isolated follicle stimulating hormone (FSH) deficiency." J Androl 1983; 4:393.

Naessens A, Foulon W, Debrucker P, Devroey D, Lauwers S: Recovery of microorganisms in semen and relationship to semen evaluation. Fertil Steril 1986; 45:101.

Nagamani M, Stuart CA, Van Dinh T: Steroid biosynthesis in the Sertoli-Leydig cell tumor: Effects of insulin and luteinizing hormone. Am J Obstet Gynecol 1989; 161:1738.

Nagamani M, Van Dinh TV, Kelver ME: Hyperinsulinemia in hyperthecosis of the ovaries. Am J Obstet Gynecol 1985; 154:384.

Navot D, Anderson TL, Droesch K, Scott RT, Kreiner D, Rosenwaks Z: Hormonal manipulation of endometrial maturation. J Clin Endocrinol Metab 1989; 68:801.

Navot D, Bergh P, Williams M, Garrisi GJ, Guzman I, Sandler B, et al.: An insight into early reproductive processes through the in vivo model of ovum donation. J Clin Endocrinol Metabol 1991; 72:408.

Page DL, De Lellis RA, Hough A: Tumors of the Adrenal. Atlas of Tumor Pathology, ser 2, fascicle 23. Washington, DC, Armed Forces Institute of Pathology, 1986.

Paus E, Fossa A, Fossa SD, Nustad K: High frequency of incomplete human chorionic gonadotropin in patients with testicular seminoma. J Urol 1988; 139:542.

Peillon F, Dupuy M, LI JY, Kujas M, Vincens M, Mowszowicz I, Derome P: Pituitary enlargement with suprasellar extension in functional hyperprolactinemia due to lactotroph hyperplasia: A pseudotumoral disease. J Clin Endocrinol Metab 1991; 73:1008.

Polson DW, Adams J, Wadsworth J, Franks S: Polycystic ovaries: A common finding in normal women. Lancet 1988; 1:870.

Properzi G, Francavilla S, Vicentini C, Cordeschi G, Galassi P, Paradiso Galatioto G, Miano L: Testicular changes after treatment with a GnRH analog (buserelin) in association with cyproterone acetate in men with prostatic cancer. Eur Urol 1989; 16:426.

Rabin D, Spitz I, Bercovici B, Bell J, Laufer A, Benveniste R, Polishuk W: Isolated deficiency of follicle-stimulating hormone. Clinical and laboratory features. N Engl J Med 1972; 287:1313.

Ranta H, Aine R, Oksanen H, Heinonen PK: Dissemination of endometrial cells during carbon dioxide hysteroscopy and chromotubation among infertile patients. Fertil Steril 1990; 53:751.

Rizk B, Aboulghar M: Modern management of ovarian hyperstimulation syndrome. Hum Reprod 1991; 6:1082.

Russell P, Bannatyne P: Surgical Pathology of the Ovaries. Edinburgh, Churchill Livingstone, 1989.

Rutgers JL, Scully RE: Pathology of the testis in intersex syndromes. Semin Diagn Pathol 1987; 4:275.

Santoro N, Filicori M, Crowley WF Jr: Hypogonadotropic disorders in men and women: Diagnosis and therapy with pulsatile gonadotropin-releasing hormone. Endocr Rev 1986; 7:11.

Schwanzel-Fukuda M, Bick D, Pfaff DW: Luteinizing hormone-releasing hormone (LHRH)-expressing cells do not migrate normally in an inherited hypogonadal (Kallmann) syndrome. Mol Brain Res 1989; 6:311.

Shenker Y, Malozowski SN, Ayers J, Grekin RJ, Barkan AL: Steroid secretion by a virilizing lipoid cell ovarian tumor: Origins of dehydroepiandrosterone sulfate. Obstet Gynecol 1989; 74:502.

Smallridge RC: Thyrotropin-secreting pituitary tumors. Endocrinol Metab Clin North Am 1987; 16:765.

Smals AGH, Kloppenborg PWC, van Haelst UJ, Lequin R, Benraad TJ: Fertile eunuch syndrome versus classic hypogonadotropic hypogonadism. Acta Endocrinol (Copenh) 1978; 87:389.

Smith KD, Steinberger E, Perloff WH: Polycystic ovarian disease (PCO). A report of 301 patients. Am J Obstet Gynecol 1965; 93:994.

Snyder PJ: Gonadotroph cell adenomas of the pituitary. Endocr Rev 1985; 6:552.

Snyder PJ: Gonadotroph cell pituitary adenomas. Endocrinol Metab Clin North Am 1987; 16:755.

Speroff L, Glass RH, Kase NG: Clinical Gynecologic Endocrinology and Infertility. Baltimore, Williams & Wilkins, 1989.

Stein IF, Leventhal ML: Amenorrhea associated with bilateral polycystic ovaries. Am J Obstet Gynecol 1985; 29:181.

Thorner MO, Vance ML, Horvath E, Kovacs K: The anterior pituitary. In Williams' Textbook of Endocrinology, 8th ed., edited by Wilson JD, Foster DW. Philadelphia, WB Saunders, 1992, p 221.

U SH, Johnson C: Metastatic prolactin-secreting pituitary adenoma. Hum Pathol 1984; 15:94.

Valenta LJ, Elias AN: Male hypogonadism due to hyperestrogenism. N Engl J Med 1986; 314:186.

Vance ML, Thorner MO: Prolactinomas. Endocrinol Metab Clin North Am 1987; 16:731.

Wentz AC: Endometrial biopsy in the evaluation of infertility. Fertil Steril 1980; 33:121.

Wentz AC: Luteal phase inadequacy. In Progress in Infertility, 3rd ed., edited by Behrman SJ, Kistner RW, Patton GW. Boston, Little, Brown, 1988, p 405.

Wilson JD, Foster DW (Eds): Williams' Textbook of Endocrinology, 8th ed. Philadelphia, WB Saunders, 1992.

Wilson JD, George FW, Griffin JE: The hormonal control of sexual development. Science 1981; 211:1278.

Witten BI, Martin SA: The endometrial biopsy as a guide to the management of luteal phase defect. Fertil Steril 1985; 44:460.

Wu FC, Butler GE, Kelnar CJ, Stirling HF, Huhtaniemi I: Patterns of pulsatile luteinizing hormone and follicle-stimulating hormone secretion in prepubertal (midchildhood) boys and girls and patients with idiopathic hypogonadotropic hypogonadism (Kallmann's syndrome): A study using an ultrasensitive time-resolved immunofluorometric assay. J Clin Endocrinol Metab 1991; 72:1229.

World Health Organization (WHO) Task Force on methods for the regulation of male fertilization: Contraceptive efficacy of testoterone-induced azoospermia in normal men. Lancet 1990; 336:955.

Wu FCW, Taylor PL, Sellar RE: LHRH pulse frequency in normal and infertile men. J Endocrinol 1989; 123:149.

Yeh J, Rebar RW, Liu JH, Yen SS: Pituitary function in isolated gonadotropin deficiency. Clin Endocrinol 1989; 31:375.

Yen SSC, Jaffe RB (Eds): Reproductive Endocrinology: Physiology, Pathophysiology and Clinical Management, 3rd ed. Philadelphia, WB Saunders, 1991.

Young RH, Scully RE: Fibromatosis and massive edema of the ovary, possibly related entities: A report of 14 cases of fibromatosis and 11 cases of massive edema. Int J Gynecol Pathol 1984; 3:153.

Young RH, Scully RE: Ovarian pathology of infertility. In Pathology of Reproductive Failure, edited by Kraus FT, Damjanov I, Kaufman N. Baltimore, Williams & Wilkins, 1991, p 104.

Young RH, Scully RE: Ovarian Sertoli-Leydig cell tumors. A clinicopathological analysis of 207 cases. Am J Surg Pathol 1985; 9:543.

Young RH, Scully RE: Ovarian sex cord-stromal tumors: Recent progress. Int J Gynecol Pathol 1982; 1:101.

Zaloudek CJ, Tavassoli FA, Norris HJ: Dysgerminoma with syncytiotrophoblastic giant cells. A histologically and clinically distinctive subtype of dysgerminoma. Am J Surg Pathol 1981; 5:361.

Zhang J, Young PH, Arseneau J, Scully RE: Ovarian stromal tumors containing lutein or Leydig cells (luteinized thecoma) and stromal Leydig cell tumor. A clinicopathologic analysis of 50 cases. Int J Gynecol Pathol 1982; 1:270.

ABNORMAL SPERMATOGENESIS

Assessment of the spermatogenic potential of the testes usually includes an analysis of ejaculated sperm, a hormonal evaluation of the hypothalamic-pituitary-testicular-adrenal axis, and a testicular biopsy. On the basis of these findings, it is possible to classify male infertility into three broad etiologic categories (Wong et al., 1978; Pesce, 1987) as:

1. Pretesticular
2. Testicular
3. Posttesticular

The common causes of male infertility are listed in the box at right. The relative frequency of various infertility problems as revealed by testicular biopsy is presented in Table 8-1. Some of these conditions have been addressed in other chapters. This chapter is limited to idiopathic testicular causes of infertility characterized by abnormal spermatogenesis. Additional data may be found in the comprehensive papers of Wong et al. (1973, 1974, 1978, 1988) and the recent review by Wheeler (1991).

GERM CELL APLASIA

The term *germ cell aplasia,* also known as Sertoli-cell–only syndrome, denotes a complete absence of germinal cells from the seminiferous tubules. The eponym *del Castillo's syndrome* commemorates the first description of that entity (del Castillo et al., 1947).

Germ cell aplasia is found in 11% to 20% of testicular biopsies performed for the evaluation of infertility (Wong et al., 1978; Levin, 1979). The etiology of germ cell aplasia remains unknown in most cases. The same histopathologic findings can be caused by many exogenous factors; the condition should be considered idiopathic only after

---

Etiologic classification of male infertility

Pretesticular causes

1. Hypothalamic hypogonadism
2. Pituitary deficiency
3. Adrenal disorders
4. Various endocrine or metabolic disorders
5. Exogenous hormones
    Androgens
    Estrogens
    Corticosteroids

Testicular causes

1. Germ cell aplasia
2. Hypospermatogenesis
3. Maturation arrest of spermatogenesis
4. Teratospermia and functional sperm defects
5. Orchitis
6. Irradiation injury
7. Cryptorchidism

Posttesticular causes

1. Congenital obstruction of ducts
2. Infection
3. Surgical ligation of ducts

Modified from Wong et al., 1978; Pesce, 1987.

Table 8-1. Relative frequency of histologic findings in testicular biopsies

Condition	Reported frequency (%)*		
	Wong et al. (1978)	Levin (1979)	Wheeler (1991)
Germ cell aplasia	10	15	16
Germ cell aplasia with focal spermatogenesis	—	6	—
Maturation arrest	43	4	11
Hypospermatogenesis	30	49	44
Klinefelter's syndrome	7	7	—
Immature testis	—	1	1
Cryptorchidism	5	—	—
Orchitis	2	—	—
Fibrosis	—	—	13
Normal histology	—	12	2
Sloughing of tubules >50%	—	—	67

Data from Wong et al. (1978); Levin (1979); and Wheeler (1991).
*The numbers are approximations and in some cases add up to more than 100 because more than one pattern was recognized in the biopsy specimen.
—, Not applicable.

Causes of germ cell aplasia, or Sertoli-cell–only syndrome

Idiopathic
Chromosomal anomalies
    Klinefelter's syndrome
    Down's syndrome
Hormonal disturbances
    Pituitary causes (FSH deficiency, hyperprolactinemia)
    Adrenogenital syndrome
Infections
    Mumps
    AIDS
Exogenous adverse effects
    Irradiation
    Chemotherapy

---

other causes of germinal epithelial destruction have been excluded (see the box above right). Sertoli-cell–only syndrome is associated with distinct hormonal changes indicative of primary testicular failure of spermatogenesis (Mičić et al., 1983).

Clinical findings

Most patients present with infertility and azoospermia (de Kretser et al., 1972). Phenotypically, they are male and have normal secondary sexual characteristics. The testes are of average size or only slightly smaller than normal. Hormonal studies typically show normal plasma luteinizing hormone (LH) and testosterone levels and elevated follicle-stimulating hormone (FSH). An association between germ cell aplasia and the HLA-B locus BW 35 has been noted (Kamidono et al., 1980). Because infertility caused by germ cell aplasia is considered irreversible, there is no treatment for it.

Pathologic findings

The seminiferous tubules have a reduced diameter and are lined by a single layer of Sertoli cells (Fig. 8-1). The Sertoli cells have well-developed cytoplasm that usually appears vacuolated. Occasionally, the cytoplasm of Sertoli cells is filled with eosinophilic granular material that stains with the periodic acid–Schiff reaction and is diastase resistant (Wong et al., 1978) (Fig. 8-2). The oval nuclei of Sertoli cells typically are located in the midportion of the cytoplasm midway between the basal lamina and the lumen of the tubule. Their longer diameter is perpendicular to the basal membrane. Some tubules may be lined by immature Sertoli cells (Nistal et al., 1982) or pseudostratified Sertoli cells with tubules that impart morphologic features reminiscent of the testes of newborn infants (Wheeler, 1991). The basement membranes of seminiferous tubules typically are thin, and there is no evidence of peritubular fibrosis. Leydig's cells appear normal.

Sertoli-cell–only syndrome may be associated with mild to moderate thickening of the basement membrane and the lamina propria of the seminiferous tubules, especially in older patients. (Peritubular fibrosis and focal hyperplasia of Leydig cells, as well as vascular changes, are indicative of testicular involution. These changes cannot be interpreted unequivocally. Some cases represent involution of functional tubules. Others are related to ischemia. In still other instances, the changes noted in the lamina propria reflect a response to an injury that has depleted the germ cells. In such cases the tubules lined with Sertoli cells may contain occasional germ cells, but the spermatogenesis is almost invariably abortive (Fig. 8-3).

Furthermore, seminiferous tubules showing germ cell aplasia may be adjacent to areas in which normal spermatogenesis occurs. Such a condition revealed on biopsy may be classified as *mixed germ cell aplasia with focal spermatogenesis* (Levin, 1979) to distinguish it from complete germ cell aplasia.

MATURATION ARREST OF SPERMATOGENESIS

Maturation arrest is an interruption of spermatogenesis preventing the formation of mature spermatozoa. The arrest can occur at any stage of spermatogenesis, but it most often affects primary spermatocytes (Wheeler, 1991). The arrest usually is complete, and all the seminiferous tubules of a given patient show the same morphologic features. The term *incomplete maturation arrest* may be used for cases that show arrest at one stage of spermatogenesis,

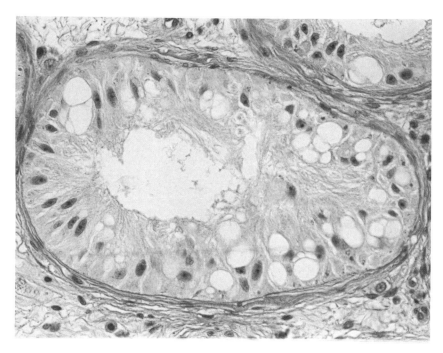

Fig. 8-1. Sertoli-cell-only syndrome. The nuclei are in the midportion of the cytoplasm and appear "wind-swept."

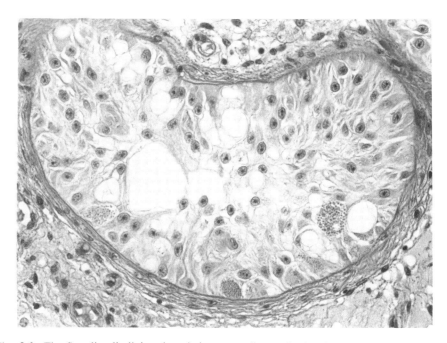

Fig. 8-2. The Sertoli cells lining the tubule appear disorganized and surround vacuolar spaces. Some cells have granular cytoplasm. There is mild peritubular fibrosis.

e.g., primary spermatocytes, and contain focally more mature cells, e.g., spermatids (Levin, 1979).

The prevalence of maturation arrest varies from institution to institution; the reported frequency is in the range of 4% to 40% (Wong et al., 1978; Levin, 1979). These differences are due to different populations of patients and nonstandardized indications for biopsies and reflect the different diagnostic criteria used in various institutions.

Clinical findings

Patients typically present with infertility and are otherwise asymptomatic. Sperm analysis usually reveals

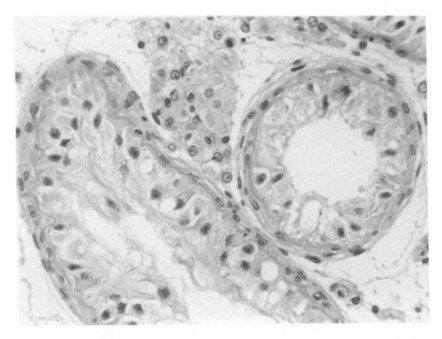

Fig. 8-3. Seminiferous tubules lined by Sertoli cells and occasional germ cells. There is however no evidence of spermatogenesis.

Causes of maturation arrest of spermatogenesis

Idiopathic
Chromosomal anomalies
    Sex chromosome defects
    Down's syndrome
Single gene defects
    Sickle cell anemia
    Cystic fibrosis
Hormonal disturbances
    Gonadotropin deficiency
    Adrenogenital syndrome
    Exogenous hormones (androgens, corticosteroids)
Infections
    Mumps
    AIDS
Exogenous adverse effects
    Irradiation (testis, hypothalamus or pituitary)
    Heat
    Chemotherapy
Trauma
    Spinal cord injury
    Pituitary or hypothalamic injury
Surgical intervention
    Vasectomy
    Hypothalamic or pituitary surgery

---

azoospermia with severe oligozoospermia. The testes are of normal size, and the secondary sex characteristics are well developed. Serum gonadotropins and testosterone levels are within normal limits, except in the most severe cases, which may be associated with elevated FSH (Wong et al., 1978). Infertility is irreversible and usually does not respond to hormonal therapy.

The cause of maturation arrest remains unclear in most instances. In addition to being idiopathic, similar morphologic features may be associated with genetic diseases, hormonal imbalances, toxic environmental influences, or infections (box at left).

Pathologic findings

Maturation arrest can occur at any stage of spermatogenesis.

Maturation arrest at the stage of spermatogonia. The seminiferous tubules contain only sparse spermatogonia. Spermatogonia are recognized by their location in the basal compartment of the tubules in contact with the basement membrane. Their nucleus has a typical appearance; it is filled with moderately dense, homogeneously distributed chromatin. There is a clearly visible nucleolus (Trainer, 1987). The Johnsen (1970) score for these lesions is 3 (Fig. 8-4).

Maturation arrest at the stage of primary spermatocytes. The seminiferous tubules contain only spermatogonia and primary spermatocytes but no secondary spermatocytes, spermatids, or spermatozoa. Primary spermatocytes have distinct nuclear features on the basis of which they can be classified into four substages:

Leptotene—Spermatocytes marked by a fine beaded arrangement of chromatin.
Zygotene—Spermatocytes marked by even more pronounced granularity of chromatin, which tends to aggregate eccentrically within the nucleoplasm.

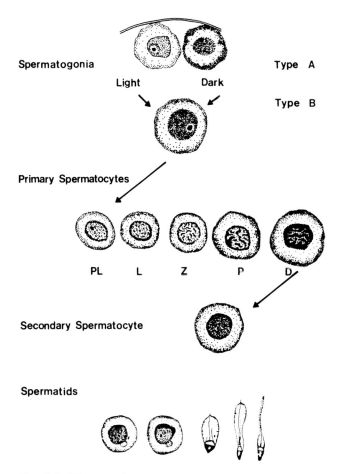

Spermatogonia

Light   Dark

Type A

Type B

Primary Spermatocytes

PL   L   Z   P   D

Secondary Spermatocyte

Spermatids

Fig. 8-4. Diagram of spermatogenesis. Abbreviations for primary spermatocytes: PL, Preleptotene; L, Leptotene; Z, Zygotene; P, Pachytene; D, Diplotene. (From Trainer TD. Histology of normal testis. Am J Surg Pathol 1987; 11:797, with permission.)

Pachytene and diplotene—Spermatocytes marked by enlarged nuclei with a coarse granular or filamentous arrangement of the chromatin.

Transition to secondary spermatocytes is marked by a decrease in nuclear size and fine dispersal of the chromatin. Secondary spermatocytes are short-lived and even under normal circumstances represent only a small fraction of all spermatogenic cells. Furthermore, secondary spermatocytes differ only slightly from round spermatids, which have nuclei of the same size and shape. However, since the maturation arrest inhibits formation of all cells beyond the diplotene stage of primary spermatocytes, this form of maturation arrest is recognized relatively easily. The Johnsen (1970) score for such lesions is 4 or 5 (Figs. 8-4 and 8-5).

Maturation arrest at the stage of secondary spermatocytes or round spermatids. This maturation arrest prevents formation of late elongated spermatids. The seminiferous tubules contain spermatogonia, spermatocytes, and/or round spermatids but no late spermatids or spermatozoa. As noted by Levin (1979), not all seminiferous tu-

bules normally contain late spermatids or spermatozoa. It is therefore important to obtain an adequate sample and to correlate the biopsy findings with the spermiogram. It also is impractical to distinguish secondary spermatocytes from early spermatids since both have round nuclei. The latter have an acrosomal notch, which can be seen on the nuclear surface of those cells that have been fortuitously sectioned through the notch and show this cytologic detail. The round nucleus of early spermatids becomes oval and then elongates to assume the shape typical of spermatozoa. Hence, late spermatids easily can be recognized and are distinct from early spermatozoa.

The seminiferous tubules typically lack elongated spermatids or spermatozoa and are filled on the luminal side with numerous round cells corresponding to secondary spermatocytes and early spermatids (Figs. 8-6 and 8-7). The Johnsen (1970) score for such lesions is 6 or 7.

HYPOSPERMATOGENESIS

Hypospermatogenesis denotes a quantitative reduction of spermatogenesis that results in oligozoospermia and decreased male reproductive capacity. The pathogenesis and etiology of this condition are poorly understood in most cases, although hypospermatogenesis may be causally related to some genetic diseases, hormonal disturbances, systemic disease, toxic substances, and physical influences from the outside world (box on p. 177).

Clinical findings

Patients are oligozoospermic and subfertile (de Kretser, 1979). In idiopathic cases, which form the majority, there are no other local or systemic symptoms. Hypospermatogenesis secondary to an identifiable disease or condition may be treated by eliminating the cause. The treatment results of idiopathic hypospermatogenesis are not encouraging. Nevertheless, since the ejaculate may contain some normal spermatozoa, it is now technically possible to collect and freeze a patient's sperm for subsequent *in vitro* fertilization.

Pathologic findings

In contrast to maturation arrest, which typically results in a blockade of sperm formation, hypospermatogenesis is associated with normal maturation of spermatogenic cells. Spermatozoa are formed but in reduced quantities, resulting in oligozoospermia of 2 million to 20 million per milliliter of semen. The germinal epithelium is hypoplastic. In some tubules there is a general, uniform thinning of the germinal epithelium, and because of this, the central lumen appears prominently dilated and empty (Fig. 8-8). In other forms of hypospermatogenesis, hypoplastic tubules are intermixed with normal tubules. In some tubules spermatogenic cells occupy only a portion of the total surface, whereas another part may contain only Sertoli's cells (Fig. 8-9). Some biopsies show hypoplastic seminiferous tu-

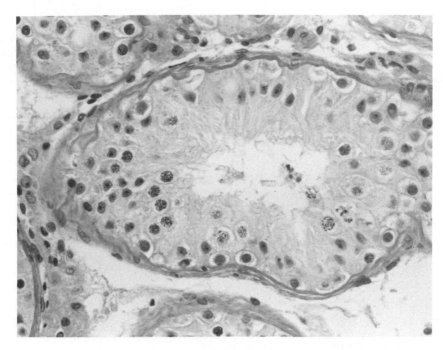

Fig. 8-5. Maturation arrest at the stage of primary spermatocytes.

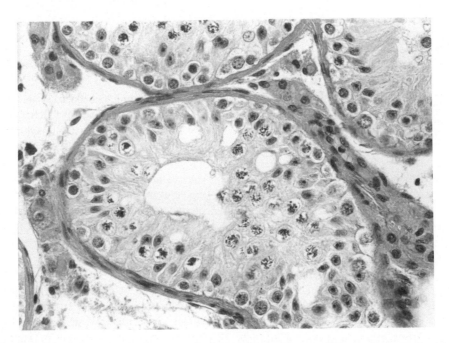

Fig. 8-6. Maturation arrest at the stage of primary spermatocytes, which can be recognized by their dispersed chromatin.

bules intermixed with hyalinized tubules (Söderström and Suominen, 1980). Such changes indicate that hypospermatogenesis may result from many causes and that the disease probably evolves through various stages or progresses to an end stage characterized by hyalinization of tubules and complete depletion of germinal epithelium.

STRUCTURAL AND FUNCTIONAL DEFECTS OF SPERMATOZOA

Structural and functional defects of spermatozoa are common in patients suffering from oligozoospermia. The seminiferous tubules of these patients may show hypospermatogenesis and various forms of reactive changes sugges-

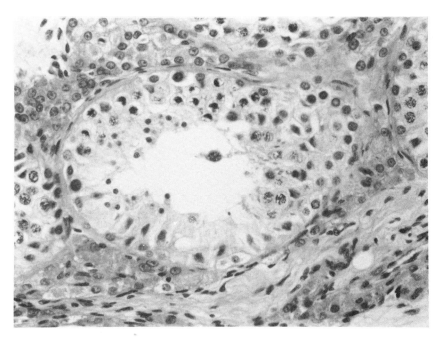

Fig. 8-7. Maturation arrest at the stage of round spermatids. All seminiferous tubules show the same degree of maturation.

Causes of tubular hyalinization and interstitial fibrosis of the testis
Idiopathic
Genetic and chromosomal diseases
Klinefelter's syndrome
Myotonic muscular dystrophy
Hormonal disturbances
Hypopituitarism
Excess of androgen
Excess of estrogen
Exogenous adverse effects
Irradiation
Chemotherapy
Vascular diseases
Atherosclerosis
Vasculitis
Torsion of the testis
Infection

tive of an injury to the seminiferous epithelium. However, in some patients there are no obvious abnormalities in the seminiferous tubules, and the reasons for the functional or structural abnormalities detected by sperm analysis remain unexplained. Varicocele is considered a cause of abnormal spermatogenesis, but the mechanism of presumptive injury remains controversial. Inadequate mobility of sperm or teratospermia that is detected in ejaculates correlates poorly with histologic findings in testicular biopsies.

TUBULAR HYALINIZATION AND INTERSTITIAL FIBROSIS

Hyalinization of seminiferous tubules and widespread interstitial fibrosis are hallmarks of end-stage testis disease and irreversible reproductive failure (Wheeler, 1991). These histologic findings are nonspecific and represent the end result of many genetic, hormonally mediated, infectious, and vascular diseases and follow metabolic, toxic, or physical injury of the testis (box on p. 179).

Hyalinization of seminiferous tubules is accompanied by a loss of germinal epithelium followed in later stages by a disappearance of Sertoli cells and obliteration of the entire lumen (Fig. 8-10). In the final stage, only outlines (so-called ghosts) of the tubules remain (Fig. 8-11). Concomitant with the changes inside the tubules there is peritubular fibrosis that spreads through the interstitial spaces. Leydig cells usually remain spared and embedded in dense, fibrous tissue, forming small groups (Fig. 8-12). The entire testis shrinks and is traversed with fibrous strands surrounding small remnants of parenchyma. Within these remnants of parenchyma, scattered tubules may show signs of spermatogenesis even in late stages of the disease. However, few of these sperm cells reach the excretory ducts because of scarring and obstruction of the tubules.

GERM CELL NEOPLASIA

Germ cell neoplasia may be considered the greatest deviation from normal spermatogenesis. Malignant transformation of spermatogonia leads to proliferation of neoplastic cells that mechanically replace the normal spermatogenic cells and elimination of the stem cell pool needed for the maintenance of spermatogenesis (Fig. 8-13). Additional adverse effects include:

1. *Compression of the normal parenchyma by mass effect*—This causes an atrophy of normal testicular

components further reducing the number of spermatogenic cells.
2. *Mechanical obstruction of sperm flow*—Intratubular tumor cells may impede the entry of sperm into the excretory ducts. The tumor mass can also compress the excretory ducts.

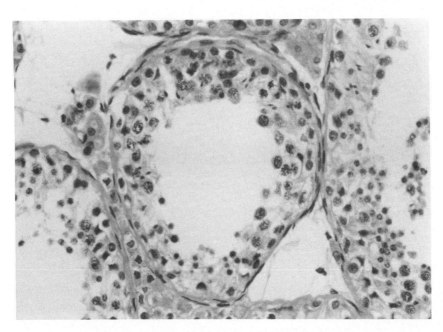

Fig. 8-8. Hypospermatogenesis. There is partial maturation arrest with only a few spermatozoa formed.

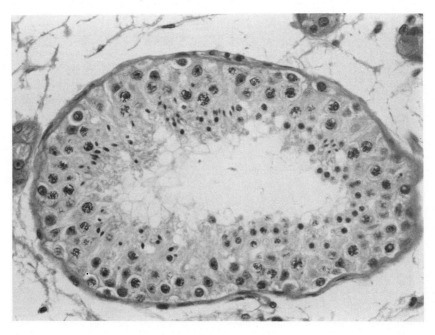

Fig. 8-9. The seminiferous tubule in hypospermatogenesis shows normal maturation of spermatogenic cells but appears "empty" and contains few spermatozoa.

3. *Damaged blood-testis barrier*—The integrity of the blood-testis barrier may be breached, adversely affecting spermatogenesis.

4. *Circulatory disturbances*—Blood flow may be compromised by tumor, adversely affecting spermatogenesis.

5. *Immune response to the tumor*—The humoral and cellular responses to tumor-specific antigens and antigens common to tumor cells and spermatogenic cells may depress spermatogenesis. Cytokines from lymphocytes and macrophages may influence the maturation of spermatogenic cells and renewal of their stem cell populations.

These hypothetical effects of germ cell tumors on spermatogenesis and the reproductive function of the testis are poorly understood albeit readily recognized in testicular biopsies (Fig. 8-14).

Clinical studies have established several facts that point to the relationship between infertility and germ cell neoplasia (Giwercman et al., 1991). These facts could be summarized as follows:

1. The prevalence of testicular cancer and infertility is increased in men with cryptorchidism as compared with men who have normally located scrotal testes (Krabbe et al., 1979; Pedersen et al., 1987). Testicular biopsies in these studies have reported a 3% to 8% prevalence of carcinoma in situ in such testes (Giwercman et al., 1989). Orchiopexy does not reduce the incidence of tumors in cryptorchid testes, and thus there is no means to prevent the development of tumors. The prevalence of tumors in cryptorchid testes correlates with the prevalence of infertility in these men. Biopsy studies performed by Giwercman et al. (1989) disclosed that the cryptorchid testes with tumors show advanced stages of spermatogenesis in only 37% of cases. One could conclude that cryptorchidism impairs spermatogenesis and favors tumorigenesis. It remains to be shown whether this is due to inherent germ cell abnormalities or to the microenvironment of cryptorchid testes. It is also possible that testicular neoplasia and

---

Causes of hypospermatogenesis

Idiopathic
Chromosomal anomalies
    Sex chromosome defects
    Down's syndrome
Hormonal disturbances
    Prolactinemia
    Adrenocortical excess
    Hypothyroidism
    Exogenous hormones (androgens, corticosteroids)
Systemic diseases
    Malnutrition
    Viral diseases
Exogenous adverse effects
    Irradiation
    Heat
    Chemotherapy
    Alcohol

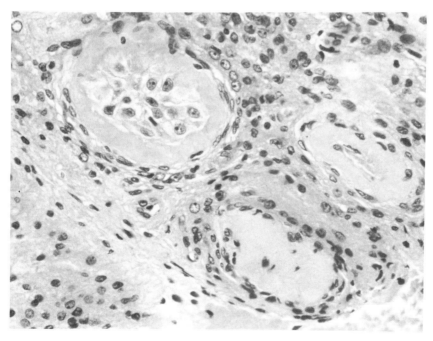

Fig. 8-10. Hyalinization of seminiferous tubules in Klinefelter's syndrome.

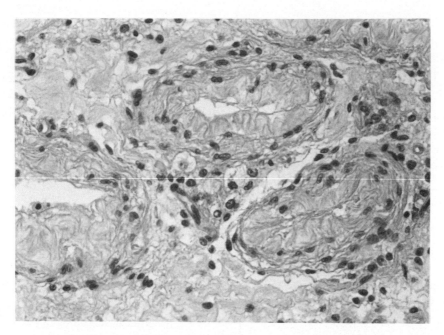

Fig. 8-11. Extensive hyalinization of seminiferous tubules.

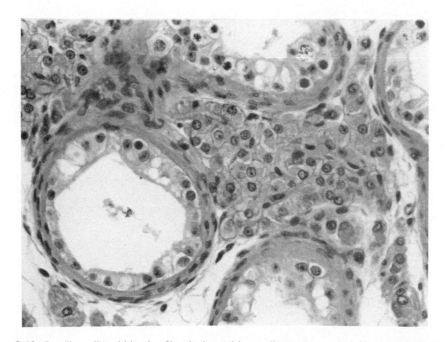

Fig. 8-12. Leydig cells within the fibrotic interstitium adjacent to a seminiferous tubule that shows atrophy.

testicular maldescent are related to the same etiologic factors that influence the development of gonocytes.

2. The prevalence of carcinoma in situ of the testis is increased in infertile men as compared with normal fertile men (Berthelsen and Skakkebaek, 1981; Pryor et al., 1983).

3. The prevalence of infertility is higher in men with testicular cancer than in age-matched controls.

4. Men with Klinefelter's syndrome and a 47,XXY karyotype suffer from infertility. At the same time an increased incidence of mediastinal germ cell tumors has been reported in these men, suggesting that this chromosomal abnormality is linked to both in-

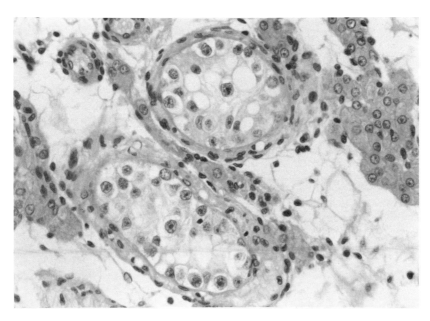

Fig. 8-13. Carcinoma *in situ* replacing the normal seminiferous epithelium.

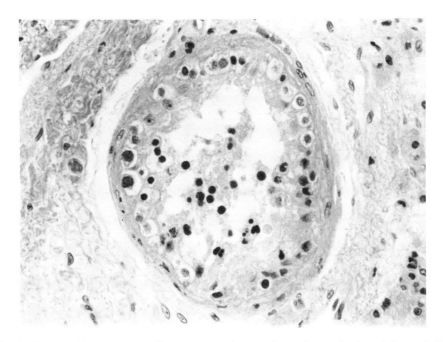

Fig. 8-14. Seminiferous tubule adjacent to a seminorma shows disorganization of the seminiferous epithelium, maturation arrest, and atypical cells.

fertility and germ cell neoplasia (Lachman et al., 1986).

5. There is increasing evidence that testicular carcinoma in situ and infertility represent inborn lesions, probably relating to early stages of gonadogenesis (Giwercman et al., 1991). However, clinical symptoms and the diagnosis of both conditions usually are delayed until adult life.

Germ cell tumors in infertile men show essentially the same features as testicular germ cell tumors in general (Damjanov, 1991). Awareness of the higher incidence of germ cell neoplasia in cryptorchid testes and infertile men has prompted a more active search for early cancer in these men and has resulted in reports of an increased incidence of carcinoma in situ (Giwercman et al., 1991). Early biopsies or screening based on noninvasive techniques promises to reduce the incidence of invasive testicular cancer by eradicating the cancer in the preinvasive stages of development. However, there is no evidence that therapy for testicular cancer improves fertility.

REFERENCES

Berthelsen JG, Skakkebaek NE: Value of testicular biopsy in diagnosing carcinoma *in situ* testis. Scand J Urol Nephrol 1981; 15:165.

Damjanov I: Pathobiology of human germ cell neoplasia. Recent Results Cancer Res 1991; 123:1.

de Kretser DM: Endocrinology of male infertility. Br Med Bull 1979; 35:187.

de Kretser DM, Burger HG, Fortune D, Hudson B, Long AR, Paulsen CA, Taft HP: Hormonal, histological and chromosomal studies in adult males with testicular disorders. J Clin Endocrinol Metab 1972; 35:392.

del Castillo EB, Trabucco A, de la Balze FE: Syndrome produced by absence of the germinal epithelium without impairment of the Sertoli or Leydig cells. J Clin Endocrinol 1947; 7:493.

Giwercman A, Bruun E, Frimodt-Moller C, Skakkebaek NE: Prevalence of carcinoma *in situ* and other histopathological abnormalities in testes of men with a history of cryptorchidism. J Urol 1989; 142:998.

Giwercman A, Müller J, Skakkebaek NE: Carcinoma *in situ* of the testis: Possible origin, clinical significance, and diagnostic methods. Recent Results Cancer Res 1991; 123:21.

Johnsen SG: Testicular biopsy score count—a method for registration of spermatogenesis in human testes: Normal values and results in 335 hypogonadal males. Hormones 1970; 1:2.

Kamidono S, Matsumoto O, Ishigani J, Nakao Y, Tsuji K: Infertility and HLA antigen-male infertility and infertile couples. Correlation between HLA antigen and infertility. Andrologia 1980; 12:317.

Krabbe S, Skakkebaek NE, Berthelsen JG, Eyben FV, Volsted P, Mauritzen K, et al: High incidence of undetected neoplasia in maldescended testes. Lancet 1979; 1:999.

Lachman MF, Kim K, Koo B-C: Mediastinal teratoma associated with Klinefelter's syndrome. Arch Pathol Lab Med 1986; 110:1067.

Levin HS: Testicular biopsy in the study of male infertility: Its current usefulness, histologic techniques, and prospects for the future. Hum Pathol 1979; 10:569.

Micic S, Micic M, Ilic V, Genbačev O, Dotlić R: Endocrine profile of 45 patients with Sertoli cell only syndrome. Andrologia 1983; 15:228.

Nistal M, Paniagua R, Abaurrea MA, Santamaria L: Hyperplasia and the immature appearance of Sertoli cells in primary testicular disorders. Hum Pathol 1982; 13:3.

Pedersen KV, Boisen P, Zetterlund CG: Experience of screening for carcinoma-*in-situ* of the testis among young men with surgically corrected maldescended testes. Int J Androl 1987; 10:181.

Pesce CM: The testicular biopsy in the evaluation of male infertility. Semin Diagn Pathol 1987; 4:264.

Pryor JP, Cameron KM, Chilton CP, Ford TF, Parkinson MC, Sinokrot J, Westwood CA: Carcinoma *in situ* in testicular biopsies from men presenting with infertility. Br J Urol 1983; 55:780.

Söderström KO, Suominen J: Human hypospermatogenesis. Histopathology and ultrastructure. Arch Pathol Lab Med 1982; 106:231.

Trainer TD: Histology of the normal testis. Am J Surg Pathol 1987; 11:797.

Wheeler JE: Histology of the fertile and infertile testis. In Pathology of Reproductive Failure, edited by Kraus FT, Damjanov I, Kaufman N. Baltimore, Williams & Wilkins, 1991, p. 56.

Wong T-W, Straus FH II, Foster LV: Cytoplasmic granular change of Sertoli cells: Two cases of Sertoli cells-only syndrome. Arch Pathol Lab Med 1988; 112:200.

Wong T-W, Straus FH II, Jones TM, Warner NE: Pathological aspects of the infertile testes. Urol Clin North Am 1978; 5:503.

Wong T-W, Straus FH II, Warner NE: Testicular biopsy in the study of male infertility. I. Testicular causes of infertility. Arch Pathol 1973; 95:151.

Wong T-W, Straus FH II, Warner NE: Testicular biopsy in the study of male infertility. II. Posttesticular causes of infertility. Arch Pathol 1973; 95:160.

Wong T-W, Straus FH II, Warner NE: Testicular biopsy in the study of male infertility. III. Pretesticular causes of infertility. Arch Pathol 1974; 98:1.

Chapter 9

PATHOLOGY OF THE CONCEPTUS AND EARLY PREGNANCY

PATHOLOGY OF THE ZYGOTE AND CLEAVAGE-STAGE EMBRYOS

Embryonic development begins at fertilization of the oocyte. The fertilized ovum or zygote undergoes several divisions while still enclosed in the zona pellucida. During these cleavage stages of embryogenesis the total size of the embryo enlarges only slightly and measurable growth begins only after the embryo has reached the blastocyst stage and has hatched from the zona pellucida (reviewed by Damjanov, 1991). As the hatching coincides with the entry of the embryo into the uterus, the embryo establishes contact with the endometrium and begins to implant (reviewed by Glasser et al., 1989; Aplin, 1991). Implantation signals and hormonal influences act on the uterus, provoking deciduation and other adaptive changes that are essential for the intrauterine stages of pregnancy.

The human zygote develops at a predictable rate (Tesarik, 1989; Tesarik and Testart, 1989). The first cleavage division occurs 24 to 28 hours after fertilization, and under optimal conditions the first three cleavage divisions are completed within the first 3 days of fertilization. In vitro fertilized ova typically are allowed to develop to the four-cell stage and then are transferred to the uterus or the fallopian tube of the biologic or surrogate mother. Success of in vitro fertilization critically depends on the quality of harvested oocytes. The quality of the oocytes is inversely proportional to the age of the donors, which correlates with reduced fertility in older women (Navot et al., 1991).

It has been estimated that more than 50% of all pregnancies end in abortion (Simpson, 1990). Most of these pregnancy losses occur before the pregnancy is clinically recognized. Spontaneous abortions interrupt approximately 15% to 20% of all clinically diagnosed pregnancies (Laferla, 1986). Using various approaches that are summarized by Boué (1988), different investigators have arrived at similar conclusions, i.e., less than one third of all conceptions result in a live birth. Only 21% to 28% of women who conceive will produce a full-term infant per interrupted menstrual cycle. From 100 ova that are fertilized in vivo, one can expect 31 live births. Even the most successful in vitro fertilization programs have less than 30% live-born children per 100 ova fertilized.

The quality of oocytes retrieved for in vitro fertilization can be assessed visually under the dissection microscope. Several grading systems have been proposed. The criteria used for choosing the best oocytes for in vitro fertilization, outlined by Hill et al. (1989), are presented in Table 9-1. The best results are obtained with mature oocytes. In vitro fertilization can be accomplished in 50% to 85% of cases but, there is only a 20% rate of live births.

Fertilization of the ovum is followed by the extrusion of the second polar body. If the polar body is not extruded, a triploid zygote will result. Alternatively, triploidy may develop after fertilization of the oocyte with two spermatozoa. Triploid embryos have a reduced developmental capacity and should be eliminated. Similarly, oocytes that

Table 9-1. Grading of Oocyte Maturity*

Grade	Cumulus Oophorus	Corona Radiata	Ooplasm	Membrana Granulosa Cells
1 Immature	Dense, compact	Adherent, compact	If visible contains germinal vesicle	Compact, aggregated
2 Nearly mature	Expanded	Slightly compact	Clear	Expanded, aggregated
3 Preovulatory, or mature	Very expanded	Radiant, visible zona pellucida	Clear	Still well aggregated
4 Postmature	Expanded with clumps	Radiant but clumped zona pellucida	Granular or dark	Small and nonaggregated
5 Atretic	Not present	Clumped, irregular	Dark	Clumped

*Based on data from Hill et al., 1989.
Reproduced from Kraus FT, Damjanov I, Kaufman N: Pathology of Reproductive Failure. Williams & Wilkins, Baltimore, 1991, with permission. ©The United States and Canadian Academy of Pathology

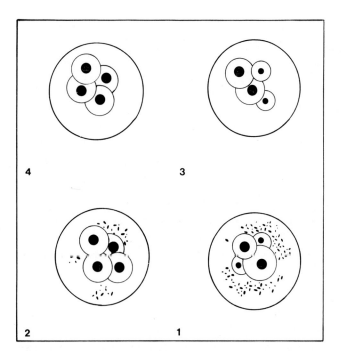

Fig. 9-1. Schematic presentation of the grading system devised by Hill et al. (1989) for the evaluation of four cell human embryos. Grade 4 is assigned to the embryos that have the best developmental potential upon transfer to the pregnant woman. (Modified from Hill GA et al. Fertil Steril 1989; 52:801, with permission of the publisher, The American Fertility Society.)

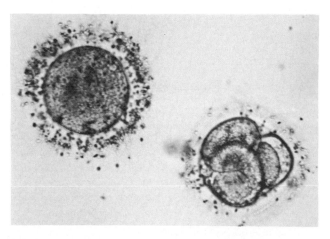

Fig. 9-2. An immature oocyte that was not fertilized adjacent to a normal four cell embryo obtained by *in vitro* fertilization.

Table 9-2. Chromosomal abnormalities in human embryos obtained by in vitro fertilization

Karyotype	Frequency of abnormalities (%)
Haploid	1.6
Diploid	21.2
Triploid	6.4
TOTAL	29.2

Data from Plachot et al., 1988.

have not been fertilized but have undergone spontaneous parthenogenetic activation are not suitable for intrauterine development. Approximately 3% to 7% of oocytes fertilized in vitro are triploid and 1.5% to 4% of oocytes undergo parthenogenetic activation (Plachot et al., 1988; Hardy et al., 1989; Dandekar et al., 1990).

Embryos ready for transfer into the uterus or the fallopian tube after in vitro fertilization could be evaluated using the criteria developed in several laboratories. The system advocated by Hill et al. (1989), which is applied to four-cell-stage embryos, takes into account the appearance of the blastomeres, their size, and the presence or absence of the detritus within the zona pellucida (Fig. 9-1). Opti-

mal results are obtained with grade 4 embryos, which are composed of equally sized blastomeres and show no evidence of degeneration. Grade 3 embryos are composed of unevenly sized blastomeres but show no evidence of fragmentation or degeneration. Grade 2 embryos are composed of equally sized blastomeres but also contain fragments and cell detritus within the zona pellucida. Grade 1 embryos are composed of unevenly sized blastomeres and cellular debris. Grade 1 embryos are least viable and are least likely to develop to term if transplanted into the uterus or fallopian tube.

Chromosomal anomalies may be found in morphologically normal as well as abnormal embryos (Plachot et al.,

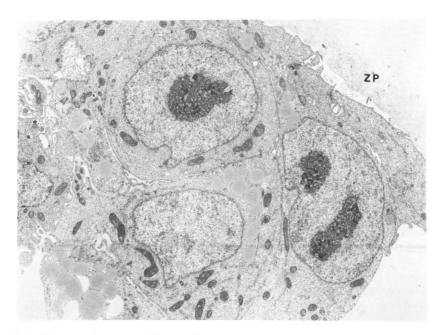

Fig. 9-3. Electron microscopy of human blastocyst stage embryo obtained by *in vitro* fertilization. Embryo showing only minor abnormalities such as an excess of lipid droplets. Zona pellucida *(ZP)* is normal. (From Hardy K, Handyside AH, Winston RML. Development 1989; 107:597, and Company of Biologists, Ltd, with permission.)

1989). A multicenter study (Plachot et al., 1988) disclosed that 26% of harvested but unfertilized oocytes and 29.2% of embryos that were obtained from various in vitro fertilization programs had chromosomal anomalies (Table 9-2). Abnormal embryos either are unsuitable for intrauterine transfer or are eliminated spontaneously after implantation. Among the morphologically abnormal diploid embryos, 32.6% had chromosomal anomalies, indicating that chromosomal anomalies may cause early detectable developmental anomalies. However, not all embryos with abnormal chromosomes can be recognized by inspection, and it was shown that 21.4% of such embryos have chromosomal anomalies. Nevertheless, even if morphologically normal embryos with chromosomal anomalies are transferred to the uterus, most of them do not develop to term. Only 0.6% of term newborns studied by Plachot et al. (1988) had chromosomal anomalies, which indicates that the remaining embryos with karyotypic defects were spontaneously aborted either by failing to implant or by spontaneously aborting.

Abnormal embryos can be recognized by light (Fig. 9-2) or electron microscopy (Figs. 9-3 to 9-6). According to Plachot et al. (1987), the most prominent features of abnormal embryos are:

1. Binucleated or anucleated blastomeres
2. Vacuolization of the cytoplasm
3. Fragmentation of the cytoplasm and formation of anucleated blebs
4. Multilobed nuclei or multinucleated blastomeres

Evaluation of zygotes and embryos is usually done by gynecologists and developmental biologists performing *in vitro* fertilization and the material is rarely if ever sent to pathologists for microscopic examination. However, in the future pathologists might become more involved in this process.

PATHOLOGY OF IMPLANTATION

The exact mechanism of implantation is not fully understood (reviewed by Glasser et al., 1987; Aplin, 1991). The morphologic aspects of normal and abnormal implantation have been described by Hertig et al. (1956), and although these descriptions were amplified in subsequent electron microscopic studies (Knoth and Larsen, 1972) or *in vitro* studies (Lindenberg et al., 1986, 1989), the mechanism of interaction between the embryo and the maternal organism still has not been elucidated.

Approximately 20% of all ova fertilized in vitro do not implant upon transfer to the uterine cavity, indicating that the failure of implantation is an important cause of reproductive failure. These failures are due in part both to embryonic and maternal factors or to dysfunction in their interplay. Currently, it is not possible to predict with certainty whether implantation will occur. Embryonic factors can be minimized by selecting good-quality embryos for implantation; maternal factors are still treated empirically.

Ectopic pregnancy

Ectopic pregnancy results from implantation of the embryo in an extrauterine site. In most cases, ectopic implan-

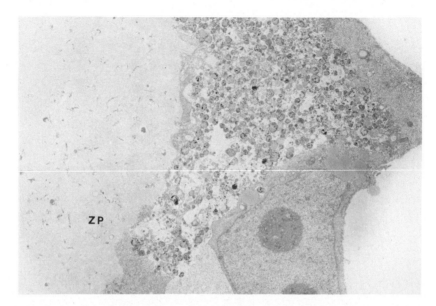

Fig. 9-4. Electron microscopy of human blastocyst stage embryo obtained by in vitro fertilization. Zona pellucida *(ZP)* contains debris and the trophoblastic cells show marked degenerative changes. (From Hardy K, Handyside AH, Winston RML. Development 1989; 107:597, and Company of Biologists, Ltd, with permission.)

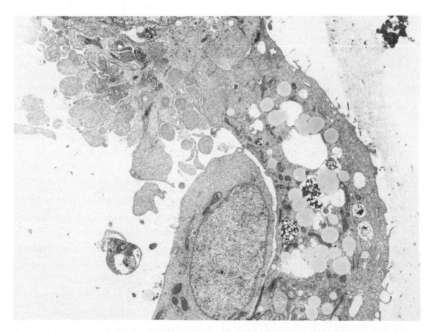

Fig. 9-5. Electron microscopy of human blastocyst stage embryo obtained by in vitro fertilization. Marked degenerative changes in the cytoplasm of the trophoblastic cell. (From Hardy K, Handyside AH, Winston RML. Development 1989; 107:597, and Company of Biologists, Ltd, with permission.)

tation occurs in the fallopian tubes and less frequently on the ovaries, on the peritoneal surface of the abdominal cavity, and in the vagina.

Incidence and etiology. The epidemiologic data reviewed by Ory (1992) indicate an increased incidence of ectopic pregnancies in the United States. Between 1970 and 1987 the number of ectopic pregnancies increased

fivefold from 17,800 to 88,000 per year. The rate increased from 4.5 to 16.8 per 1000 pregnancies and was comparable for all groups of women registered during this period.

The etiology of ectopic pregnancy remains elusive. Risk factors include a history of pelvic inflammatory disease, tubal adhesions, and other pelvic pathologic pro-

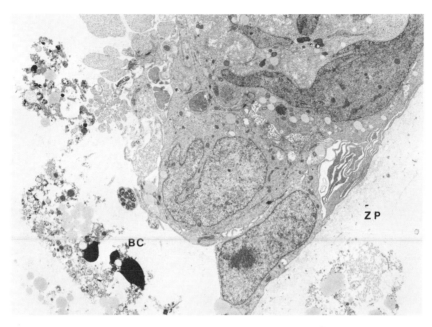

Fig. 9-6. Electron microscopy of human blastocyst stage embryo obtained by in vitro fertilization. Abnormal blastocyst contains cellular detritus in the blastocele cavity *(BC)* and zona pellucida *(ZP)*. (From Hardy K, Handyside AH, Winston RML. Development 1989; 107:597, and Company of Biologists, Ltd, with permission.)

Risk factors for ectopic pregnancy

Pelvic inflammatory disease
Salpingitis isthmica nodosa
Previous ectopic pregnancy
Infertility
Surgery
    Pelvic surgery
    Appendectomy
    Tubal surgery (tubal ligation with reanastomosis, lysis
        of tubal adhesions)
Exposure to diethylstilbestrol in utero

---

cesses that could affect tubal patency and tubal peristalsis, thus causing interference with the normal passage of zygote through the fallopian tube. Tubal pathology is considered to be the most common cause, but in 70% of women the fallopian tubes are histologically normal (Pauerstein et al., 1986). Nordenskjold and Ahlgren (1991) identified as the most important risk factors previous ectopic pregnancy, tuboplasty, gynecologic laparotomies, salpingitis, and appendectomy. The risk factors for ectopic pregnancy are listed in the box above. One or more of these risk factors were found in 76.5% of affected women and in 23% of controls.

Clinical and laboratory findings. Advances in clinical biochemistry and ultrasonography have made it possible to recognize ectopic pregnancies at an early stage. In early stages of pregnancy an ectopic pregnancy may be indistinguishable from a normal uterine pregnancy. Typical clinical symptoms associated with extrauterine pregnancy usually appear during weeks 6 to 10 of gestation. In addition to the usual signs of pregnancy, symptoms may include abdominal pain, abdominal tenderness, vaginal bleeding, adnexal tenderness, or an adnexal mass palpable on gynecologic examination (Weckstein, 1985). Tenesmus, dizziness, loss of consciousness, orthostatic hypotension, and fever usually are associated with rupture of the fallopian tube and hemorrhage. Death due to paroxysmal exsanguination is rare today.

Major advances in the diagnosis and treatment of ectopic pregnancies that help immensely in retaining fertility after an ectopic pregnancy were made possible by the introduction of human chorionic gonadotropin (hCG) radioimmunoassays capable of detecting hCG in concentrations of 0.01 ng/ml; high-resolution ultrasonography, which can visualize very early gestational sacs; and laser laparoscopy, which, in well-trained hands, can eliminate the pregnancy with minimal surgical insult.

The serum concentrations of hCG are most useful for monitoring the pregnancy. During early normal pregnancy, serum concentrations of hCG double every 1.98 days (Kadar et al., 1981), and since this highly predictable increase does not occur in abnormal pregnancies, an increase of less than 66% over 48 hours is indicative of either an ectopic or an abnormal uterine pregnancy. Ultrasonography, which is the most efficient method of confirming the presence or absence of an intrauterine preg-

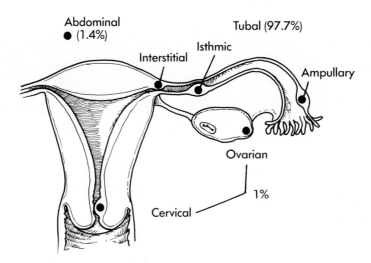

Fig. 9-7. The most common sites of ectopic pregnancy according to Breen, 1970.

nancy, together with the hormonal data virtually secures the diagnosis. Laparoscopy is confirmatory.

Ultrasonographic proof of an intrauterine pregnancy does not exclude the coexistence of an ectopic pregnancy. Combined pregnancies in the uterus and in an ectopic site occur at a rate of 1 in 4000 (Bello et al., 1986). The rate of combined pregnancies is increased after in vitro fertilization and occurs in the range of 1 in 100 pregnancies (Molloy et al., 1990; Dimitry et al., 1990).

Ectopic pregnancies may be treated by laparoscopic surgery with preservation of the fallopian tube, salpingocentesis, surgical resection of the involved segment of the tube with reanastomosis, or complete salpingectomy (Leach and Ory, 1989). Treatment with methotrexate, followed by serial hCG measurement and ultrasonographic monitoring, is widely used and is becoming an acceptable alternative to surgery (Brown et al., 1991).

Infertility is a common sequela of ectopic pregnancy, occurring after at least 30% of such pregnancies (Ory, 1992). It has been estimated that at least 30 percent of ectopic pregnancies will entail infertility (Ory, 1992). However, in many women ectopic pregnancy is preceded by prolonged periods of involuntary infertility, suggesting that infertility and ectopic pregnancy are related to the same etiologic factors. In these women infertility usually persists after the ectopic pregnancy is successfully treated.

Pathologic findings. Breen (1970) reviewed data on 654 patients and noted that 97.7% of ectopic pregnancies were tubal, 1.4% were abdominal, and less than 1% ovarian or cervical (Fig. 9-7).

Ectopic pregnancy has many histologic features in common with normal intrauterine pregnancy (Budowick et al., 1980). After the nidation of the embryo among the folds of the fallopian tube, the trophoblastic cells invade the wall of the tube, causing tissue destruction, hemorrhage, and deposition of fibrin. This causes tubal distention and rupture (Fig. 9-8).

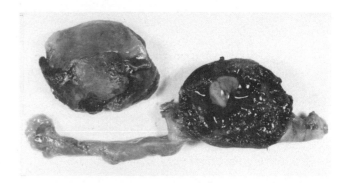

Fig. 9-8. Tubal pregnancy. The fallopian tube ruptured and had to be resected.

The blastocyst may implant on the ovary or the surface of the peritoneum in the same manner (Fig. 9-9). In some cases the peritoneal pregnancy represents secondary implantation of placental fragments from a ruptured tubal pregnancy. Tissue invasion of the trophoblast is associated with a weak decidual reaction in the fallopian tubes and almost no decidual reaction in the ovary or on the peritoneum.

Among placental cells one can distinguish cytotrophoblastic, syncytiotrophoblastic, and intermediate trophoblastic cells (O'Connor and Kurman, 1988). Morphologically, these cells are identical to those in orthotopic implantation sites.

Ectopic pregnancy may provoke major hemorrhage, and unless prompt hemostasis is achieved, massive hemoperitoneum may ensue with a lethal outcome. Other complications include local tissue destruction, calcification of the necrotic tissue, or fetal remnants. Many ectopic pregnancies are, however, spontaneously aborted or resorbed without major consequences or complications (Garcia et al., 1987). After surgical removal of the gestational sac from the fallopian tube, some trophoblastic tissue may remain (Pauerstein et al., 1986). This trophoblastic tissue may

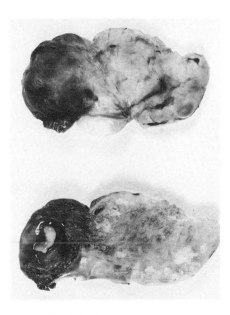

Fig. 9-9. Ovarian pregnancy.

proliferate and cause additional tissue destruction and hemorrhage. The symptoms of ectopic pregnancy recur in such cases within 2 weeks and are associated with elevated levels of serum hCG. Treatment with methotrexate usually is used with very good results (Rose and Cohen, 1990).

Spontaneous abortion

Spontaneous abortion or miscarriage is defined as an early involuntary termination of pregnancy with expulsion of the embryo before it has reached viability (Stirrat, 1990; McBride, 1991). Although the exact definition of *abortus* varies from state to state, the term generally is used for pregnancies less than 20 weeks and fetuses weighing less than 500 g.

Incidence. The incidence of spontaneous pregnancies is unknown because of underreporting and because many clinically are unrecognized or mistaken for delayed menstruation or metrorrhagia. It has been estimated that at least 15% of clinically recognized pregnancies end in abortions (Laferla, 1986); the true incidence could be much higher.

Preclinical abortions. Preclinical abortions usually are unrecognized unless special efforts have been taken to monitor the early pregnancy, as is typically done with *in vitro* fertilization. According to Acosta et al. (1990), the diagnosis of preclinical abortion is acceptable if the following criteria are met:

1. Fertilization was successfully performed and the embryo was transferred to the mother without technical difficulties.
2. Transient and synchronous elevation of serum β-hCG, estradiol, and progesterone has been documented during the 13 days after hCG was administered.

<table>
<tr><td>

Causes of spontaneous abortions

Fetal factors

Chromosomal anomalies
Lethal genes
Mutations
Developmental anomalies

Placental Factors

Placental anomalies
Hydatidiform mole

Maternal factors

Anatomic anomalies
Endocrine insufficiency
Immune disorders

Infections
External adverse influences

Alcohol
Drugs
Radiation
Surgery

</td></tr>
</table>

3. Vaginal bleeding occurs within the first 14 days after the missed menstrual period, i.e., 28 days after oocyte aspiration and fertilization. Using these strict criteria, it was shown that certain women fall into a group called "the preclinical abortion group" and have a tendency to abort at a higher rate than other women. Causative factors are not well defined.

Recurrent abortion. Recurrent abortion, also known as habitual abortion, is defined as pregnancy loss with three or more consecutive gestations (Stirrat, 1990). In these women, one can distinguish a primary group composed of women who have lost all previous pregnancies and a second group composed of women who have had at least one successful pregnancy. The probability that a third miscarriage will occur after two previous pregnancies have ended in abortions is in the range of 17% to 35%. For women who have had three or more miscarriages, the chances of aborting subsequent pregnancies are between 25% and 46% (Stirrat, 1990).

Etiology. The etiology of spontaneous abortions is complex, and although many risk factors have been identified, the cause of abortion usually is obscure. Two general categories have been defined: those factors pertaining to the conceptus and those operating in the maternal organism. These can be further subdivided into several subsets listed in the box above.

Clinical findings. On the basis of history and gynecologic clinical data, it is customary to recognize six categories of spontaneous abortion: threatened, inevitable, incomplete, complete, missed, and septic (McBride, 1991).

Table 9-3. Causes of vaginal bleeding before the 20th week of pregnancy in 1549 women studied by Cavanaugh et al. (1964)

Diagnosis	Frequency (%)
Threatened abortion	14
Inevitable and incomplete abortion	61
Complete abortion	13
Septic abortion	4
Missed abortion	2
Hydatidiform mole	1
Tubal pregnancy	5
TOTAL	100

Table 9-4. Chromosomal abnormalities detected in 2743 spontaneous abortions studied by Creasy (1988)

Chromosomal abnormality	Frequency (%)
Trisomy	52
Sex chromosome monosomy	20
Polyploidy	21
Structural abnormality	3.5
Mosaicism	3
Other	0.5
TOTAL	100

Modified from Creasy MR. In Beard RW, Sharp F (Eds). Early Pregnancy Loss. New York, Springer Verlag, 1988, by permission.

Table 9-3 lists the frequency of occurrence of each category (Cavanaugh et al., 1964).

Pathologic findings. The pathologic aspects of spontaneous abortions were analyzed systematically by Hertig and Sheldon (1943), who attributed pregnancy loss primarily to the abnormal conceptus. More detailed analysis, summarized by Boué (1988) and Kalousek (1991), confirmed those data and showed that spontaneous abortions are related in most instances to chromosomal anomalies, developmental defects in the morphogenesis of the embryo, abnormal implantation, and abnormal placentogenesis and less often to anatomic, functional, or immune abnormalities of the mother.

On the basis of gross examination, one can determine whether an embryo shows growth disorganization, is morphologically normal, or shows growth disorganization or localized defects (Kalousek, 1991). Among the aborted conceptuses that are well enough preserved to make possible a complete evaluation, approximately 48% show growth disorganization, 20% are morphologically normal, and 16% have localized defects; the remaining 16% are fragmented and degenerated (Kalousek, 1991). Growth disorganization (GD) can be classified further into four categories:

GD1—The most severe failure of embryonic development. The embryonic sac contains no embryo at all and is filled with mucoid material. The amnion is closely apposed to the chorion, which has few villi. These chorionic villi appear hydropic and are lined by attenuated trophoblast cells.

GD2—Abnormal development, which profoundly affects the embryo. The embryo is transformed into a 1-mm to 4-mm nodule lying within an attached embryo directly to the internal surface of the amnion or through a short body stalk. A yolk sac may be seen attached to the embryo. The chorionic villi are underdeveloped and resemble those in GD1 conceptuses.

GD3—Development is abnormal, but the embryo is better developed, though still not fully organized.

The embryo lacks external features of a human body but shows retinal pigmentation in the cephalic area.

GD4—Developmental disorder resulting in general retardation of embryonic development. Although the embryo shows the typical external signs of body formation, various parts are disproportionately formed and some parts are either missing or unrecognizable. Localized defects are less commonly detected in these embryos and early fetuses than growth disorganization. In addition to malformations, which are detectable on external gross examination, other common malformations include central nervous system, cardiovascular, and alimentary tract anomalies (Kalousek, 1991). These grossly disorganized embryos frequently have chromosomal abnormalities, which range from 73% in GD2 embryos to 37% in GD4 embryos (Kalousek, 1991). Among the chromosomal anomalies, the most common are trisomies, sex chromosomal monosomies, and polyploidy; structural chromosomal anomalies are less common (Table 9-4). Embryos with only localized embryonic defects as well as normal embryos may have chromosomal abnormalities.

GESTATIONAL TROPHOBLASTIC DISEASE

Gestational trophoblastic disease (GTD) denotes several developmental and proliferative disorders of the placenta, including hydatidiform mole, choriocarcinoma, and related disorders (Kurman, 1991) as listed in the box on p. 191.

Incidence and pathogenesis

Hydatidiform mole occurs in the United States in 1 in 1000 to 2000 pregnancies but is two to five times more common in Southeast Asia (Buckley, 1984). Choriocarcinoma occurs in 1 in 20,000 pregnancies. Most choriocarcinomas develop after molar pregnancy, but they may be a complication of normal as well as ectopic pregnancies.

The etiology of GTD is not clear, and the risk factors have not been fully defined. Cytogenetic studies show that

Gestational trophoblastic disease

Hydatidiform mole
    Complete
    Partial
Choriocarcinoma
Placental site trophoblastic tumor
    Exaggerated placental site
    Placental site nodule or plaques

Modified from Kurman RJ. In Kraus FT, Damjanov I, Kaufman N (Eds). Pathology of Reproductive Failure. Baltimore, Williams and Wilkins, 1991, by permission. © The United States and Canadian Academy of Pathology.

complete hydatidiform moles are diploid, whereas partial moles usually are triploid (Szulman and Surti, 1978). Chromosomes in the complete hydatidiform moles are of paternal origin, indicating that the maternal chromosomes have been lost. This process of fertilization, called *androgenesis,* results in degeneration of the conceptus early in pregnancy. The placenta develops abnormally and gives rise to the hydatidiform mole. Studies of triploid partial hydatidiform moles have shown that the cells of this lesion contain one maternal set of chromosomes and two paternal sets, which indicates that the ovum was fertilized by two spermatozoa. In addition to the molar changes involving the placenta, partial hydatidiform moles contain fetal parts. Chromosomal studies of choriocarcinoma and placental site trophoblastic tumors have not contributed to the understanding of the pathogenesis of these lesions.

Clinical findings

The symptoms of GTD vary. An abnormal pregnancy can be diagnosed readily in most patients with partial and complete hydatidiform moles (Szulman and Surti, 1984). Choriocarcinoma develops either subsequent to hydatidiform mole or after abortion and normal pregnancy (Olive et al., 1984). All patients with GTD have elevated serum levels of hCG, which is an important marker for monitoring the progress and regression of the disease. The prognosis for patients with hydatidiform mole is excellent, whereas the prognosis for those with choriocarcinoma depends on the extent of the disease (Mortakis and Braga, 1990).

Pathologic findings

Hydatidiform moles are characterized by massive hydropic transformation of the chorionic villi that gives the placenta a grapelike appearance. In a complete hydatidiform mole, all the villi have undergone hydropic transformation, whereas in a partial mole some villi appear normal and others are swollen. Fetal parts may be seen in the partial hydatidiform mole. The placental site trophoblastic tumors do not have any distinct gross morphologic features and appear as solid masses of tissue intermixed with clotted blood.

Microscopic findings are typical. In hydatidiform moles the stromal component of chorionic villi appears edematous and acellular, whereas the trophoblastic cells show signs of proliferation and nuclear atypia. Choriocarcinomas are composed of solid sheets of cytotrophoblastic cells admixed with multinucleated giant trophoblastic cells and intermediate trophoblasts. Placental site trophoblastic tumors consist predominantly of intermediate trophoblasts. Immunochemically, the syncytiotrophoblastic cells react with antibodies to hCG and the intermediate trophoblast with antibodies to human placental lactogen (Kurman, 1991).

REFERENCES

Acosta AA, Ochninger S, Hammer J, Muasher IIM, Jones DL. Preclinical abortions: Incidence and significance in the Norfolk in vitro fertilization program. Fertil Steril 1990; 53:673.

Aplin JD: Implantation, trophoblast differentiation and haemochorial placentation: Mechanistic evidence *in vivo* and *in vitro.* J Cell Sci 1991; 99:681.

Bello GV, Schonholz D, Moshirpur J, Jeng DY, Berkowitz RL. Combined pregnancy: the Mount Sinai experience. *Obstet Gynecol Surv.* 1986; 41:603.

Boué A: Spontaneous abortions and cytogenetic abnormalities. In Behrmans J, Kistner RW, Patton GW, editors: Progress in Infertility, 3rd ed, Boston, 1988, Little and Brown, p. 783.

Breen JL: A 21 year survey of 654 ectopic pregnancies. Am J Obstet Gynecol 1970; 106:1004.

Brown DL, Felker RE, Stovall TG, Emerson DS, Ling FW. Serial endovaginal sonography of ectopic pregnancies treated with methotrexate. Obstet Gynecol. 1991; 77:406.

Buckley JD: The epidemiology of molar pregnancy and choriocarcinoma. Clin Obstet Gynecol 1984; 27:153.

Budowick M, Johnson TR Jr, Genadry R, Parmley TH, Woodruff JD: The histopathology of the developing tubal ectopic pregnancy. Fertil Steril 1980; 34:169.

Cavanaugh D, Fleisher A, Ferguson JH: Inevitable and incomplete abortion. Am J Obstet Gynecol 1964; 90:216.

Creasy MR: The cytogenetics of spontaneous abortion in humans. In Early Pregnancy Loss, edited by Beard RW, Sharp F, New York, Springer-Verlag, 1988, p 293.

Damjanov I: Pathobiology of fertilization, embryonic cleavage, and implantation. In Pathology of Reproductive Failure, edited by Kraus FT, Damjanov I, Kaufman N. Baltimore, Williams & Wilkins, 1991, p 32.

Dandikar PV, Martin MC, glass RH: Polypronuclear embryos after in vitro fertilization. Fertil Steril, 1990; 53:510.

Dimitry ES, Subak-Sharpe R, Mills M, Margara R, Winston R. Nine cases of heterotopic pregnancies in four years of in vitro fertilization. *Fertil Steril.* 1990 53:107.

Glasser SR, Julian J, Mani SK, Mulholland H, Munir MI, Lampelo S, Soares MJ: Blastocyst-endometrial relationship: Reciprocal interactions between uterine epithelial and stromal cells and blastocysts. Trophoblast Res 1989; 5:8.

Glasser SR, Julian J, Munir MI, Soares MJ: Biological markers during early pregnancy: Trophoblastic signals of the peri-implantation period. Environ Health Perspect 1987; 74:129.

Garcia AJ, Aubert JM, Sama J, Josimovich JB. Expectant management of presumed ectopic pregnancies. *Fertil Steril.* 1987; 48:395.

Hardy K, Handyside AH, Winston RML: The human blastocyst: Cell number, death and allocation during late preimplantation development *in vitro.* Development 1989; 107:597.

Hertig AT, Rock J, Adams EC: A description of 34 human ova within the first 17 days of development. Am J Anat 1956; 98:435.

Hertig AT, Sheldon WH: Minimal criteria to prove prima facie case of traumatic abortion or miscarriage. Ann Surg 1943; 117:596.

Hill GA, Brodie BL, Herbert CM, Rogers BJ, Herbert CM III, Osteen KG, Wentz AC: The influence of oocyte maturity and embryo quality on pregnancy rate in a program for in vitro fertilization. Fertil Steril 1989; 52:801.

Kadar N, Caldwell BV, Romero R: A method of screening for ectopic pregnancy and its indications. Obstet Gynecol. 1981; 58:162.

Kadar N, DeVore G, Romer R. Discriminatory hCG zone: its use in the sonographic evaluation for ectopic pregnancy. Obstet Gynecol. 1981; 58:156.

Kalousek DK: Pathology of abortion: Chromosomal and genetic correlations. In Pathology of Reproductive Failure, edited by Kraus FT, Damjanov I, Kaufman N. Baltimore, Williams & Wilkins, 1991, p 228.

Knoth M, Larsen JF: Ultrastructure of human implantation site. Acta Obstet Gynecol Scand 1972; 51:385.

Krantz SG, Gray RH, Damewood MD, Wallach EE: Time trends in risk factors and clinical outcome of ectopic pregnancy. Fertil Steril 1990; 54:42.

Kurman RJ: Pathology of trophoblast. In Pathology of Reproductive Failure, edited by Kraus FT, Damjanov I, Kaufman N. Baltimore, Williams & Wilkins, 1991, p 195.

Laferla JJ: Spontaneous abortion. Clin Obstet Gynecol 1986; 13:105.

Lauritsen JG: Aetiology of spontaneous abortion. A cytogenetic and epidemiological study of 288 abortuses and their parents. Acta Obstet Gynecol Scand 1976; 52(Suppl):1.

Leach RL, Ory SJ: Modern management of ectopic pregnancy. J Reprod Med. 1989; 34:324.

Lindenberg S, Hyttel P, Lenz S, Holmes PV: Ultrastructure of the early human implantation in vitro. Hum Reprod 1986; 1:533.

Lindenberg S, Hyttel P, Sjogren A, Greve T: A comparative study of attachment of human, bovine and mouse blastocysts to uterine epithelial monolayer. Hum Reprod 1989; 4:446.

McBride WZ: Spontaneous abortion. Am Fam Physician 1991; 43:175.

Molloy D, Deambrosis W, Keeping D, Hynes J, Harrison K, Hennessey J: Multiple-sited (heterotopic) pregnancy after in vitro fertilization and gamete intrafallopian transfer. Fertil Steril. 1990; 53:1068

Mortakis AE, Braga CA. "Poor Prognosis" metastatic gestational trophoblastic disease: The prognostic significance of the scoring system in predicting chemotherapy failure. Obstet Gynecol 1990; 76:272.

Navot D, Bergh PA, Williams MA, Garrisi GJ, Guzman I, Sandler B, Grunfeld L: Poor oocyte quality rather than implantation failure as a cause of age-related decline in female fertility. Lancet 1991; 337:1375.

Nordenskjold F, Ahlgren M: Risk factors in ectopic pregnancy. Results of a population-based case-control study. Acta Obstet Gynecol Scand 1991; 70:575.

O'Connor DM, Kurman RJ: Intermediate trophoblast in uterine curettings in the diagnosis of ectopic pregnancy. Obstet Gynecol 1988; 72:665.

Olive DL, Lurain JR, Brewer JI: Choriocarcinoma associated with term gestation. Am J Obstet Gynecol 1984; 148:711.

Ory SJ: New options for diagnosis and treatment of ectopic pregnancy. JAMA 1992; 267:534.

Pauerstein CJ, Croxatto HB, Eddy CA, Ramzy I, Walters MD: Anatomy and pathology of tubal pregnancy. Obstet Gynecol. 1986; 67:301

Plachot M: Chromosome analysis of spontaneous abortions after IVF. A European survey. Hum Reprod 1989; 4:425.

Plachot M, Mandelbaum J, Junca AM, Cohen J, Salat-Baroux J, Da Lage C: Morphologic and cytologic study of human embryos obtained by in vitro fertilization. In Future Aspects in Human In Vitro Fertilization, edited by Feichtinger W, Kemeter P, Berlin, Springer-Verlag, 1987, p 267.

Plachot M, Mandelbaum J, Junca A-M, de Grouchy J, Salat-Baroux J, Cohen J: Cytogenetic analysis and developmental capacity of normal and abnormal embryos after IVF. Hum Reprod 1989; 4(Suppl):99.

Plachot M, Veiga A, Montagut J, de Grouchy J, Calderon G, Lepretre S, et al.: Are clinical and biological IVF parameters correlated with chromosomal disorders in early life: A multicentric study. Hum Reprod 1988; 3:627.

Rose PG, Cohen SM: Methotrexate therapy for persistent ectopic pregnancy after conservative laparoscopic management. Obstet Gynecol. 1990; 76:947.

Simpson JL: Incidence and timing of pregnancy losses: Relevance to evaluating safety of early prenatal diagnosis. Am J Med Genet 1990; 35:165.

Stirrat GM: Recurrent miscarriage. I. Definition and epidemiology. Lancet 1990; 336:673.

Stray-Pedersen B, Stray-Pedersen S: Etiologic factors and subsequent reproductive performance in 195 couples with a prior history of habitual abortion. Am J Obstet Gynecol 1984; 148:140.

Szulman AE, Surti U: The syndromes of hydatidiform mole. I. Cytogenetic and morphologic correlations. Am J Obstet Gynecol 1978; 131:665.

Szulman AE, Surti U: The syndromes of partial and complete molar gestation. Clin Obstet Gynecol 1984; 27:172.

Tesarik J: Developmental control of human preimplantation embryos: A comparative approach. J In Vitro Fertil Embryo Transf 1988; 5:347.

Tesarik J: Involvement of oocyte-coded message in cell differentiation control of early human embryos. Development 1989; 105:317.

Tesarik J, Testart J: Human sperm-egg interactions and their disorders: Implications in the management of infertility. Hum Reprod 1989; 4:729.

Weckstein LN: Current perspective on ectopic pregnancy. Obstet Gynecol Surv 1985; 40:259.

INDEX

Figures are indicated by *f*; tables are indicated by *t*.

Seminal vesicles—cont'd
  rectal palpation of, 11
  variations in size and shape of, 92*f*
Seminiferous tubules
  diameter of, 20
  evaluation of changes involving, 22
  hyalinization of, 177, 180*f*
    causes of, 179
    in Klinefelter's syndrome, 179*f*
  hypospermatogenesis in, 178*f*
  immature, in Kallmann's syndrome, 71f
  seminoma adjacent to, 181*f*
  semiquantitative scoring system for, 18
  Sertoli cells in, 19*f*, 20*f*
  size and structure of, 17
  spermatids in with maturation arrest, 175
Seminoma
  adjacent to seminiferous tubule, 181*f*
  germ cell, 150-151
  seminiferous tubules adjacent to, 151*f*
Seminoma dysgerminoma, 58
Serologic studies, in infertile female, 26
Sertoli cell index (SCI), in classification of testes, 85-86
Sertoli-cell-only syndrome, 171, 173*f*
  causes of, 172*t*
  pathologic findings in, 172
Sertoli cell ratio (SCR), 20
Sertoli cells, 19*f*
  AMH secretion by, 45-46
  disorganized, 173*f*
  in seminiferous tubules, 19*f*, 20*f*
  tumor of, 150, 151*f*
Sertoli-Leydig cell tumors, 153
Serum antisperm antibodies, in unexplained infertility, 27
Sex, clinical determination of, 49
Sex chromosomes
  abnormalities of, 49-61
    without gonadal changes, 61
  diagram of, 44*f*
  function of, 44-45
Sex-cord stromal tumors, 152-153
Sex-determining region on chromosome Y (SRY), 44-45
Sex hormone-binding globulin (SHBG), low levels of, 155
Sexual ambiguity
  in 5-α-reductase deficiency, 69-70
  with mixed gonadal dysgenesis, 59
Sexual development, normal, 43-49
Sexual differentiation
  abnormalities of, 49-61
  female, 46*f*
  genetic anomalies of, 49
  normal, 43-49
  processes determining, 43
Sexual dimorphism, 48
Sexual function, nutrition and, 4
Sexual maturation
  changes during, 48
  precocious, with Leydig cell tumors, 149-150
Sexually transmitted disease, history of in infertile male, 7-8
Social history
  in infertile female, 24
  and male infertility, 9
Sperm
  coagulation of, 11
  mechanical obstruction of flow of, 178

Sperm—cont'd
  morphology of, 12-13
  most common abnormalities of, 13
  motility and viability of, 12
  physical properties of, 11
  tail abnormalities of, 13
Sperm analysis, 11-15
  in maturation arrest of spermatogenesis, 173-174
  routine parameters of, 11
Sperm counts, 11
  in assessment of sperm quality, 11-12
  effect of age at treatment for cryptorchidism on, 84*t*
  in patients with cryptorchidism, 83*t*
Sperm granulomas
  early, 128*f*
  with vasectomy, 128
Spermarche, 48
Spermatids, round, maturation arrest at stage of, 18*f*, 175, 177*f*
Spermatoceles, 90
Spermatocytes
  classification of, 174-175
  maturation arrest at stage of primary, 19, 174-175, 176*f*
  maturation arrest at stage of secondary, 175
  maturation arrest of, 174-175
Spermatogenesis, 18
  abnormal, 171-182
  arrest of with radiation therapy, 131
  depression of, 8
  diagram of, 175*f*
  germ cell tumors affecting, 150
  lack of in postpubertal cryptorchid testis, 86*f*
  maturation arrest of, 172-173
    causes of, 174
    clinical findings in, 173-174
    pathologic findings in, 174-175
    at stage of primary spermatocytes, 19, 174-175, 176*f*
    at stage of round spermatids, 175, 177*f*, 186
  with postpubertal hypothalamic and pituitary lesions, 140
  theories of varicocele influence on, 133
Spermatogenic cells, lack of, 52
Spermatogenic maturation, scoring of, 20-21
Spermatogonia, maturation arrest at, 174
Spermatozoa
  assessment of ratio of normal to abnormal, 13
  classes of, 15*f*
  common abnormalities of, 12
  diagrammatic presentation of abnormalities of, 15*f*
  morphology of, 13
    normal and abnormal, 14*f*
  structural and functional defects of, 176-177
Spinnbarkeit, 25
Splenic choristomas, 90
Splenic gonadal fusion, 100
SRY mutations, 57
Sterility, definition of, 2
Sterilization
  reversal of, 135
  tubal, 135
Steroid hormones
  increased production of in ovary with polycystic ovary syndrome, 155
  metabolic block in synthesis of, 62
  synthesis of, 62*f*
Streak gonads
  of mixed gonadal dysgenesis, 58*f*
  in Turner syndrome, 54*f*, 55-56